# Handbook of Poultry Parasites

## Edited by

## Tanmoy Rana

*Department of Veterinary Clinical Complex*
*West Bengal University of Animal & Fishery Sciences*
*Kolkata, India*

# Handbook of Poultry Parasites

Editor: Tanmoy Rana

ISBN (Online): 979-8-89881-123-5

ISBN (Print): 979-8-89881-124-2

ISBN (Paperback): 979-8-89881-125-9

Published by Bentham Science Publishers Pte. Ltd. Singapore, in collaboration with Eureka Conferences, USA. All Rights Reserved.

First published in 2025.

need for a court order if at any point you breach any terms of this License Agreement. In no event will any delay or failure by Bentham Science Publishers in enforcing your compliance with this License Agreement constitute a waiver of any of its rights.

3. You acknowledge that you have read this License Agreement, and agree to be bound by its terms and conditions. To the extent that any other terms and conditions presented on any website of Bentham Science Publishers conflict with, or are inconsistent with, the terms and conditions set out in this License Agreement, you acknowledge that the terms and conditions set out in this License Agreement shall prevail.

**Bentham Science Publishers Pte. Ltd.**
No. 9 Raffles Place
Office No. 26-01
Singapore 048619
Singapore
Email: subscriptions@benthamscience.net

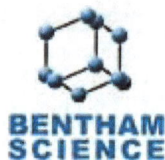

**BENTHAM SCIENCE**

# CONTENTS

*P.N. Bashetti* and *Debolina Dattaray*

# FOREWORD

Poultry production is one of the most significant sectors in the global agricultural economy, providing an essential source of protein through meat and eggs. As the demand for poultry products continues to grow, so does the need to understand and address the challenges that threaten the health and productivity of poultry flocks. Among these challenges, parasitic infections stand out as a persistent and pervasive problem that affects poultry worldwide, with substantial impacts on animal welfare, food safety, and economic sustainability.

The "Handbook of Poultry Parasites" is an indispensable resource that addresses this critical issue with clarity, depth, and scientific rigor. This book provides comprehensive insights into the various parasites that infect poultry, including their biology, epidemiology, diagnosis, control, and management. It covers a wide range of parasites, from protozoa and helminths to ectoparasites, each of which poses unique threats to poultry health.

What sets this handbook apart is its balanced approach, combining foundational knowledge with practical applications. It serves not only as a reference for veterinarians, poultry health specialists, and researchers but also as a practical guide for poultry producers and farm managers. The book emphasizes integrated pest management strategies, highlighting the importance of prevention, monitoring, and judicious use of treatments to minimize the impact of parasites while reducing the risk of resistance.

In an era marked by increasing concerns over antimicrobial resistance, food safety, and sustainable agriculture, this handbook is timely and relevant. It provides the tools and knowledge needed to develop effective, sustainable, and science-based strategies for managing parasites in poultry, ensuring that poultry production remains both profitable and responsible.

I commend the authors and contributors for their dedication to this project and for their valuable contributions to the field of poultry health. This handbook is a testament to their expertise and commitment to advancing our understanding of parasitic infections in poultry and their management.

I am confident that this book will become a vital reference for all those involved in poultry health and production. It will undoubtedly contribute to improving poultry welfare, enhancing productivity, and ensuring the sustainability of poultry farming around the world.

**Peter Ibrahim Rekwot**
National Animal Production Research Institute
Ahmadu Bello University
Zaria, Kaduna State
Nigeria

# PREFACE

POULTRY generally suffers from many parasitic diseases, and the object of this book is to present to poultry-keepers the information about life histories of these pests, so that protection may be successfully ensured. Poultry products are valuable protein sources throughout the globe and the poultry commercial industry, especially Commercial Production Systems (CPS) gained continuous growth during 20-30 years. On the other hand, the traditional scavenging rural systems are also exploited with low growth and serious nutritional, management, and constraints of diseases. The parasite can cause harm in poultry developing countries with the declined productivity of backyard poultry. The handbook describes useful updated information on the pathogenic parasites of economic consequences and also elaborately describes the procedure as well as techniques for the epidemiological study, diagnosis, treatment, and control. The book is structured interestingly for routine application in research institutes, field laboratories, and universities. The book describes the characteristics and habits of the parasites in relation to the occurrence of many diseases. The book guides poultry-breeders, and fanciers in distinguishing and coping with poultry parasites that can cause them serious loss. As most of the birds are grown in more concentrated/confinement areas, new disease problems may appear and old ones sometimes reoccur simultaneously. Proper treatment, management, and sanitation can reduce disease or parasite problems at an early stage. The book is an invaluable resource for both veterinarians in training and in practice for gathering knowledge about the parasitic diseases of poultry. The contributors are well-specialized in their knowledge for writing the individual chapter. This book is especially intended for farmers, industry specialists, practitioners, academics, researchers, veterinarians, and DVM graduate students engaged with a special interest in poultry health, and management. It is assumed that a wide circulation of the handbook can accelerate the standardization and enhancement of diagnostic capacity, treatment, and effective disease control programmes. I hope that this book serves as a new paradigm for the stimulus to further research in clarifying the pathomechanisms, diagnosis, and treatment of parasitic diseases of poultry. I expect that the reader will observe this book interestingly with updated information about the diseases. The book can utilize the knowledge in research and teaching to the new generation. I always welcome constructive feedback and encouragement from my veterinarian colleagues all over the world.

**Tanmoy Rana**
Department of Veterinary Clinical Complex
West Bengal University of Animal & Fishery Sciences
Kolkata, India

# ACKNOWLEDGEMENTS

I would like to convey my regards and sincere gratitude to the Hon'ble Vice Chancellor, West Bengal University of Animal & Fishery Sciences, Kolkata, India for providing me an opportunity to edit the book. I am also extremely grateful to all contributors who helped me by submitting their respective chapter/s at the proper time. I also convey my warmest thanks to all departmental colleagues for giving me wonderful thoughts, extreme energy, and bits of knowledge for editing the book. This book could not have been written without the understanding and support of Bentham Science Publishers. Therefore, a big "thanks" to all of the people at Bentham who worked as a team to get it into the final form. I am really grateful to the clients who have confidence in my abilities to allow me to treat poultry. I also acknowledge and thank all veterinary practitioners, researchers, and academicians whose works are highly cited profusely throughout the text of the book. Last, but not the least, I am indebted to my family for the expanse of time spent on editing of the book.

# List of Contributors

| | |
|---|---|
| **Alok Kumar Singh** | Department of Veterinary Parasitology, College of Veterinary Science & Animal Husbandry, Kuthuliya, Rewa, Rewa 486001, Madhya Pradesh, India |
| **Amna Shakoor** | Department of Anatomy, Faculty of Veterinary Science, University of Agriculture, Faisalabad 38040, Pakistan |
| **Anupam Brahma** | Faculty of Veterinary and Animal Sciences, Institute of Agricultural Sciences, Banaras Hindu University, Varanasi 221005, Uttar Pradesh, India |
| **Amit Kumar Jaiswal** | Department of Veterinary Parasitology, COVSc & AH, Uttar Pradesh Pandit Deen Dayal Upadhyaya pashu Chikitsa Vigyan Vishwavidyalaya Evam Go Anusandhan Sansthan (DUVASU), Mathura 281001, Uttar Pradesh, India |
| **Bhavanam Sudhakara Reddy** | Department of Veterinary Parasitology, College of Veterinary Science, Sri Venkateswara Veterinary University, Proddatur 516360, Andhra Pradesh, India |
| **Clement Akotsen-Mensah** | Integrated Pest Control Program, Alabama Cooperative Extension System, Alabama A & M University, Normal, Albama, USA |
| **C. Sreedevi** | Department of Veterinary Parasitology, NTR College of Veterinary Science, Sri Venkateswara Veterinary University, Gannavaram 521102, Andhra Pradesh, India |
| **Debolina Dattaray** | Department of Veterinary Pharmacology and Toxicology, Institute of Veterinary Science and Animal Husbandry, Siksha 'O' Anusandhan University, Bhubaneswar, Odisha, India |
| **Felix Uchenna Samuel** | Animal Science Program, Alabama Cooperative Extension System, Alabama A & M University, Normal, Alabama, USA |
| **Furqan Munir** | Department of Parasitology, Faculty of Veterinary Science, University of Agriculture, Faisalabad 38040, Pakistan |
| **Gaurav Kumar Verma** | COVSc & AH, Uttar Pradesh Pandit Deen Dayal Upadhyaya pashu Chikitsa Vigyan Vishwavidyalaya Evam Go Anusandhan Sansthan (DUVASU), Mathura 281001, Uttar Pradesh, India |
| **H. Srinivas Naik** | Department of Veterinary Pathology, College of Veterinary Science, Sri Venkateswara Veterinary University, Proddatur 516360, Andhra Pradesh, India |
| **Ibrahim Abdul Mohammed** | Poultry Research Program, National Animal Production Research Institute, Shika-Zaria, Nigeria |
| **Jinu Manoj** | Department of Veterinary Public Health & Epidemiology, College Central Laboratory, Lala Lajpat Rai University of Veterinary and Animal Sciences, Hisar 125004, Haryana, India |
| **Jayalakshmi Jaliparthi** | Department of Veterinary Parasitology, SKPP AHP, S.V.V.U, Ramachandrapuram, Andhra Pradesh, India |
| **Krishnendu Kundu** | Department of Veterinary Parasitology, Faculty of Veterinary and Animal Sciences, Institute of Agricultural Sciences, Banaras Hindu University, Varanasi 221005, Uttar Pradesh, India |

| | |
|---|---|
| **Kamlesh A. Sadariya** | Department of Veterinary Pharmacology and Toxicology, College of Veterinary Science and Animal Husbandry, Kamdhenu University, Anand, Gujarat, India |
| **Kale Chandrakant Dinkar** | Department of Veterinary Parasitology, COVSc & AH, Uttar Pradesh Pandit Deen Dayal Upadhyaya pashu Chikitsa Vigyan Vishwavidyalaya Evam Go Anusandhan Sansthan (DUVASU), Mathura 281001, Uttar Pradesh, India |
| **Manoj Kumar Singh** | Department of Livestock Production and Management, College of Veterinary and Animal Sciences, Sardar Vallabhbhai Patel University of Agriculture and Technology, Meerut 250110, Uttar Pradesh, India |
| **Muhammad Tahir Aleem** | Department of Pharmacology, Shantou University Medical College, Shantou 515041, China |
| **Mukesh Shakya** | Department of Veterinary Parasitology, College of Veterinary Sciences & A.H., Nanaji Deshmukh Veterinary Science University, Mhow, Indore 453446, Madhya Pradesh, India |
| **Nanga Divyasree** | Department of Veterinary Parasitology, College of Veterinary Science, Sri Venkateswara Veterinary University, Proddatur 516360, Andhra Pradesh, India |
| **Nidhi S. Choudhary** | Department of Medicine, College of Veterinary Sciences & A.H Nanaji Deshmukh Veterinary Science University, Mhow, Indore 453446, Madhya Pradesh, India |
| **P.N. Bashetti** | Divison of Veterinary Pathology, IVRI, Izatnagr, Uttar Pradesh, India |
| **Pradeep Kumar** | Department of Veterinary Parasitology, Uttar Pradesh Pandit Deen Dayal Upadhyaya Pashu Chikitsa Vigyan Vishwavidyalaya Evam Go-Anusandhan Sansthan, Mathura 281001, Uttar Pradesh, India |
| **P. Ramadevi** | Department of Veterinary Parasitology, C.V.Sc, S.V.V.U, Garividi, Andhra Pradesh, India |
| **Poojasree Alli** | Department of Veterinary Parasitology, C.V.Sc, P.V.N.R.T.V.U, Rajendranagar, Hyderabad, Telangana, India |
| **R.L. Rakesh** | Department of Veterinary Parasitology, Veterinary College, Hassan, KVAFSU, Bidar, Hassan 573202, India |
| **Renu Singh** | Department of Veterinary Pathology, Uttar Pradesh Pandit Deen Dayal Upadhyaya Pashu Chikitsa Vigyan Vishwavidyalaya Evam Go-Anusandhan Sansthan, Mathura 281001, Uttar Pradesh, India |
| **R.S. Ghasura** | College of Veterinary Science & A.H, Kamdhenu University, Anand, Gujarat, India |
| **Rupam Sachan** | Department of Veterinary Parasitology, COVSc & AH, Uttar Pradesh Pandit Deen Dayal Upadhyaya pashu Chikitsa Vigyan Vishwavidyalaya Evam Go Anusandhan Sansthan (DUVASU), Mathura 281001, Uttar Pradesh, India |
| **Sivajothi Sirigireddy** | Department of Veterinary Parasitology, College of Veterinary Science, Sri Venkateswara Veterinary University, 516360, India |
| **Saroj Kumar** | Department of Veterinary Parasitology, Faculty of Veterinary and Animal Sciences, Institute of Agricultural Sciences, Banaras Hindu University, Varanasi 221005, Uttar Pradesh, India |

| | |
|---|---|
| **Shahbaz Ul Haq** | Department of Pharmacology, Shantou University Medical College, Shantou 515041, China |
| **Shailesh K. Bhavsar** | Department of Veterinary Pharmacology and Toxicology, College of Veterinary Science and Animal Husbandry, Kamdhenu University, Anand, Gujarat, India |
| **S.T. Parmar** | College of Veterinary Science & A.H, Kamdhenu University, Anand, Gujarat, India |
| **S.V. Mavadiya** | College of Veterinary Science & A.H, Kamdhenu University, Anand, Gujarat, India |
| **Souti Prasad Sarkhel** | Faculty of Veterinary and Animal Sciences, Institute of Agricultural Sciences, Banaras Hindu University, Varanasi 221005, Uttar Pradesh, India |
| **Tanmoy Rana** | Department of Veterinary Clinical Complex, West Bengal University of Animal & Fishery Sciences, Kolkata, India |
| **Tamanna H. Solanki** | Department of Veterinary Pharmacology and Toxicology, College of Veterinary Science and Animal Husbandry, Kamdhenu University, Anand, Gujarat, India |
| **Vaidehi N. Sarvaiya** | Department of Veterinary Pharmacology and Toxicology, College of Veterinary Science and Animal Husbandry, Kamdhenu University, Anand, Gujarat, India |
| **Vandeep Chahuan** | College of Veterinary Science & A.H, Kamdhenu University, Anand, Gujarat, India |
| **Vivek Agrawal** | Department of Veterinary Parasitology, College of Veterinary Sciences & A.H., Nanaji Deshmukh Veterinary Science University, Mhow, Indore 453446, Madhya Pradesh, India |
| **V. Gnani Charitha** | Department of Veterinary Parasitology, College of Veterinary Science, Sri Venkateswara Veterinary University, Proddatur 516360, Andhra Pradesh, India |
| **V. C. Rayulu** | YSR Administrative building, Sri Venkateswara Veterinary University, Tirupati 517502, Andhra Pradesh, India |
| **Yellay Praneetha** | Department of Veterinary Parasitology, College of Veterinary Science, Sri Venkateswara Veterinary University, Proddatur 516360, Andhra Pradesh, India |

# CHAPTER 1

# Introduction

**Sirigireddy Sivajothi[1,*], Tanmoy Rana[2], Bhavanam Sudhakara Reddy[1], Nanga Divyasree[1] and Yellay Praneetha[1]**

*[1] Department of Veterinary Parasitology, College of Veterinary Science, Sri Venkateswara Veterinary University, Proddatur 516360, Andhra Pradesh, India*

*[2] Department of Veterinary Clinical Complex, West Bengal University of Animal & Fishery Sciences, Kolkata, India*

**Abstract:** Poultry now constitutes 30% of global meat consumption, with a rising demand observed worldwide. However, parasites pose a significant challenge in both large-scale commercial poultry operations and small backyard flocks, leading to considerable economic losses. Nematode and cestode worm infections in chickens can result in decreased egg production, weight loss, growth impediments, and weakness. Parasitic infestations in poultry are widespread, regardless of the rearing method used, and can severely affect production outcomes. In confinement systems, parasites have short life cycles and routes of direct transmission, such as *Heterakis gallinarum*, *Ascaridia galli*, *Eimeria spp.*, and *Capillaria spp.* thrive more easily. On the other hand, free-range or backyard rearing creates opportunities for parasites that depend on intermediate hosts to complete their life cycles. It is important to understand that parasitism in poultry impacts the entire flock, and the health of an individual bird is of less economic significance compared to the overall impact on flock productivity.

**Keywords:** Diseases, Infection, Infestation, Parasites, Parasitism, Poultry.

## INTRODUCTION

Various factors, including infectious agents, toxins, and nutritional deficiencies, significantly influence farm performance, thereby affecting the local poultry industry [1]. In addition, poultry is vulnerable to a variety of common diseases, including endoparasites, ectoparasites, infectious bronchitis, Marek's disease, fowl cholera, salmonellosis, infectious coryza, fowl pox, avian encephalomyelitis, among others. These health challenges can significantly impact poultry production and the sustainability of the industry. Controlling infectious diseases is essential for preserving poultry health, and diagnostic methods are critical for identifying disease causes and evaluating the effects of pathogens on the host [2].

* **Corresponding author Sirigireddy Sivajothi:** Department of Veterinary Parasitology, College of Veterinary Science, Sri Venkateswara Veterinary University, Proddatur 516360, Andhra Pradesh, India; E-mail: sivajothi579@gmail.com

Although the core principles of disease diagnostics remain consistent, the landscape of poultry diseases is continually evolving, with new pathogens being discovered and deeper insights gained into epidemiology and disease mechanisms. At the same time, innovative technologies have emerged to detect and characterize infectious agents [3]. However, traditional methods, such as pathogen isolation and characterization through functional assays and studies, remain essential in the diagnostic process. These classical approaches complement new technologies, providing a more complete understanding of poultry health and disease management.

In poultry medicine, the diagnostic approach has shifted from focusing on individual birds to evaluating the health of entire flocks [4]. Flocks are considered "healthy" when they perform according to their genetic potential and show no clinical signs of disease [4]. On-farm diagnostic activities involve regular sampling and investigations as part of health control programs, often aligned with national or international efforts targeting specific parasitic diseases. Samples collected on-site may be tested immediately using rapid antigen tests or sent to laboratories for further analysis, including ELISA and PCR. Field veterinarians play a key role in diagnostic surveillance, and gathering epidemiological data to support flock management. Routine sample collection, such as feces, serum, and mucosal swabs, focuses on confirming flock health status and monitoring vaccine effectiveness [5]. The data generated through these diagnostic processes enable informed decision-making to optimize both flock health and production outcomes.

In field settings, diagnostic procedures are initiated promptly when flock health is compromised, typically indicated by rising morbidity or mortality rates. Investigations begin with the collection of a detailed case history, including relevant information about the flock, management practices, and the characteristics of the infection or disease [6]. This involves recording details such as the type and origin of the birds, their age, routine medications, vaccination protocols, history of diseases, husbandry practices, and standard operating procedures for feeding, watering, ventilation, and lighting systems. Additionally, hygiene and biosecurity measures are documented [7]. In addition, production parameters, morbidity and mortality statistics, the duration of observed signs or problems, and any epidemiological links to other production sites are carefully documented. This comprehensive information serves as the basis for the next diagnostic steps, enabling a systematic approach to identifying and resolving flock health issues [8].

On the farm, diagnostic procedures begin with the clinical examination of both flocks and individual birds at various disease stages, as well as their products, such as feces and eggs. These assessments are carried out by experienced poultry workers and veterinarians who have a deep knowledge of what defines a healthy flock and environment. While clinical evaluations are thorough, they can be time-consuming and labor-intensive. Unfortunately, they may not always identify diseases, particularly subclinical infections, which can be difficult to diagnose accurately [9]. The manifestation of infectious diseases can vary greatly, ranging from subtle subclinical symptoms to severe clinical illness. This variability is influenced by factors such as the causative agent, host characteristics, and environmental conditions, making diagnosis more challenging. Common clinical signs often include non-specific indicators like apathy, ruffled feathers, and decreased appetite, which can be associated with a wide array of diseases [10]. Specific signs may also be present, indicating particular disorders, such as enteric, respiratory, or neurologic issues. In certain cases, signs may be pathognomonic, serving as unique indicators of a specific disease, such as those observed in histomonosis [11].

Post-mortem investigations, whether performed on the farm or in a laboratory, are essential diagnostic procedures designed to identify gross pathological changes in organs and tissues. These investigations assist in determining a tentative cause of impaired performance and clinical signs. By integrating a detailed case history, a comprehensive assessment of clinical signs, and careful post-mortem examinations, the range of presumptive diagnoses can be narrowed. This process lays the groundwork for selecting suitable laboratory methods to further confirm and refine the diagnosis [12].

## Protozoa

The primary protozoa are predominantly from the phylum Apicomplexa, encompassing genera such as *Eimeria spp., Leucocytozoon spp., Haemoproteus spp., Toxoplasma spp., Sarcocystis spp.*, and *Cryptosporidium spp.* Additionally, flagellates like *Histomonas spp., Trypanosoma spp., Trichomonas spp., Chilomastix spp.*, and *Hexamita spp.*, as well as amoeba including *Entamoeba spp.* and *Endolimax spp.*, are commonly found. Recently, a microsporidian known as *Encephalitozoon cunicule* has also been reported in chickens [13].

## Coccidiosis

Coccidia unquestionably stands out as the most significant parasite affecting poultry, with widespread distribution, high frequency of occurrence, and substantial economic repercussions [14]. Although mortality from coccidiosis is effectively managed with anticoccidial medications, the poultry industry continues to face significant losses due to reduced weight gain, decreased feed efficiency, and treatment costs. To highlight the economic sensitivity of the industry, even a slight improvement in feed efficiency, such as a reduction of 0.01

kg of feed required per kg of gain, could save the U.S. poultry sector over $70 million, based on recent production figures [15].

Coccidiosis, caused by the protozoan *Eimeria spp.*, is a prevalent ailment in poultry. Nine distinct species of *Eimeria* (Fig. **1** and Table **1**) have been identified as infecting chickens: *Eimeria acervulina, Eimeria brunetti, Eimeria maxima, Eimeria mitis, Eimeria necatrix, Eimeria praecox, Eimeria tenella, Eimeria mivati,* and *Eimeria hagani*. The impact of infection can range from weight loss to high mortality, depending on the species or strain involved [16]. Each *Eimeria* species presents different levels of severity and unique clinical characteristics, highlighting the importance of accurately identifying the species impacting the flock. Precise identification is essential for effective monitoring and control of coccidiosis, as well as for determining the most suitable treatment strategies [17].

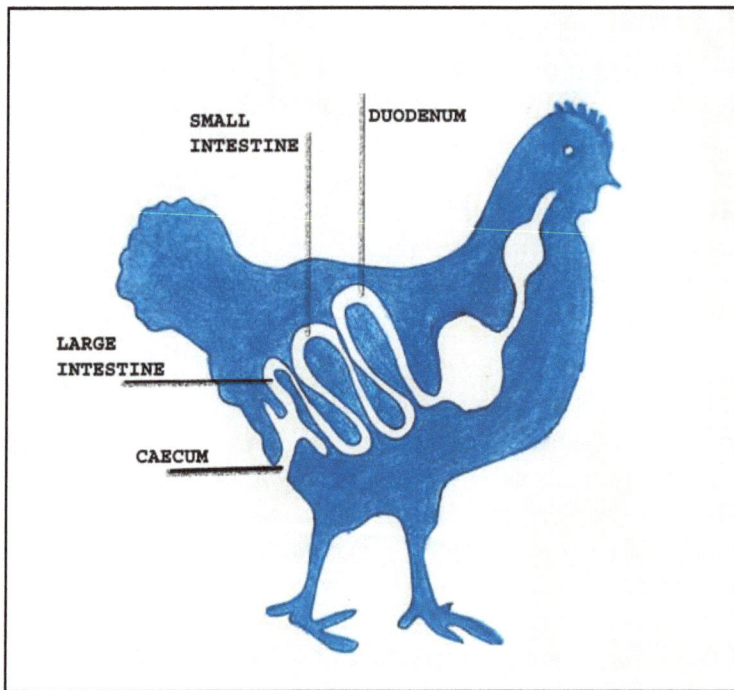

**Fig. (1).**  Different regions of the digestive tract of poultry affected by nine *Emieria spp.*

Avian coccidia from the genus *Eimeria* displays notable host specificity, with pheasants, chickens, Japanese quail, turkeys, and bobwhite quail each hosting distinct species. Poultry producers are primarily focused on the potential issues that any species can cause when present in large numbers. Some species may require higher inoculation doses to cause significant problems [18].

**Table 1. Different regions of the digestive tract of poultry affected by nine *Emieria* spp.**

| Parasites in Digestive tract (*Eimeria* spp) | Region of Digestive tract | | | |
|---|---|---|---|---|
| | **Small Intestine** | **Duodenum** | **Caecum** | **Large Intestine** |
| ***Eimeria* spp** | *Eimeria necatrix* | *Eimeria acervulina* | *Eimeria tenella* | *Eimeria brunetti* |
| - | *Eimeria maxima* | *Eimeria mivati* | - | - |
| | - | *Eimeria hagani* | - | - |
| | - | *Eimeria praecox* | - | - |
| | - | *Eimeria mitis* | - | - |

All avian *Eimeria* species lead to weight loss, increased feed conversion ratios, loss of skin pigmentation, and reduced egg production. The widespread presence of coccidia in poultry production units of all sizes is due to the remarkable reproductive capacity of these intracellular parasites. Each ingested oocyst can produce hundreds of thousands of infective oocysts in the feces within 7 to 12 days [19]. Transmission between farms is facilitated by the movement of personnel and equipment, and new farms can harbor the parasite within weeks of introducing poultry [20].

## The Digestive Tract of other Protozoa

Among the protozoa that affect the digestive tract (Fig. **2**), *Histomonas meleagridis* infections can occasionally become a significant economic concern, particularly in turkeys, but also in chickens and, on rare occasions, game birds. The role of the earthworms and cecal worm, *Heterakis gallinarum* in transmission, along with the necessity of specific bacterial flora for pathogenicity, is well documented [21]. Mortality rates can be significantly high, particularly in turkeys, chukar partridge, and ruffed grouse. *Cryptosporidium* presents serious challenges in certain poultry species [22], with *C. meleagridis* infections in turkeys leading to diarrhea and mild mortality [23]. Another species, *C. baileyi*, infects both the respiratory tracts and digestive of turkeys and chickens [24].

## Blood and Tissue Protozoa

These blood parasites (Table **2**) are primarily prevalent among birds inhabiting tropical regions. In chickens, the most significant genera of haemoparasites include *Haemoproteus spp.*, *Leucocytozoon spp.*, and *Plasmodium spp.*. *Leucocytozoon spp.*, which infects the tissue cells and blood of internal organs, with transmission facilitated by various dipteran intermediate hosts like simuliid flies and *Culicoides midges* in areas of residency. Infection rates can reach up to 100% in some regions [25]. The primary species include *L. simondi* (found in ducks and geese), *L. caulleryi* (in chickens), and *L. smithi* (in turkeys), although additional species have been identified [26]. *L. smithi* notably led to the failure of a large-scale turkey production endeavor in South Carolina's sandhill areas and coastal plains [27].

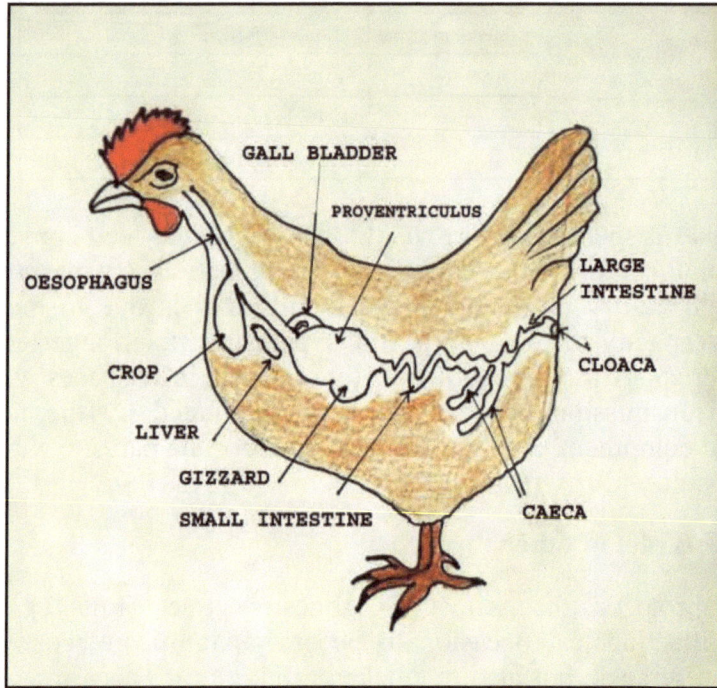

**Fig. (2).** Digestive tract of poultry.

**Table 2. Blood parasites of poultry and vectors.**

| Blood Parasites | Vectors |
| :---: | :---: |
| *Haemoproteus* spp. | Midges<br>Hippoboscid flies |
| *Aegyptynella* spp. | *Argas persicus* |
| *Leucocytozoon* spp. | Midges<br>Blackflies |
| *Plasmodium* spp. | *Culex* mosquitoes |
| *Trypanosoma* spp. | Biting insects<br>Red mites |

120 species of *Haemoproteus* have been discussed from birds, they generally pose minimal problems [28]. Sarcosporidiosis can be a significant concern in waterfowl, and many bird species are susceptible to *Toxoplasma* infections. With

limited or no effective medications available for these infections, prevention remains the primary control method. Although over 65 species of *Plasmodium* have been cited in birds, avian *Plasmodium* species primarily develop in mosquitoes from the *Culex* and *Aedes* genera, with occasional development in *Anopheles*. Among the most pathogenic for domestic fowl are *Plasmodium gallinaceum*, *P. juxtanucleare,* and *P. durae*, which can lead to mortality rates exceeding 90% [29].

## Nematodes

Nematodes stand out as the predominant and consequential helminth species found in poultry, with over 50 distinct species identified [30]. Among these, a majority inflict pathological harm upon their hosts. Belonging to the phylum Nemathelminthes and the class Nematoda, these parasitic worms in poultry exhibit a characteristic unsegmented, cylindrical body shape. Their exterior may feature various textures, such as circular annulations, smoothness, longitudinal striations, or cuticular ornamentations like plagues or spines [31]. All nematodes have an alimentary tract and display distinct sexes. Their life cycles can be direct or indirect, with the latter often involving intermediate hosts [2]. Among breeders, nematodes, or roundworms (Table **3**), reign as the most prevalent internal parasites. This group comprises *Ascaridia galli* (found in the intestine), *Heterakis gallinarum* (residing in the ceca), and various *Capillaria species* (occupying the crop and intestine), which traverse the digestive tract. Additionally, the *Syngamus trachea*, commonly known as the gape worm, resides in the lungs and trachea. These nematodes typically have elongated spindle shapes and range in color from off-white to creamy yellow [5]. Distinct species further define their habitats within the avian body. *Capillaria contorta* infests the crop, while *Capillaria obsignata* targets the intestine. *Ascaridia galli* primarily inhabits the jejunum, whereas *Heterakis gallinarum* resides in the cecum. *Tetrameres americana*, a spherical nematode measuring 3 mm, resides beneath the mucosa of the proventriculus. Meanwhile, *Cheilospirura hamulosa,* a 2.5 cm long nematode, is found beneath the mucosa, specifically within the koilin layer of the ventriculus [7, 9].

## Cestodes

Tapeworms, belonging to the phylum Platyhelminthes and class Cestoda, are internal parasites commonly found in poultry. These hermaphroditic organisms have flat, elongated bodies made up of segments and lack both an alimentary tract and a body cavity. Poultry tapeworms can reach lengths of 30 to 50 cm [22, 24]. They have a distinct scolex, or head, followed by a neck. The rest of the body, known as the strobila, is made up of numerous proglottids, or segments, that develop from the neck. Each segment contains a set of reproductive organs, with the number varying among species. As these segments mature, the ones furthest from the neck detach from the body. Gravid segments, filled with numerous eggs, release their contents into the environment through the host's feces [17, 18].

**Table 3. Common nematode parasites of poultry.**

| S.No. | Name of the Nematode | Definitive host | Intermediate Host | Predilection site |
|-------|---------------------|-----------------|-------------------|-------------------|
| 1 | *Ascaridia galli* | Chicken | Direct | Small intestine |
| 2 | *Capillaria caudinflata* | Chicken | Earthworms | Small intesstine |
| 3 | *Capillaria contorta* | Chicken | None or Earthworms | Mouth, Oesophagus, Crop |
| 4 | *Capillaria obsignata* | Chicken | Direct | Small intestine, caeca |
| 5 | *Heterakis gallinarum* | Chicken | Direct | Caeca |
| 6 | *Oxyspirura mansoni* | Chicken | Cockroaches | Eye |
| 7 | *Strongyloides avium* | Chicken | Direct | Caeca |
| 8 | *Syngamus trachea* | Chicken | None or Earthworms | Trachea |
| 9 | *Tetameres americana* | Chicken | Grass-hopperss, cockroaches | Proventriculus |
| 10 | *Trichostrongylus tenuis* | Chicken | Direct | Caeca |

Poultry raised in free-range environments are vulnerable to cestode (tapeworm) infections. These tapeworms have indirect life cycles that depend on intermediate hosts, such as earthworms, beetles, flies, ants, or grasshoppers, to complete their development. As a result, infections are rare in indoor systems. The extensive diversity of tapeworms affecting domesticated poultry and wild birds includes over 1,400 species; however, the pathogenicity of most of these species remains unclear. Many are benign or cause only mild pathogenic effects, while only a few induce severe reactions in the host [5, 9].

The most frequently identified cestodes in diagnoses include:

• *Davainea proglottina*: A 4 mm cestode residing in the duodenum.
• *Choanotaenia infundibulum*: A 25 cm cestode found in the distal duodenum and jejunum.
• *Raillietina tetragona*: A 25 cm cestode inhabiting the distal jejunum.
• *Raillietina echinobothridia*: A 30 cm cestode located in the jejunum, leading to the formation of nodular granulomas and catarrhal enteritis [6, 9].

Cestodes (Table **4**) depend on intermediate hosts such as insects, crustaceans, earthworms, or snails to complete their life cycle (Fig. **3**). In poultry farming, various types of birds, including floor layers, breeders, and broilers, can contract *Raillietina cesticillus* by ingesting its intermediate host, small beetles that breed in the contaminated litter. In unscreened houses, cage layers may ingest *Choanotaenia infundibulum via* house flies, which serve as its intermediate host. Additionally, litter beetles nearby can also act as intermediate hosts. Notably, there have been recorded instances of over 3,000 microscopic tapeworms of the species *Davainea proglottina* found in a single bird [8].

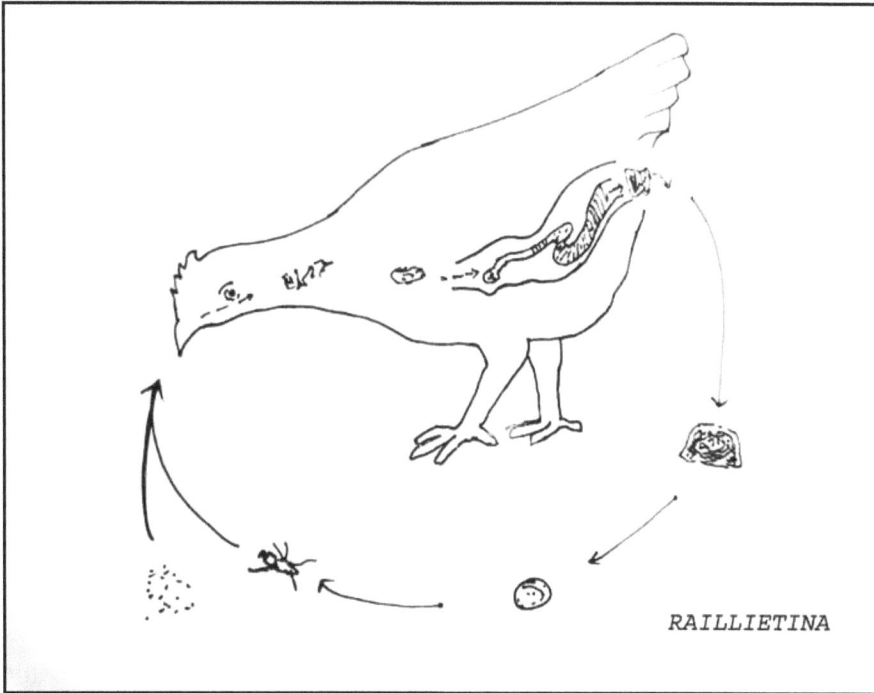

**Fig. (3).** Lifecycle of Cestodes.

**Table 4. Cestodes of poultry.**

| Parasite | Host | Intermediate host or life cycle | Organ infected | Pathogenicity |
|---|---|---|---|---|
| *Choanotaenia infundibulum* | Chicken | Houseflies | Upper intestine | Moderate |
| *Davainea proglattina* | Chicken | Slugs, snails | Duodenum | Severe |
| *Raillietina cesticillus* | Chicken | Beetles | Duodenum, jejunum | Mild |
| *Raillietina echinobothrida* | Chicken | Ants | Lower intestine | Severe, nodule |
| *Raillietina tetragona* | Chicken | Ants | Lower intestine | Severe |

Many species of slugs and snails serve as intermediate hosts for cestode parasites, with reports indicating that over 1,500 infective parasites can be recovered from a single slug [12]. While the gastrointestinal tract of domestic fowl offers a favorable environment for various cestode parasites, those belonging to the genus *Raillietina* are the most widely distributed avian helminth parasites globally. Among them, *R. echinobothrida* is particularly significant due to its prevalence and pathogenicity, especially in domestic fowl, *Gallus domesticus* [17].

The cestode infests the small intestine, leading to stunted growth in young chickens, emaciation in adults, and reduced egg production in hens [14]. A high prevalence and significant variation in cestode infections were found particularly in indigenous poultry compared to exotic breeds [12]. They attributed this discrepancy to potential shortcomings in the management practices of indigenous layers. Various cestode parasites, including *Raillietina tetragona, R. echinobothrida, R. cesticillus,* and *Choanotaenia infundibulum*, were encountered [17]. Among them, *Hymenolepis carioca* emerged as the most prevalent, while *R. cesticillus* was the least common.

**Other Helminths**

Acanthocephalans, also known as spiny-headed worms, and trematodes, commonly referred to as flukes, are rarely found in poultry. In many instances, acanthocephalans appear in their larval forms, indicating accidental infections and the resulting pathology is typically mild. While more than 500 species of trematodes have been documented in birds, approximately 20 are considered potentially hazardous to poultry. Most trematode species exhibit broad host specificity, so diagnosticians may encounter either adult or larval metacercaria in various tissues or cavities, particularly in poultry from backyard flocks or pet birds [30, 31]. One of the more commonly encountered trematodes is *Prostogonimus* spp., known as the oviduct fluke. This fluke relies on two intermediate hosts: snails and dragonflies. Once it reaches adulthood in the oviduct, it significantly reduces egg production [9, 17].

**Ectoparasites**

Various arthropods are the primary ectoparasites affecting poultry (Table **5**), including bugs, lice, mites, fleas, and ticks. The extent and nature of these infestations are greatly influenced by the production methods employed. In the United States, modern high-density production units have resulted in a notable prevalence of the northern fowl mite, *Ornithonyssus sylviarum*, in breeder and layer houses [12]. However, these production systems have also decreased the occurrence of lice infestations (due to fewer bird ages on the same farm) and chicken mites (because of reduced hiding places). In contrast, in countries like Denmark, such production methods have led to increased infestations of *Dermanyssus gallinae*. Detecting ectoparasites is generally easier for those that live directly on the bird, such as northern fowl mites, lice, hard ticks, and sticktight fleas, compared to those that only feed on the bird temporarily, such as bedbugs, chicken mites, and soft ticks [19].

**Table 5. Ectoparasites and their preferred sites of infestation in free-range poultry.**

| Type | Host | Parasite species | Predilection sites |
|---|---|---|---|
| **Fleas** | Chickens | *Echidnophaga gallinacea* | Head, eyes, comb, and wattles. |
| **Mites** | Chickens | *Cnemidocoptes mutans, Dermanyssus gallinae* | Fetlock joint and planter /distal surface of the foot, on the skin. |
| **Soft ticks** | Chickens | *Argas persicus* | Under the wing base. |
| **Hard ticks** | Chickens | *Rhipicephalus spp nymph* | On the skin. |
| **Lice** | Chickens and pigeons | *Menopon gallinae* | On the skin and feathers. |
| **-** | Chickens and Pigeons | *Menacanthus stramineus* | On the skin and feathers of chickens and pigeons. |
| **Flies** | Pigeons | *Pseudolynchia canariensis* | On the skin and feathers (pigeons). |

## Insects

Among ectoparasites, only chewing lice (Fig. **4**) of the order Mallophaga are known to infect birds. Domestic birds have reported over 40 species, with relatively low host specificity. However, lice can pose significant pathogenic risks, particularly in young birds. The sticktight flea, *Echidnophaga gallinacea*, is found across a wide range of birds and mammals. Its adults typically cluster on the host's head, with groups numbering up to 100. This flea is distinctive among poultry fleas because its mouthparts are deeply penetrated in the skin, rendering the adult sessile. In contrast, other adult fleas of mammals and birds intermittently feed on poultry [25].

The common human bedbug, *Cimex lectularius*, is known to infest poultry, sometimes in significant numbers, resulting in detrimental effects on production. While numerous *Diptera* species, such as midges, mosquitoes, gnats, and stable flies, feed on poultry, a few are typically considered significant by parasitologists, as they act as intermediate hosts for other parasites [12].

Black flies, belonging to the family Simuliidae, play a crucial role in transmitting *Leucocytozoon* spp. to poultry, including ducks and turkeys. Biting midges, such as *Culicoides* spp., act as intermediate hosts for *Haemoproteus nettionis*, which infects domestic ducks in Canada. Various genera of mosquitoes are also capable of transmitting avian *Plasmodium* spp. Additionally, the pigeon fly, known as the hippoboscid fly or louse fly (*Pseudolynchia canariensis*), poses significant threats to nestling pigeons and transmits *Haemoproteus columbae*, that causes a malarial-like exhibition of disease in pigeons. Notably, this fly has an unusual life cycle, with larvae maturing inside the female and pupating immediately upon being ejected [17].

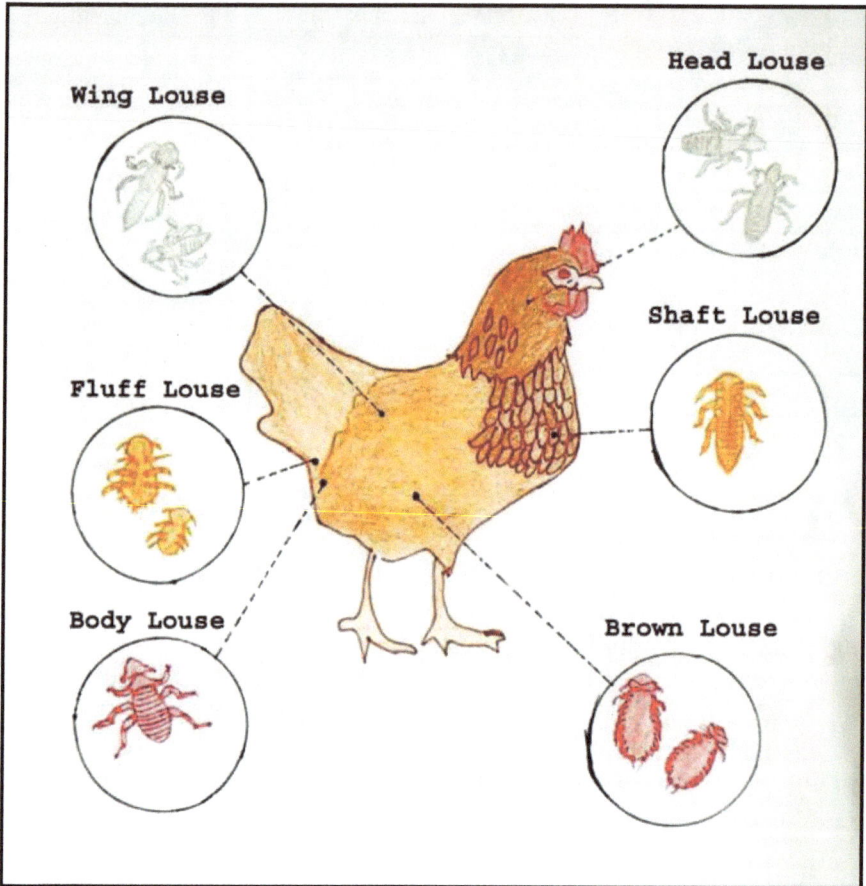

**Fig. (4).** Lice infestation in poultry.

## Arachnids

The northern fowl mite is the most prevalent and important ectoparasite affecting poultry [11]. In severe infestations, feathers may darken, particularly around the vent area. In warmer regions worldwide, the tropical fowl mite often replaces the northern fowl mite, exhibiting similarly severe pathology. Although the chicken mite, also known as the red mite or roost mite (*Dermanyssus gallinae*), is relatively rare in caged-layer operations in the U.S., it is common on breeder farms and is found in 60% of layer systems in Denmark. Mite infestations can lead to reduced egg production and may increase feed costs by 1 to 6 cents per dozen eggs laid. Furthermore, mite infestations can be fatal to both young and adult birds. Additionally, during heavy infestations, mites may leave the birds to attack poultry workers or infest nearby dwellings [22].

Various mites can be found on or within the respiratory system, quills, air sacs, and subcutaneous tissue of poultry. Among these, larval chiggers are particularly notable due to their economic impact. In turkeys, these larvae are attached to the skin, often in clusters, resulting in prominent abscesses. This can lead to downgrading during processing, as the skin lesions should be trimmed. Soft-bodied ticks of the genus *Argas* are the primary concern among poultry ticks, although various species of hard ticks may also intermittently feed on poultry [5, 7]. Blood loss caused by the feeding activities of soft tick larvae and nymphs can lead to fatal anemia. Furthermore, the fowl tick has been associated with the transmission of various diseases, including spirochetosis, piroplasmosis, rickettsial infections, and other bacterial diseases, which are of significant concern worldwide.

## CONTROL MEASURES

### Management

In the absence of effective medications for many parasitic infections in poultry, management practices become the primary method of control. This typically involves disrupting the parasite's life cycle by preventing birds from encountering intermediate or transport hosts and minimizing contact with contamination sources, such as feces, through the use of caging. Furthermore, implementing good sanitation practices, such as promptly removing dead birds and restricting the pathway of equipment and personnel, is crucial in reducing the incidence of parasitic infections [11, 13].

Removing contaminated litter and disinfecting the area can be highly beneficial when parasite levels become excessive. It is essential to avoid housing birds of different ages close together, as older birds can act as reservoirs, infecting younger ones. This principle also applies to parasites that can cross species barriers; for example, turkeys can serve as reservoirs for gapeworm in pheasants, and *vice versa* for histomoniasis. For several years, it was determined that management practices had a very limited effect on reducing coccidiosis due to the resilience of oocysts, which can survive for long periods and resist most disinfectants [14]. However, over the past decade, significant advancements in ventilation as well as nipple watering systems have enhanced litter conditions, making them less conducive to the survival as well as sporulation of coccidial oocysts. As a result, exposure levels in modern broiler houses have significantly decreased. For histomoniasis, the most effective control method is preventing poultry from accessing the earthworms and eggs of cecal worms. Controlling earthworm populations in dirt-floor pens has often proven to be an effective strategy [19].

## Chemotherapy

Chemotherapy, including anticoccidials, anthelmintics, and insecticides, has long been the cornerstone of preventing and controlling parasitic infestation in poultry. When introduced, these compounds demonstrated high efficacy and affordability, particularly given the substantial benefits they provided. Prophylactic use of anticoccidial drug treatment in feed continues to be the primary method for preventing coccidiosis [22].

The main challenge with this prevention and controlling method is the development of parasitic resistance to all available medications. The effectiveness of modern anticoccidials varies depending on the severity of exposure; for instance, some drugs, such as ionophores, maintain their efficacy even when coccidia exposure is mild [25]. However, if conditions change and exposure levels rise, these drugs often struggle to control resistant coccidia populations. Such populations tend to remain consistent within farms but can vary significantly between different complexes. Conducting sensitivity testing at very moderate to very high exposure levels is the only reliable way to determine the resistance profile of a specific complex [28].

The efficacy at lower levels of exposure in the field does not guarantee effectiveness if the challenge intensifies. Therefore, carefully selecting an anticoccidial program is crucial for slowing the development of resistance [29]. Strategies such as shuttle programs—using different medications throughout the grow-out period that can help delay and, in some cases, even prevent the emergence of resistance [30].

The trend in the commercial poultry industry depends on highly effective drug development in combating parasitic resistance in poultry. For example, some highly effective anticoccidials, such as arprinocid, have been withdrawn from the market due to widespread resistance caused by overuse. Additionally, anticoccidials that work against *Eimeria* species in chickens and turkeys may not be effective against coccidia species found in game birds. Furthermore, nitroimidazoles (such as dimetridazole, ipronidazole, or ronidazole) have proven highly effective in controlling histomoniasis; however, their removal from the market in the U.S. poses a potential hazard for isolated flocks once again [31].

The availability of drugs for treating helminth infections is scarce, primarily due to the small market size and the severity of the issue, which do not justify the rising costs associated with developing and securing regulatory approval for new drugs. In the U.S., anthelmintics had been wisely approved only for major nematodes such as *Ascaridia, Capillaria, Heterakis,* and *Syngamus,* the latter of which is classified under a minor use program [32]. However, even for these species, new compounds are lacking, with none anticipated in the near future. Currently, only Hygromycin B, piperazine, and thiabendazole are approved for use in poultry to control these species, and even these options come with significant restrictions [19, 33].

Drug resistance has been observed with all compounds, with piperazine exhibiting particularly significant resistance. Several other drugs have demonstrated efficacy in the infections against both common and less prevalent nematode species experimentally, including pyrantel, mebendazole, citrin, fenbendazole, tetramisole, levamisole, and disophenol. In contrast, only a few modified drugs have been determined for controlling trematodes and cestodes, and none are currently approved for use in poultry in the U.S. However, fenbendazole and levamisole have shown effectiveness against these parasites [22, 32].

## Immunity

Vaccination is a crucial tool for controlling most viral and bacterial diseases in poultry. However, immunity has a limited role in parasite control, except in the case of coccidiosis. Interest in immunity as a means to prevent economic losses from coccidiosis is increasing due to rising drug resistance. The host's ability to mitigate the severity of a challenge infection largely depends on its capacity to mount an immune response. This process involves a complex interplay of internal factors, including the levels and activity of cytokines, hormones, leukocytes, gut-associated lymphoid tissues, macrophages, and antigen presentation [27, 32].

There is increasing evidence that many of the recently developed commercial poultry lines have been bred for maximum growth and feed efficiency, often compromising their ability to develop rapid and consistent immunity [22]. A significant factor affecting an animal's response to vaccination or infection is the complex interplay among nutritional status, the immune system, and the disease organism [15, 33]. There is competition between the immune system and production (growth) systems, along with competition for nutrients [17, 32]. The proper response to a parasitic infection/infestation places increased demands on nutritional status, which may be not adequate to trigger the immune response with an infection of coccidiosis affecting all stages of nutrient utilization [24]. Consequently, coccidial infections can have detrimental effects on viral or bacterial vaccination programs in poultry.

In the initial efforts to mitigate the effects of coccidiosis in commercial poultry operations, a live virulent vaccine called Coccivac (American Scientific Laboratories, Millsboro, DE) was used in breeders. This vaccine delivered live oocysts through the drinking water during the birds' early life. The development of immunity depended on the successful cycling of low levels of coccidia in the litter, allowing for gradual and increasing exposure over time [27, 32].

In the past, exposures that were either too high or less led to poor immunity or clinical disease, resulting in economic losses. Approximately ten years ago, efforts were made to enhance the consistency of the initial dose delivered to individual chicks by switching from water-based delivery to spraying oocysts onto the feed. Improvements were later achieved by administering the vaccine *via* eye spray at the hatchery. Initially, this method was limited to protecting "heavy" broilers. More recently, promising results have been observed with the Immucox (Vetech Laboratories, Rockwood, Ont., Canada) live vaccine, which uses a gel to suspend the oocysts, providing a very consistent dose through ingestion of the gel [21, 23].

Significant efforts have been focused on developing live attenuated vaccines through embryo passage of coccidia or by selecting strains with shortened life cycles (precocious lines). Recently, two live attenuated vaccines—Paracox (Schering-Plough Animal Health, Middlesex, UK) and Livacox (Biopharm, Research Institute of Biopharmacy and Veterinary Drugs, Prague, Czech Republic)—are available in Europe and South America. These vaccines are primarily used in replacement and breeding flocks [17, 33].

While these vaccines are highly effective in breeders with mild exposure to coccidia oocysts, a significant drawback is that they cannot be used alongside medications. As a result, if birds face severe exposure to coccidia, they remain susceptible to wild strains while immunity is gradually developed through the cycling parasites. Although research into subunit vaccines continues to be a major focus, commercial products have yet to materialize despite ongoing efforts [11, 33].

Immunization trials applying antigens derived from recombinant proteins, parasite products, or parasite fractions, have demonstrated that partial immunity though not complete can be achieved against coccidial challenges [12, 32]. Several factors influencing outcomes include the bird line used, the type of adjuvant, the timing and route of immunization, and the combinations of antigens. Battery-type trials have produced more promising results than experiments on floor pens. Future prevention and control of coccidiosis may evolve an integrated approach that combines management practices, vaccines as well as targeted use of medications. In contrast, controlling other parasitic diseases will depend on traditional methods, such as destroying the life cycle and the judicious application of the few remaining antiparasitic agents.

## CONCLUDING REMARKS

Poultry flocks can be affected by a range of external and internal parasites. A heavy infestation can pose serious health risks, diminish performance, and negatively impact animal welfare, potentially leading to death. Additionally, the presence of these parasites can adversely affect egg or meat production. Therefore, it is crucial to monitor and control the flock for any signs of parasites. Implementing environmental management practices can help prevent the entry of external birds and support overall parasite control efforts.

## REFERENCES

[1]     Abdul M, Begum N, Dey AR, Paran S, Zahangir MA. Prevalence of blood protozoa in poultry in tangail, Bangladesh. J Agric Vet Sci 2014; 7(7): 55-60.

[2]     Belete A, Addis M, Ayele M. Review on major gastrointestinal parasites that affect chickens. J Biol Agric Healthc 2016; 6(11): 11-21. Available from: www.iiste.org

[3]     Adriano EA, Cordeiro NS. Prevalence and intensity of *Haemoproteus columbae* in three species of wild doves from Brazil. Mem Inst Oswaldo Cruz 2001; 96(2): 175-8.
[http://dx.doi.org/10.1590/S0074-02762001000200007] [PMID: 11285493]

[4]     Ybañez RHD, Resuelo KJG, Kintanar APM, Ybañez AP. Detection of gastrointestinal parasites in small-scale poultry layer farms in Leyte, Philippines. Vet World. 2018 Nov;11(11):1587-1591.
[http://dx.doi.org/10.14202/vetworld.2018.1587-1591.]

[5]     Arends JJ. External parasites and poultry pests. In: Calnek BW, Barnes HJ, Beard CW, McDougald LR, Saif YM, Eds. Diseases of Poultry. 10th ed. Ames, Iowa: Iowa State University Press 1997; pp. 785-813.

[6]     Cook ME ,Miller CC, Park Y, Pariza M. Nutritional control of immune-induced depression of food intake and growth. Poult Sci. 1993l;72(7):1301-5.
[http://dx.doi.org/10.3382/ps.0721301.]

[7]     Current WL. Cryptosporidiosis. In: Calnek BW, Barnes HJ, Beard CW, McDougald LR, Saif YM, Eds. Diseases of Poultry. 10th ed. Ames, Iowa: Iowa State University Press 1997; pp. 883-90.

[8]     Danforth HD. Use of live oocysts-based vaccines in avian coccidial control. In: Shirley MW, Tomley FM, Freeman BM, Eds. 7th Int. Cocci. Conf. Clere Print. Newbury, Berks, UK. 1996; pp. 95-6.

[9]     Essam A, Elmishmishy B, Hammad E, Elwafa SA, Abbas I. Occurrence and molecular characterization of *Cryptosporidium* oocysts in chickens from Egypt, and a meta-analysis for *Cryptosporidium* infections in chickens worldwide. Vet Parasitol Reg Stud Reports. 2025 Jan;57:101169.
[http://dx.doi.org/10.1016/j.vprsr.2024.101169]

[10]    Danforth HD. Use of live oocyst vaccines in the control of avian coccidiosis: experimental studies and field trials. Int J Parasitol 1998; 28(7): 1099-109.
[http://dx.doi.org/10.1016/S0020-7519(98)00078-2] [PMID: 9724881]

[11]    Forrester DJ, Foster GW, Morrison JL. Leucocytozoon toddi and *Haemoproteus tinnunculi* (Protozoa: Haemosporina) in the Chimango caracara (*Milvago chimango*) in Southern Chile. Mem Inst Oswaldo Cruz 2001; 96(7): 1023-4.
[http://dx.doi.org/10.1590/S0074-02762001000700024] [PMID: 11685273]

[12]    Kenneth S. Overview of Helminthiasis in Poultry, the merk veterinary manual. Gondar City, Northwest Ethiopia Veterinary Medicine Research and Report 2021; 12: 217-8. Available from: http://www.mercmanuals.com/vet/nematode_and_cestod    e_infection/overview-of-helminthosis-in-poultry.html.Factors

[13]    Klassing KC. Interaction between nutrition and infectious disease in broiler chickens. Proc. 26th Nat. Mtg. Poultry Hlth.. Processing, DPI, Georgetown, DE. 1991; pp. 97-106.

[14]    Lawal RJ, Yusuf BZ, Dauda J, Gazali YA, Biu AA. Ectoparasites infestation and its associated risk factors in village chickens (*Gallus gallus domesticus*) in and around potiskum, Yobe State, Nigeria. J Anim Husb Dairy Sci 2017; 1(1): 8-19.
[http://dx.doi.org/10.22259/2637-5354.0101002]

[15]    Leeson S, Summer JD. Internal parasites: Broiler breeder production, 1st published by nottingham university press in 2000 and digitally reprinted in 2009 from broiler breeder production, university books. Guelp Onta Canada 2009; c: 104-6.

[16]    Luka SA, Ndams IS. Short communication report: Gastrointestinal parasites of domestic chicken *gallus-gallus domesticus* linnaeus 1758 in Samaru, Zaria Nigeria. Sci World J 2010; 2(1): 27-9.
[http://dx.doi.org/10.4314/swj.v2i1.51723]

[17]    Martynova-VanKley A, Syvyk A, Teplova I, Hume M, Nalian A. Rapid detection of avian *Eimeria* species using denaturing gradient gel electrophoresis. Poult Sci 2008; 87(9): 1707-13.
[http://dx.doi.org/10.3382/ps.2008-00098] [PMID: 18753436]

[18]    McDougald L, Swayne D, Saif Y, Barnes H, Fadly A, Glisson J. Diseases of Poultry, Iowa USA. Blacwell. Publishing Company 2003; 11: 72-961.

[19]    McDougald LR, Reid WM. Coccidiosis. In: Calnek BW, Barnes HJ, Beard CW, McDougald LR, Saif YM, Eds. Diseases of Poultry. 10th ed. Ames, Iowa: Iowa State University Press 1997; pp. 865-83.

[20]    Sparagano OA, George DR, Harrington DW, Giangaspero A. Significance and control of the poultry red mite, *Dermanyssus gallinae* Annu Rev Entomol. 2014; 59: pp. 447-66.
[http://dx.doi.org/10.1146/annurev-ento-011613-162101]

[21]    Permin A, Hansen JW. The Epidemiology. Diagnosis and control of poultry parasites: An FAO handbook 2003; 8: 5-43.

[22]    Reetz J. Naturally-acquired microsporidia (*Encephalitozoon cuniculi*) infections in hens. Tierarztl Prax 1993; 21(5): 429-35.
[PMID: 8248903]

[23]    Reid WM, McDougald LR. Cestodes and trematodes. In: Calnek BW, Barnes HJ, Beard CW, McDougald LR, Saif YM, Eds. Diseases of Poultry. 10th ed. Ames, Iowa: Iowa State University Press 1997; pp. 850-64.

[24]    Ruff MD. External and internal factors affecting the severity of avian coccidiosis. In: Barta JR, Fernando MA, Eds. Proc. 6th Int. Cocci. Conf. Miffitt Print Craft. Guelph, Ont., Canada. 1993; pp. 73-9.

[25]    Ruff MD, Allen PC. Pathology of coccidial infections. In: Long PL, Ed. Coccidiosis of Man and Domestic Animals. Boca Raton, FL: CRC Press 1990; pp. 263-80.

[26]    Ruff MD, Danforth HD. Resistance of coccidia to medications. Proc XX World's Poult Cong World's Poult Sci Assoc. New Delhi, India. 1996; pp. 427-30.

[27]    Ruff MD, Norton RA. Nematodes and Acanthocephalans. In: Calnek BW, Barnes HJ, Beard CW, McDougald LR, Saif YM, Eds. Diseases of Poultry. 10th ed. Ames, Iowa: Iowa State University Press 1997; pp. 815-50.

[28]    Simon M. Emeritus. Enteric diseases. In: Handbook on poultry diseases. American Soybean Association 2005; 2: 133-43.

[29]   Suhail R, Tanveer S, Ahad S. Review article global significance of epidemiology, immunodiagnostics and histopathology of cestode parasites in fowl (*Gallus gallus*). Int J Curr Res 2013; 5(6): 1426-8.

[30]   Sychra O, Harmat P, Literák I. Chewing lice (*Phthiraptera*) on chickens (*Gallus gallus*) from small backyard flocks in the eastern part of the Czech Republic. Vet Parasitol 2008; 152(3-4): 344-8.
[http://dx.doi.org/10.1016/j.vetpar.2008.01.001] [PMID: 18280661]

[31]   Weber GM. Optimum use of anticoccidial products for efficacious prevention of poultry coccidiosis. In: Shirley MW, Tomley FM, Freeman BW, Eds. 7th Int. Cocci. Conf. Clere Print. Newbury, Berks, UK. 1997; pp. 51-2.

[32]   Jilo SA, Abadula TA, Abadura SZ, Gobana RH, Hasan LA, Nair SP. Review on epidemiology, pathogenesis, treatment, control and prevention of gastrointestinal parasite of poultry. Int J Vet Sci Anim Husb 2022; 7(5): 26-34.
[http://dx.doi.org/10.22271/veterinary.2022.v7.i5a.439]

[33]   Snyder RP, Guerin MT, Hargis BM, Page G, Barta JR. Monitoring coccidia in commercial broiler chicken flocks in Ontario: Comparing oocyst cycling patterns in flocks using anticoccidial medications or live vaccination. Poult Sci 2021; 100(1): 110-8.
[http://dx.doi.org/10.1016/j.psj.2020.09.072] [PMID: 33357673] [PMCID: PMC7772663]

# CHAPTER 2

# Seasonal Dynamics in Parasitic Diseases

**Felix Uchenna Samuel[1,*], Clement Akotsen-Mensah[2]** and **Ibrahim Abdul Mohammed[3]**

[1] *Animal Science Program, Alabama Cooperative Extension System, Alabama A & M University, Normal, Alabama, USA*

[2] *Integrated Pest Control Program, Alabama Cooperative Extension System, Alabama A & M University, Normal, Albama, USA*

[3] *Poultry Research Program, National Animal Production Research Institute, Shika-Zaria, Nigeria*

**Abstract:** Seasonal dynamics play a crucial role in the epidemiology and prevalence of parasitic diseases in poultry, influencing transmission patterns, host susceptibility, and environmental conditions. This abstract provides an overview of the seasonal variation observed in parasitic diseases affecting poultry populations and highlights the implications for disease management and control strategies. Seasonal factors, including temperature, humidity, rainfall, and photoperiod, can influence the survival, development, and transmission of parasitic pathogens, such as helminths, protozoa, and ectoparasites. Additionally, seasonal changes in host behavior, immune function, and reproductive status may impact susceptibility to parasitic infections and disease outcomes. Understanding the seasonal dynamics of parasitic diseases in poultry is essential for implementing targeted preventive measures, such as strategic deworming, parasite monitoring, and environmental management practices, to mitigate the risk of disease outbreaks and minimize production losses. Furthermore, seasonal variation in parasite populations underscores the importance of integrated approaches to disease control, including vaccination, biosecurity, and sustainable management practices, tailored to the specific epidemiological context and environmental conditions. By considering seasonal factors in disease management strategies, poultry producers can optimize health outcomes, improve welfare standards, and enhance the overall productivity and profitability of poultry production systems.

**Keywords:** Disease management, Environmental factors, Epidemiology, Parasitic diseases, Poultry, Seasonal dynamics.

* **Corresponding author Felix Uchenna Samuel:** Animal Science Program, Alabama Cooperative Extension System, Alabama A & M University, Normal, Alabama, USA; E-mail: felixsam75@yahoo.com

Tanmoy Rana (Ed.)

# INTRODUCTION

Poultry serves as the primary source of animal protein globally [1]. According to data from the USDA, chicken meat production reached 102.9 million tons in January 2020, marking a 3.9% increase from the previous year [2]. This upward trend in production is significant, especially considering projections that the global population will reach approximately nine billion by 2050, emphasizing the urgent need for sustainable and safe protein production. In intensive poultry farming systems, where birds are kept in close proximity and at high stocking densities, stress levels, and disease prevalence tend to be elevated. As a result, any disease that compromises the efficiency of such production systems poses a potential threat to the global food supply chain [3].

Seasonal dynamics in parasitic diseases of poultry encompass a broad spectrum of interactions between environmental factors, parasite life cycles, host physiology, and management practices [4]. A good understanding of these dynamics is important for effective disease prevention, control, and management in poultry production systems. Parasitic diseases represent an important obstacle in the poultry industry, exerting profound effects on health, welfare, and productivity on a global scale. These diseases, caused by different kinds of parasites, pose multifaceted challenges to poultry producers, impacting both economic viability and animal well-being. Parasites, ubiquitous in the environment, have a remarkable ability to adapt and proliferate, exploiting diverse ecological niches to perpetuate their life cycles [5]. However, their prevalence and intensity are not static but undergo dynamic fluctuations influenced by a multitude of factors, prominently including seasonal variations in environmental conditions. Seasonal changes, encompassing shifts in temperature, humidity, precipitation, and other environmental parameters, play a pivotal role in shaping the epidemiology of parasitic diseases in poultry. These environmental factors directly impact parasite survival, development, and transmission dynamics, exerting a profound influence on disease prevalence and severity [6]. For instance, warmer temperatures may accelerate the growth and multiplication of parasites, promoting their transmission within poultry flocks. Conversely, colder temperatures may hinder parasite development but facilitate their persistence in environmental reservoirs, perpetuating the risk of infection. Likewise, humidity levels significantly influence the viability of parasite stages outside the host, with higher humidity favoring survival and transmission. Precipitation patterns, by altering environmental moisture levels, can create conducive breeding grounds for parasite vectors, exacerbating the risk of transmission to poultry [7].

Moreover, host-related factors such as immune status, age, and management practices further modulate susceptibility to parasitic infections. Immune function, influenced by genetics, nutrition, and prior exposure, plays a critical role in determining the host's ability to resist parasite invasion and mount an effective immune response. Age-related differences in immune competence and physiological susceptibility can render certain poultry populations more vulnerable to parasitic diseases, particularly young or immune-compromised individuals. Furthermore, management practices, including housing conditions, sanitation protocols, and biosecurity measures, profoundly impact the risk of parasite exposure and transmission within poultry flocks [8].

## ENVIRONMENTAL FACTORS INFLUENCING SEASONAL DYNAMICS

Environmental factors play a crucial role in influencing the seasonal dynamics of poultry diseases. These factors encompass various elements of the environment, including temperature, humidity, precipitation, and other ecological parameters, which directly impact the survival, transmission, and prevalence of pathogens affecting poultry (Fig. **1**) [9]. The various factors are explained;

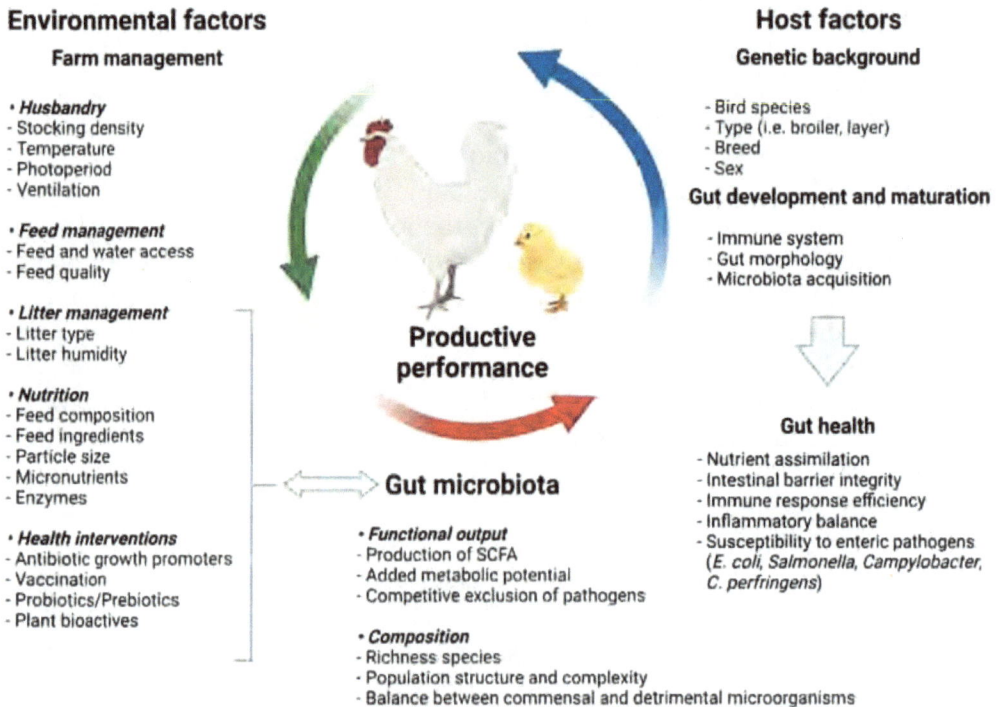

**Fig. (1).** Factors influencing parasite infection in poultry by Shehata *et al.* [15].

## Temperature

Temperature plays a pivotal role in shaping the dynamics of infectious diseases, exerting profound effects on both pathogens and their host organisms within poultry populations. The influence of temperature extends across various aspects of pathogen biology and host physiology, dictating the development, reproduction, and survival of pathogens, as well as modulating the immune response and metabolic processes of the host [10]. Many pathogens exhibit temperature-dependent life cycles, with optimal temperature ranges for growth and multiplication. Warmer temperatures create favorable conditions for pathogen replication and development, accelerating their life cycle and increasing the rate of transmission. Pathogens such as bacteria, viruses, and parasites thrive in warm environments, where enzymatic reactions and metabolic processes are more efficient, facilitating their proliferation within poultry flocks. Elevated temperatures can also enhance the survival and stability of certain pathogens outside the host, prolonging their persistence in the environment and increasing the risk of transmission to susceptible hosts [11]. However, colder temperatures can impede pathogen growth and replication, slowing down their life cycle and reducing transmission rates. However, cold temperatures may also enhance pathogen survival in the environment or within host organisms, as some pathogens can enter a dormant or resistant state to withstand adverse conditions [12]. For example, certain bacterial and viral pathogens may form protective structures, such as spores or lipid envelopes, to survive in cold environments and remain infectious for extended periods. As a result, seasonal fluctuations in temperature can influence the timing and intensity of disease outbreaks in poultry populations, with warmer seasons typically associated with increased disease prevalence and transmission rates. In addition to affecting pathogens directly, temperature also impacts the physiology and immune response of poultry hosts. High temperatures can induce stress responses in birds, compromising their immune function and making them more susceptible to infections. Conversely, cold temperatures can suppress immune function and metabolic activity, further increasing the risk of disease. Seasonal variations in temperature can therefore exacerbate the susceptibility of poultry hosts to infections, particularly during periods of temperature extremes [13].

## Humidity

Humidity levels wield considerable influence over the viability and transmission of pathogens, particularly those transmitted *via* environmental routes such as water or air. The moisture content in the air not only affects the survival of pathogens outside the host but also dictates their ability to persist in the environment and ultimately infect susceptible hosts. Understanding the role of humidity in pathogen dynamics is crucial for elucidating disease transmission patterns and implementing effective control measures within poultry production systems [14].

Higher humidity levels create an environment conducive to pathogen survival and proliferation outside the host. Pathogens such as bacteria, viruses, and fungi thrive in moist conditions, where they can remain viable for extended periods. Elevated humidity prolongs the persistence of pathogens in the environment, increasing the likelihood of transmission to susceptible hosts. For example, waterborne pathogens, including various strains of bacteria and parasites, can survive and propagate in water sources with high humidity levels, posing a significant risk to poultry health. Similarly, airborne pathogens, such as certain viruses and fungi, can remain suspended in the air for longer durations under humid conditions, enhancing their potential for transmission between birds [15]. Conversely, low humidity levels pose challenges for pathogen survival and transmission, particularly for organisms sensitive to desiccation. Dry environments can lead to the desiccation and inactivation of pathogens, reducing their viability and limiting their ability to infect hosts. Some pathogens may form protective structures, such as spores or cysts, to withstand adverse environmental conditions, but prolonged exposure to low humidity levels can still impair their survival [16]. As a result, poultry diseases transmitted *via* environmental routes may exhibit reduced prevalence and transmission rates in regions with low humidity, mitigating the risk of outbreaks within poultry populations. Seasonal changes in humidity further modulate the prevalence and spread of poultry diseases, particularly those with environmental transmission routes. Variations in humidity levels throughout the year, influenced by factors such as temperature, rainfall, and geographical location, can impact the dynamics of pathogen transmission within poultry production systems. For instance, regions experiencing high humidity during certain seasons may observe increased incidences of waterborne diseases, as pathogens thrive in moist environments [17]. Conversely, areas with low humidity levels may experience fluctuations in disease prevalence, with reduced transmission rates during drier periods.

## Precipitation

Precipitation patterns influence environmental moisture levels, creating suitable habitats for parasite development and propagation. Heavy rainfall can lead to water accumulation in pastures, poultry litter, and other environments, creating breeding sites for parasites and their vectors. Increased precipitation can also facilitate the survival and dispersal of infective parasite stages, contributing to higher infection rates in poultry flocks. Conversely, prolonged drought conditions may reduce parasite transmission by limiting the availability of water sources for vector breeding and parasite development [18].

## Seasonal Migration of Wild Birds

Seasonal migration of wild birds can introduce new parasites and pathogens to poultry flocks, contributing to seasonal fluctuations in disease prevalence. Migratory birds may serve as reservoir hosts for parasites such as coccidia, nematodes, and ectoparasites, which can be transmitted to domestic poultry during their seasonal movements. The timing and routes of bird migration can influence the introduction and spread of parasites in poultry-producing regions, highlighting the importance of biosecurity measures and surveillance programs [19].

## COMMON PARASITIC DISEASES AND SEASONAL PATTERNS

## Coccidiosis

The poultry industry faces various parasitic diseases, which can result in significant chronic losses without manifesting apparent clinical symptoms. In the United States, the annual costs associated with coccidiosis are estimated to exceed USD 127 million, while in China, they surpass USD 73 million. Coccidiosis alone accounts for 30% of the total expenditure on pharmacological control measures for all potential poultry diseases. Coccidiosis, caused by protozoan parasites of the genus *Eimeria*, is one of the most economically significant parasitic diseases affecting poultry worldwide [18]. There are seven species of *Eimeria* implicated in coccidiosis in chickens, with *E. tenella* being the most significant in broilers. The other species include *E. acervuline, E. brunetti, E. maxima, E. necatrix, E. praecox*, and *E. mitis*. Each species exhibits unique pathogenicity and targets different segments of the intestinal tract. *Eimeria* infection results in the destruction of host mucosal cells, leading to increased cell permeability and the leakage of nutrients and proteins [6]. Consequently, this impairs the digestion and absorption of proteins and other nutrients, directly contributing to both subclinical and clinical manifestations of coccidiosis Coccidiosis poses substantial challenges to the poultry industry, resulting in significant economic losses due to reduced growth rates, increased mortality, and costs associated with treatment and prevention measures. The seasonal dynamics of coccidiosis play a crucial role in its epidemiology, influencing the prevalence, severity, and management of the disease within poultry populations [7].

## Life Cycle of Eimeria Species

The life cycle of *Eimeria* in poultry typically involves both external (sporogony) and internal phases within the host, where both sexual (schizogony and gametogenic) and asexual reproductive stages occur. Oocysts, which are capsules containing parasite eggs and have protective walls, are shed in the feces in an unsporulated state and are non-infectious until they sporulate outside the host environment [11]. Sporulation typically requires warmth and oxygen and occurs throughout 24 to 48 hours, depending on environmental conditions. Each sporulated oocyst contains four sporocysts, each containing two sporozoites. This direct life cycle begins with oral infection from active oocysts during the infectious transmission stage. Sporocysts are released through the mechanical action of the gizzard, while sporozoites are released through the action of bile and protein-degrading enzymes in the small intestine [14].

These eukaryotic, host-specific, single-celled protozoa infiltrate the intestinal tissue of the host, rapidly multiplying and damaging gastrointestinal cells. This process impairs food absorption and can result in the development of diarrhea and hemorrhage if left untreated. Even in mild cases, gastrointestinal lesions caused by the proliferation of parasites in epithelial cells often facilitate secondary infections, worsening the overall health of the animal (Fig. **2**). At least seven species of *Eimeria* have been identified as parasites of intestinal epithelial cells in chickens. While the pathophysiology of *Eimeria spp.* infection varies, *Eimeria tenella*, *Eimeria necatrix*, and *Eimeria brunetti* are particularly virulent and can cause severe disease outbreaks in poultry. Among broiler chickens, three economically significant species of *Eimeria*, namely *Eimeria acervulina*, *Eimeria maxima*, and *Eimeria tenella*, are of utmost importance. Upon initial exposure to the infectious agent, young animals quickly develop immunity, which protects them from subsequent infections. However, there is no cross-immunity among different *Eimeria* species, and recurrent episodes of the disease may occur [14].

## Factors Influencing Seasonal Dynamics of Coccidiosis

The various factors influencing seasonal dynamics are elaborated (Mesa-Pineda *et al.*) [10]

### *Temperature and Humidity*

Temperature and humidity are key environmental factors influencing the sporulation and survival of Eimeria oocysts in the environment. Warmer temperatures and higher humidity levels create favorable conditions for oocyst sporulation and persistence, promoting the transmission of coccidiosis within poultry flocks. Seasonal variations in temperature and humidity can therefore impact the prevalence and intensity of coccidiosis outbreaks, with peak transmission occurring during warmer, wetter months.

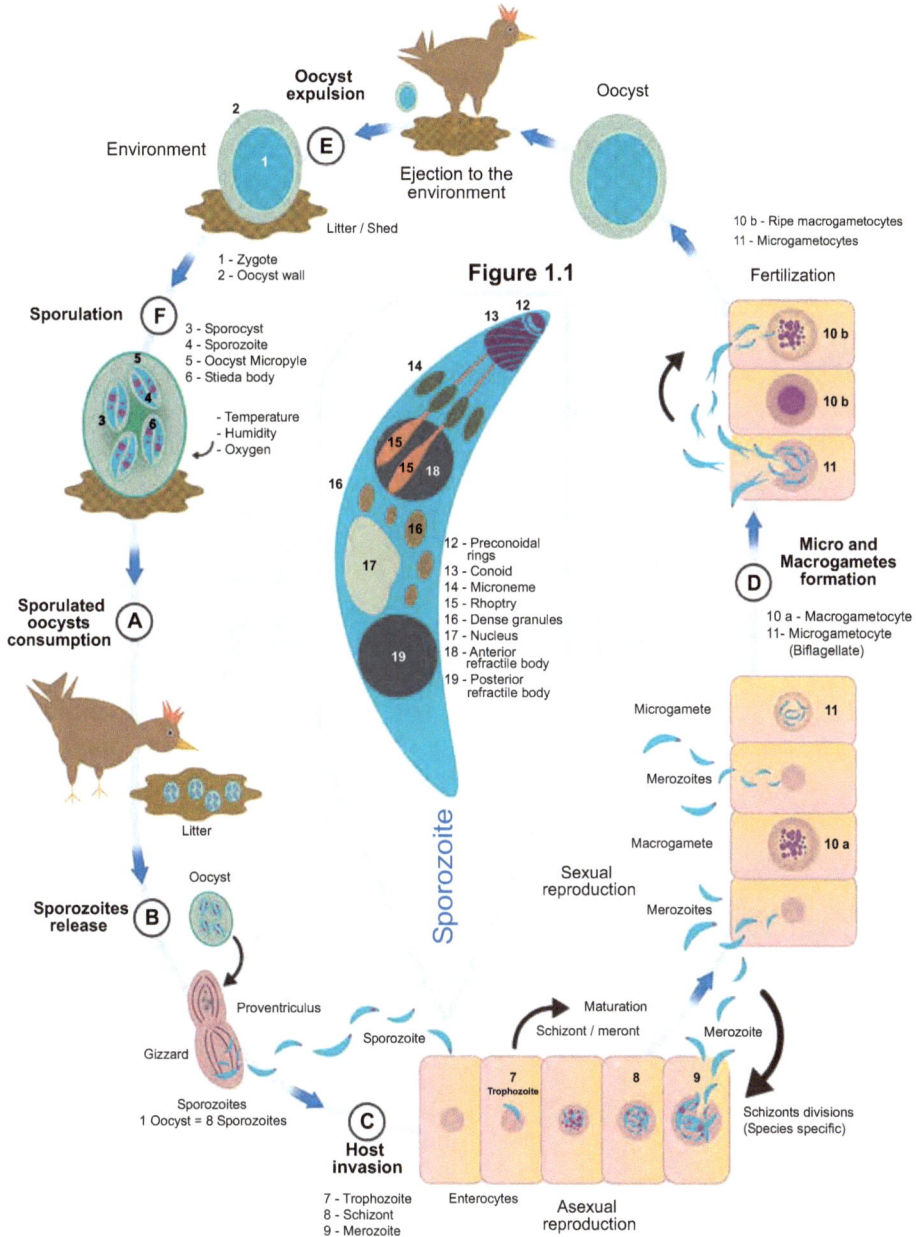

**Fig. (2).** Chicken coccidiosis: From the parasite life cycle to control of the disease (Mesa-Pineda *et al.* [10]).

## Litter Management Practices

Litter management practices, such as moisture control, litter replacement, and sanitation protocols, can influence the risk of coccidiosis in poultry houses. Wet and caked litter provides an ideal substrate for oocyst sporulation and survival, increasing the likelihood of environmental contamination and subsequent infection. Proper litter management, particularly during periods of high humidity, is essential for minimizing the risk of coccidiosis outbreaks and maintaining poultry health [11].

## Poultry Density and Stress

Poultry density and stress levels can impact the susceptibility of birds to coccidiosis and the severity of disease outbreaks. High stocking densities and overcrowded conditions can exacerbate stress, compromising immune function and increasing the risk of coccidiosis transmission. Seasonal fluctuations in poultry density, such as during peak production periods or in response to market demand, can influence the prevalence of coccidiosis within poultry populations [13].

## Immune Status of Birds

The immune status of birds plays a critical role in determining susceptibility to coccidiosis and the severity of clinical disease. Immunosuppression, caused by factors such as concurrent infections, nutritional deficiencies, or management stressors, can increase the susceptibility of birds to *Eimeria* infection and exacerbate disease outcomes. Seasonal variations in immune function, influenced by factors such as age, genetics, and environmental stressors, can impact the prevalence and severity of coccidiosis outbreaks in poultry flocks [17].

## Seasonal Patterns of Coccidiosis

Seasonal factors like temperature and humidity can influence the sporulation of the oocysts in the environment, impacting the transmission and prevalence of coccidiosis. Warmer, more humid conditions tend to favor faster sporulation. The seasonal dynamics of coccidiosis outbreaks are complex, as they depend on factors like the survival of oocysts during host diapause/dormancy periods, the ability of the parasites to spread horizontally between hosts, and the development of host immunity [15].

## Spring and Summer

Coccidiosis outbreaks are commonly observed during the spring and summer months, coinciding with warmer temperatures and higher humidity levels. These conditions create favorable environments for oocyst sporulation and transmission, leading to increased disease prevalence in poultry flocks. Additionally, the seasonal influx of new birds, such as chicks or pullets, during peak production periods can contribute to the spread of coccidiosis within poultry houses.

## Fall and Winter

In temperate regions, coccidiosis outbreaks may decline during the fall and winter months, as cooler temperatures and lower humidity levels inhibit oocyst sporulation and survival in the environment. However, coccidiosis can still occur year-round in regions with mild climates or in poultry houses with controlled environmental conditions. Additionally, stressors associated with winter management practices, such as changes in lighting or ventilation, may predispose birds to coccidiosis infection [9].

## Management Strategies for Seasonal Control

This is elaborated below (Liana, *et al.*) [8];

1. **Litter Management**: Implementing effective litter management practices, such as regular removal of wet or soiled litter, maintaining proper moisture levels, and using litter amendments or treatments, can help reduce the risk of coccidiosis transmission within poultry houses. Proper ventilation and air circulation can also aid in drying litter and minimizing oocyst survival [8].
2. **Biosecurity Measures**: Strict biosecurity measures, including controlling access to poultry houses, disinfecting equipment and footwear, and implementing quarantine protocols for new birds, are essential for preventing the introduction and spread of coccidiosis within poultry flocks. Biosecurity measures should be reinforced during periods of increased disease risk, such as during peak production or when environmental conditions are conducive to oocyst transmission [12].
3. **Vaccination and Medication:** Vaccination and medication are important tools for controlling coccidiosis in poultry flocks, particularly during periods of high disease pressure. Live attenuated vaccines or coccidiostats can be administered to birds to stimulate immunity or prevent clinical disease. However, proper timing and administration protocols should be followed to ensure optimal vaccine efficacy and minimize the risk of drug resistance [12].
4. **Nutritional Management:** Optimal nutrition is essential for maintaining the health and resilience of poultry flocks against coccidiosis. Providing balanced diets with adequate levels of vitamins, minerals, and amino acids can support immune function and reduce the impact of stressors on birds. Nutritional supplements or feed additives may also be utilized to enhance gut health and improve resistance to coccidiosis infection [17].

## Gastrointestinal Nematodes

Gastrointestinal nematodes, also known as roundworms, are a significant concern for the poultry industry worldwide. These parasitic worms, including species from the genera *Ascaridia, Heterakis*, and *Capillaria*, can infect a wide range of domestic and wild avian hosts, causing clinical disease, reduced growth rates, and even mortality in severe cases. The prevalence and seasonal dynamics of these nematode infections are closely tied to environmental factors, particularly temperature and moisture levels, which influence the survival and infectivity of the parasite's eggs and larvae [11].

*Ascaridia*: *Ascaridia galli* is a large roundworm that infects the small intestine of chickens and other poultry species. Adult worms can cause mechanical damage to the intestinal mucosa, leading to enteritis, poor nutrient absorption, and decreased feed efficiency. Clinical signs of *Ascaridia* infection may include diarrhea, weight loss, and poor growth rates in affected birds.

*Heterakis*: *Heterakis gallinarum* is a nematode species that infects the ceca of poultry, including chickens and turkeys. While adult worms typically do not cause significant clinical disease, they serve as intermediate hosts for the poultry parasite *Histomonas meleagridis*, which causes blackhead disease. *Heterakis* infection can contribute to the transmission of blackhead disease in poultry flocks [15].

*Capillaria*: *Capillaria* species, also known as hairworms, are small nematodes that infect the digestive tract of poultry. These parasites primarily inhabit the crop, esophagus, and proventriculus, causing inflammation, hemorrhage, and tissue damage. Severe *Capillaria* infections can lead to reduced growth rates, anemia, and mortality in affected birds.

### *Factors Influencing Seasonal Dynamics*

The prevalence and intensity of gastrointestinal nematode infections in poultry are influenced by a complex interplay of environmental, host, and parasite-related factors.

### *Environmental Factors*

Temperature and moisture levels are the primary environmental factors that affect the survival and development of nematode eggs and larvae in the poultry house environment. Warmer temperatures and higher humidity levels generally favor the survival and infectivity of nematode stages, leading to increased prevalence during the summer and fall seasons [17].

A study conducted in the Kashmir valley found that the prevalence of gastrointestinal nematodes was significantly higher during the summer and fall seasons compared to the winter and spring seasons. The researchers attributed this seasonal pattern to the favorable environmental conditions for the development and transmission of the parasites. Similarly, a study in India reported that the prevalence of gastrointestinal nematodes in backyard poultry was significantly associated with precipitation and the presence of seasonal rainfall.

The increased moisture in the environment can facilitate the dispersal and survival of nematode eggs and larvae, contributing to higher infection rates during the rainy seasons.

## *Host-related Factors*

The age and immune status of the poultry host can also influence the prevalence and intensity of gastrointestinal nematode infections. Young birds, particularly chicks and pullets, are more susceptible to nematode infections due to their underdeveloped immune systems. As the birds age and acquire natural immunity through repeated exposure, the prevalence and severity of nematode infections may decrease [8].

The seasonal influx of new, susceptible birds, such as chicks or pullets, during peak production periods, can contribute to the increased prevalence of gastrointestinal nematodes within poultry houses. This is particularly relevant in production systems where new birds are regularly introduced into the flock, as the naive hosts provide a suitable environment for the parasites to thrive and spread.

## *Parasite-related Factors*

The life cycle and transmission dynamics of the nematode parasites also play a role in their seasonal patterns. Gastrointestinal nematodes, such as *Ascaridia*, *Heterakis*, and *Capillaria*, have direct life cycles, where the eggs or larvae are shed in the host's feces and can directly infect new hosts through the fecal-oral route [7].

The ability of nematode eggs to survive and persist in the poultry house environment, even during periods of host dormancy or diapause, can contribute to the recurrence of infections in subsequent seasons. The eggs may remain viable in the litter or on equipment, serving as a source of infection for new, susceptible birds.

Additionally, the potential for horizontal transmission of nematode parasites between birds within a flock, as well as the introduction of new parasite species or strains through the movement of birds or contaminated equipment, can influence the seasonal dynamics of gastrointestinal nematode infections [6].

### Seasonal Patterns of Gastrointestinal Nematode Infections

The seasonal patterns of gastrointestinal nematode infections in poultry have been well-documented in various studies. In general, the prevalence and intensity of these parasitic infections tend to be higher during the warmer, more humid months of the year, particularly in the summer and fall seasons. The increased moisture in the environment during the rainy seasons can facilitate the dispersal and survival of nematode eggs and larvae, leading to higher infection rates.

In contrast, the cooler, drier conditions during the winter months often inhibit the development and survival of nematode eggs and larvae, resulting in a lower prevalence of gastrointestinal nematode infections in poultry flocks. However, it is important to note that high relative humidity alone does not necessarily translate to increased disease prevalence, as the temperature factor is also crucial [5].

### Seasonal Dynamics of Gastrointestinal Nematodes

The seasonal dynamics of gastrointestinal nematode infections in poultry are influenced by environmental factors, particularly temperature and moisture levels. These factors impact the survival, development, and infectivity of nematode eggs and larvae in the environment, ultimately influencing the risk of infection for poultry flocks.

**Temperature:** Temperature plays a crucial role in the development and survival of nematode eggs and larvae in the environment. Warmer temperatures accelerate the development of nematode eggs and larvae, leading to increased infectivity and transmission rates. In contrast, colder temperatures can slow down the development of nematode parasites, reducing the risk of infection during the winter months [4].

**Moisture Levels:** Moisture levels in the environment also affect the survival and transmission of gastrointestinal nematodes. Higher humidity levels provide optimal conditions for egg and larval development, increasing the risk of infection for poultry flocks. Conversely, drier conditions can inhibit the development and survival of nematode parasites, reducing the overall burden of infection in poultry.

### Management Strategies for Seasonal Control

Implementing effective management strategies is essential for controlling gastrointestinal nematode infections in poultry and minimizing their impact on health and productivity. Seasonal approaches, tailored to the specific challenges posed by temperature and moisture fluctuations, can help reduce nematode burdens in poultry flocks [3].

**Pasture Rotation:** Rotational grazing practices can help reduce the risk of nematode infection in free-range and pasture-raised poultry systems. Rotating poultry to different pasture areas periodically can minimize exposure to infective larvae, allowing contaminated areas to undergo natural degradation and reducing the overall nematode burden in the environment.

**Sanitation Measures:** Maintaining clean and dry housing facilities is essential for preventing the buildup of nematode larvae and reducing the risk of infection in confined poultry flocks. Regular removal of bedding material, thorough cleaning of equipment, and proper waste management practices can help minimize environmental contamination and break the nematode life cycle [2].

**Deworming Programs:** Implementing deworming programs is an important component of nematode control in poultry flocks. Anthelmintic medications, such as benzimidazoles, imidazothiazoles, and macrocyclic lactones, can be administered orally or through feed to target adult worms and larvae in the digestive tract. Deworming schedules may be adjusted seasonally to coincide with periods of increased nematode transmission risk [1].

**Nutritional Supplementation**: The inclusion of certain feed additives, such as organic acids, essential oils, or probiotics, can enhance the birds' intestinal health and immune response, potentially mitigating the impact of gastrointestinal nematode infections.

These nutritional supplements may improve the birds' ability to withstand and recover from nematode infestations, particularly during periods of high disease pressure [11].

**Genetic Selection and Breeding**: Selecting and breeding poultry with enhanced genetic resistance to gastrointestinal nematodes can be a long-term strategy for reducing the prevalence and impact of these parasites. Identifying and propagating genetic markers associated with nematode resistance can help develop more resilient poultry lines.

**Integrated Pest Management**: Adopting an integrated pest management (IPM) approach, which combines multiple control strategies, can be an effective way to manage gastrointestinal nematodes in poultry. This may include a combination of the aforementioned strategies, as well as the use of biological control agents, such as nematode-trapping fungi or predatory mites.

## MONITORING AND SURVEILLANCE

Regular monitoring of flock health, including routine fecal sampling and diagnostic testing, can help producers identify emerging nematode issues and implement timely interventions. This information can also be used to guide the implementation of seasonal control measures and optimize the use of anthelmintic treatments [15].

### Ectoparasites

Ectoparasites such as mites, lice, and fleas can infest poultry year-round, but their prevalence may increase during warmer months. Ectoparasites are organisms that live on the outer surface of their host's body, feeding on blood, skin, or other bodily fluids. In poultry production, ectoparasites can cause significant economic losses due to reduced productivity, increased mortality, and the cost of control measures. The seasonal dynamics of ectoparasites in poultry are influenced by environmental factors such as temperature, humidity, and daylight length, as well as management practices and host susceptibility [10].

### *Seasonal Patterns of Ectoparasites*

Ectoparasites in poultry exhibit distinct seasonal patterns in their abundance, activity, and prevalence. These patterns are influenced by various factors, including environmental conditions, host availability, and the life cycle of the ectoparasite species. While specific seasonal dynamics may vary depending on the region and local climate, several general trends can be observed across different geographical areas [9].

### *Spring*

Spring marks the beginning of the ectoparasite season in many regions, as temperatures rise and environmental conditions become more favorable for ectoparasite development and reproduction. Warmer temperatures stimulate ectoparasite activity and increase the rate of egg hatching and larval development. Additionally, increased daylight length during the spring months may enhance ectoparasite breeding and dispersal, leading to higher infestation rates in poultry flocks.

### *Summer*

Summer is typically the peak season for ectoparasite infestations in poultry, as temperatures reach their highest levels and humidity levels remain elevated. These warm and humid conditions provide ideal breeding grounds for ectoparasites such as mites, lice, and fleas. Poultry housed outdoors or in poorly ventilated environments are particularly susceptible to ectoparasite infestations during the summer months. Increased host activity and reduced grooming behavior may also contribute to higher ectoparasite burdens in poultry flocks during this time [12].

## *Fall*

As temperatures begin to cool in the fall, ectoparasite activity may decline, and infestation rates may decrease in some regions. However, certain ectoparasite species may continue to thrive in moderate temperatures, particularly in indoor poultry production systems where environmental conditions can be controlled. Fall is also a critical time for ectoparasite control measures, as reducing infestations before winter can help prevent carryover into the next season.

## *Winter*

Winter is generally considered a low season for ectoparasite infestations in poultry, as cold temperatures and reduced humidity levels create less favorable conditions for ectoparasite survival and reproduction. However, certain ectoparasite species may persist in indoor poultry facilities, where environmental conditions remain relatively stable. Additionally, winter can be a challenging time for ectoparasite control, as freezing temperatures may limit the effectiveness of certain treatment methods [15].

## *Factors Influencing Seasonal Dynamics*

Several factors influence the seasonal dynamics of ectoparasite in poultry, including:

1. **Temperature**: Temperature plays a crucial role in ectoparasite development, activity, and survival. Warmer temperatures accelerate ectoparasite reproduction and development, leading to higher infestation rates in poultry flocks during the spring and summer months. In contrast, colder temperatures can suppress ectoparasite activity and reduce infestation rates, particularly in outdoor poultry production systems [11].
2. **Humidity:** Humidity levels affect ectoparasite survival and reproduction, with higher humidity favoring the proliferation of certain species. Increased humidity levels during the spring and summer months provide ideal conditions for ectoparasite breeding and development, leading to higher infestation rates in poultry flocks. Conversely, lower humidity levels in the fall and winter may inhibit ectoparasite activity and reduce infestation rates, especially in regions with dry climates.
3. **Daylight Length:** Daylight length influences ectoparasite breeding and activity patterns, with longer daylight hours during the spring and summer months

promoting ectoparasite reproduction and dispersal. Increased daylight length may stimulate mating behavior and egg laying in certain ectoparasite species, leading to higher infestation rates in poultry flocks. Conversely, shorter daylight hours in the fall and winter may slow ectoparasite activity and reduce infestation rates, particularly in species that are sensitive to photoperiod [4].

4. **Host Availability:** Host availability plays a crucial role in ectoparasite population dynamics, with higher host densities leading to increased ectoparasite infestations. Poultry housed in crowded or densely populated environments are more susceptible to ectoparasite infestations, particularly during peak production periods when flock sizes are larger. Management practices that reduce host availability, such as frequent rotation of outdoor grazing areas or maintaining optimal stocking densities, can help mitigate ectoparasite infestations in poultry flocks.

## *Control Strategies for Seasonal Ectoparasites*

Implementing effective control strategies is essential for managing seasonal ectoparasites in poultry and minimizing their impact on health and productivity. These strategies may include:

1. **Environmental Management**: Maintaining clean and dry housing conditions is essential for reducing ectoparasite infestations in poultry flocks. Regular removal of bedding material, thorough cleaning of equipment, and proper waste management practices can help minimize ectoparasite breeding grounds and reduce the risk of infestation. Additionally, improving ventilation and reducing humidity levels in poultry facilities can create less favorable conditions for ectoparasite survival and reproduction [5].

2. **Biological Control Agents:** Biological control agents, such as predatory mites or parasitic wasps, can be used to target specific ectoparasite species in poultry flocks. These natural enemies prey on or parasitize ectoparasites, reducing their numbers and limiting their impact on poultry health and productivity. Biological control agents can be introduced into poultry facilities or outdoor grazing areas to help suppress ectoparasite populations and prevent infestations.

3. **Chemical Treatments:** Chemical treatments, including insecticides and acaricides, are commonly used to control ectoparasite infestations in poultry. These treatments may be applied directly to poultry or their living environments to target ectoparasites at different life stages. However, care must be taken to select appropriate chemical agents and follow label instructions to minimize risks to poultry, humans, and the environment. Additionally, rotating between different classes of chemicals can help prevent the development of resistance in ectoparasite populations.

4. **Host Management:** Implementing good host management practices is essential for reducing the risk of ectoparasite infestations in poultry flocks. This may include providing adequate nutrition and veterinary care to maintain optimal host health and immunity. Regular grooming and inspection of poultry for signs of ectoparasite infestations can help detect problems early and prevent widespread outbreaks. Additionally, segregating or culling infected individuals can help reduce the spread of ectoparasites within poultry flocks [7].

## PROTOZOAN PARASITES OF POULTRY

Protozoan parasites are unicellular organisms belonging to various taxonomic groups, including the phyla Sarcomastigophora, Apicomplexa, Ciliophora, Amoebozoa, and Microsporidia. Among these parasites, *Giardia* and *Cryptosporidium* are two significant genera known to cause enteric diseases in birds. While the seasonal dynamics of protozoan parasites in poultry are not as extensively studied as those of other parasites, such as helminths, seasonal variations in environmental conditions can still influence their prevalence and transmission dynamics. This chapter provides an overview of protozoan parasites in poultry, focusing on *Giardia* and *Cryptosporidium*, and discusses the potential impact of seasonal variations on their epidemiology [9].

### *Giardia* in Poultry

*Giardia* is a genus of flagellated protozoan parasites known to infect the gastrointestinal tract of birds, including poultry. Infection with *Giardia* can lead to a condition known as giardiasis, characterized by diarrhea, weight loss, and reduced feed efficiency. While giardiasis is more commonly associated with mammals, such as dogs and humans, poultry can also be affected by certain species of *Giardia*.

### *Cryptosporidium* in Poultry

*Cryptosporidium* is a genus of apicomplexan protozoan parasites known to infect the gastrointestinal tract of birds, including poultry. Infection with Cryptosporidium can lead to a condition known as cryptosporidiosis, characterized by diarrhea, abdominal pain, and dehydration. While cryptosporidiosis is more commonly associated with mammals, such as calves and lambs, poultry can also be affected by certain species of *Cryptosporidium* [11].

### Seasonal Dynamics of Protozoan Parasites in Poultry

Seasonal variations in environmental conditions, such as temperature, humidity, and rainfall, can influence the prevalence and transmission dynamics of protozoan parasites in poultry. While the seasonal patterns of protozoan parasites in poultry are less well-documented compared to other parasites, such as helminths, these environmental factors can still play a role in shaping their epidemiology [12].

## Temperature

Temperature is a critical factor influencing the survival and development of protozoan parasites in poultry. Warmer temperatures are generally more conducive to the growth and reproduction of protozoa, leading to increased infection rates in poultry flocks. Conversely, colder temperatures can inhibit protozoan development and transmission, resulting in lower infection rates during the winter months.

## Humidity

Humidity levels also play a significant role in the survival and transmission of protozoan parasites in poultry. Higher humidity levels create more favorable conditions for protozoan survival and dissemination, leading to increased infection rates in poultry flocks. Conversely, lower humidity levels can inhibit protozoan transmission, resulting in lower infection rates during periods of drought or low rainfall.

## Rainfall

Rainfall can influence the prevalence and transmission dynamics of protozoan parasites in poultry by affecting environmental conditions and the availability of intermediate hosts. Heavy rainfall can create moist environments conducive to protozoan survival and transmission, leading to increased infection rates in poultry flocks. Conversely, drought conditions can reduce the availability of water sources and intermediate hosts, resulting in lower infection rates [10].

## Control and Prevention of Protozoan Parasites in Poultry

Effective control and prevention measures are essential for managing protozoan parasite infections in poultry and minimizing their impact on poultry health and productivity. While seasonal variations in environmental conditions can influence the prevalence and transmission dynamics of protozoan parasites, implementing improved hygiene practices, water sanitation, and regular monitoring can help prevent protozoan infections in poultry, regardless of seasonal variations [15].

**Biosecurity Measures**: Implementing strict biosecurity measures is essential for preventing the introduction and spread of protozoan parasites in poultry flocks. Biosecurity protocols should include measures such as restricting access to contaminated areas, disinfecting equipment and footwear, and preventing the introduction of infected birds or animals into poultry facilities.

**Sanitation Protocols**: Maintaining clean and hygienic poultry facilities is essential for minimizing the risk of protozoan parasite infections in poultry flocks. Regular cleaning and disinfection of housing facilities, equipment, and feeders can help reduce environmental contamination and prevent the buildup of parasite oocysts or cysts [13].

**Parasite Control Programs**: Implementing parasite control programs is essential for managing protozoan parasite infections in poultry flocks. These programs may involve the use of chemotherapeutic agents, such as coccidiostats or anticoccidial drugs, to control coccidiosis in poultry. Additionally, deworming programs may be implemented to control other protozoan parasites, such as *Histomonas* or *Trichomonas* species, in poultry flocks.

**Vaccination**: Vaccination is an effective strategy for preventing protozoan parasite infections in poultry flocks. Several live and inactivated vaccines are available for preventing coccidiosis in chickens and turkeys. Vaccination programs should be tailored to the specific needs of each poultry flock and may involve the use of multiple vaccine strains to provide broad-spectrum protection against different Eimeria species [12]

## GENERAL CONTROL MEASURES FOR PARASITIC DISEASES OF POULTRY

The various measures are outlined (Rajesh *et al*) [14].

### Biosecurity Measures

Implementing strict biosecurity measures is paramount for safeguarding the health and well-being of poultry flocks by preventing the introduction and spread of parasitic diseases. Biosecurity protocols encompass a comprehensive set of practices and procedures designed to minimize the risk of pathogen transmission within and between poultry facilities. These measures are essential for maintaining a disease-free environment and ensuring the productivity and profitability of poultry operations [10].

One fundamental aspect of biosecurity is controlling access to poultry facilities and restricting movement between different areas to prevent the introduction of pathogens. Access should be limited to authorized personnel only, and visitors should be required to follow strict biosecurity protocols, such as wearing dedicated footwear and protective clothing and undergoing disinfection procedures upon entry and exit. Additionally, vehicles and equipment entering the premises should be thoroughly cleaned and disinfected to prevent the inadvertent introduction of parasites or other pathogens [9].

Disinfection plays a crucial role in biosecurity, as it helps eliminate pathogens from the environment and prevent their spread within poultry facilities. Regular cleaning and disinfection of equipment, housing facilities, and other high-touch surfaces are essential to reduce the risk of contamination. Disinfectants should be carefully selected based on their efficacy against specific parasites and applied according to manufacturer recommendations to ensure optimal results.

Footwear and clothing can serve as vehicles for the transmission of parasites between poultry houses, so it is essential to implement strict hygiene protocols for personnel working in or entering poultry facilities. Dedicated footwear and clothing should be provided for use within poultry houses, and personnel should change into clean attire upon entering and exiting. Additionally, hand hygiene practices, such as regular hand washing and the use of hand sanitizers, should be emphasized to minimize the risk of pathogen transmission *via* contaminated hands [8].

Preventing the introduction of infected birds or animals into poultry facilities is critical for maintaining biosecurity and preventing the spread of parasitic diseases. Poultry producers should source birds from reputable suppliers with robust health monitoring programs to minimize the risk of introducing parasites or other pathogens. Quarantine measures should be implemented for new arrivals to allow for observation and testing before integration into the main flock, reducing the risk of introducing infectious agents [7].

In addition to external biosecurity measures, internal biosecurity practices are also essential for preventing the spread of parasitic diseases within poultry facilities. These may include measures such as separating different age groups of birds, implementing strict hygiene protocols for handling eggs and chicks, and regularly monitoring flock health and performance for signs of parasitic infection. Veterinary oversight is essential for developing and implementing effective biosecurity protocols tailored to the specific needs and risks of each poultry operation [5].

Training and education are crucial components of successful biosecurity programs, as they ensure that all personnel understand their roles and responsibilities in maintaining biosecurity and preventing the spread of parasitic diseases. Regular training sessions should be conducted to review biosecurity protocols, reinforce best practices, and address any emerging threats or challenges. By fostering a culture of biosecurity awareness and compliance, poultry producers can minimize the risk of parasitic disease outbreaks and protect the health and productivity of their flocks.

## Sanitation Protocols

Maintaining clean and hygienic poultry facilities is paramount for minimizing the risk of parasitic diseases and ensuring the health and welfare of poultry flocks. Proper sanitation practices are essential for reducing environmental contamination and preventing the buildup of parasite eggs, larvae, or cysts in poultry litter. This chapter explores the importance of maintaining clean and hygienic poultry facilities and discusses best practices for cleaning, disinfection, and waste management to mitigate the risk of parasitic diseases [11].

### *Importance of Clean and Hygienic Poultry Facilities*

Cleanliness and hygiene are fundamental aspects of poultry management, as they play a crucial role in preventing the spread of pathogens, including parasitic organisms, within poultry facilities. A clean and hygienic environment not only promotes the health and well-being of poultry but also contributes to improved productivity, efficiency, and profitability of poultry operations. By minimizing the risk of disease transmission and maintaining optimal conditions for growth and development, clean poultry facilities support the overall success and sustainability of poultry production [13].

### *Cleaning and Disinfection Practices*

Regular cleaning and disinfection of housing facilities, equipment, and feeders are essential components of effective biosecurity protocols in poultry operations. These practices help to remove organic matter, debris, and microbial contaminants from surfaces, reducing the risk of pathogen transmission and disease outbreaks. Proper cleaning and disinfection procedures should be followed to ensure thorough and effective sanitation of poultry facilities.

### *Cleaning Procedures*

Cleaning involves the removal of visible dirt, organic matter, and debris from surfaces using water, detergent, and mechanical scrubbing. It is the first step in the sanitation process and is essential for preparing surfaces for disinfection. Cleaning should be conducted regularly, ideally on a daily or weekly basis, depending on the level of soiling and usage of the facility. Surfaces to be cleaned include housing facilities (*e.g.*, floors, walls, nesting boxes), equipment (*e.g.*, feeders, waterers, incubators), and other high-touch surfaces [19].

### Disinfection Procedures

Disinfection involves the application of chemical agents to surfaces to kill or inactivate microorganisms, including bacteria, viruses, fungi, and parasites. Disinfectants should be selected based on their efficacy against specific pathogens and compatibility with the materials being treated. Common disinfectants used in poultry facilities include quaternary ammonium compounds, chlorine-based compounds, peroxygen compounds, and aldehydes. Disinfection should be conducted after cleaning and allowed to dry completely before reintroducing birds or equipment into the treated area [10].

### Waste Management Practices

Effective waste management is essential for preventing the buildup of organic matter and microbial contaminants in poultry litter, which can serve as reservoirs for parasitic eggs, larvae, or cysts. Proper waste management practices involve the timely removal and disposal of soiled bedding material, manure, and other organic waste from poultry facilities. Waste should be collected and stored in designated areas away from housing facilities to minimize the risk of contamination. Composting or other waste treatment methods may be employed to further reduce the microbial load and prevent the spread of pathogens [8].

### Parasite Control Programs

These programs typically involve the use of various strategies aimed at preventing, controlling, and eliminating parasitic infections. This chapter explores the importance of parasite control programs in poultry production and discusses strategies for prevention and control, including the use of chemotherapeutic agents, vaccination programs, and integrated pest management approaches [6].

### Importance of Parasite Control Programs

Parasitic diseases can have significant economic implications for the poultry industry, leading to decreased productivity, increased mortality, and the need for costly treatment and control measures. Implementing parasite control programs is essential for minimizing the impact of parasitic infections on poultry flocks and maintaining optimal health and performance. These programs help to prevent disease outbreaks, reduce production losses, and ensure the sustainability and profitability of poultry operations.

### Chemotherapeutic Agents

Chemotherapeutic agents, such as anthelmintic drugs and acaricides, are commonly used to control helminth and arthropod parasites in poultry flocks.

These agents work by targeting specific parasites or groups of parasites, either killing them outright or inhibiting their growth and reproduction. Anthelmintic drugs, for example, are effective against internal parasites such as roundworms and tapeworms, while acaricides are used to control external parasites such as mites and lice [11].

## *Anthelmintic Drugs*

Anthelmintic drugs are commonly used to control nematode and cestode parasites in poultry flocks. These drugs work by disrupting the parasite's nervous system, muscle function, or metabolism, leading to paralysis and death. Commonly used anthelmintic drugs in poultry include benzimidazoles (*e.g.*, albendazole, fenbendazole), avermectins (*e.g.*, ivermectin), and praziquantel. These drugs are typically administered orally or *via* feed or water, and treatment regimens may need to be repeated periodically to maintain efficacy.

## *Acaricides*

Acaricides are chemical agents specifically designed to control arthropod parasites such as mites and lice in poultry flocks. These agents work by interfering with the parasite's nervous system, respiration, or reproductive processes, leading to death or impaired reproduction. Commonly used acaricides in poultry production include pyrethroids (*e.g.*, permethrin, cypermethrin), organophosphates (*e.g.*, dichlorvos), and carbamates (*e.g.*, carbaryl). Acaricides are typically applied as sprays, dust, or dips to poultry housing facilities and equipment, and treatment may need to be repeated periodically to maintain efficacy.

## *Vaccination Programs*

Vaccination programs are an effective strategy for preventing protozoan parasite infections in poultry flocks. Vaccines stimulate the bird's immune system to produce protective antibodies against specific parasites, thereby preventing infection or reducing the severity of disease. Vaccination programs may be implemented for parasites such as *Eimeria* species, which cause coccidiosis in poultry. Live attenuated or recombinant vaccines are commonly used for coccidiosis control, and birds may be vaccinated *via* drinking water, spray, or oral administration [10].

## *Integrated Pest Management (IPM)*

Integrated pest management (IPM) approaches combine multiple control strategies to manage parasitic organisms and reduce the risk of infestation in poultry facilities. IPM programs may include a combination of biological, chemical, and cultural control methods aimed at disrupting the parasite's life cycle and minimizing its impact on poultry health and productivity. Common IPM strategies for poultry parasites include habitat modification, sanitation practices, biological control agents, and targeted chemical treatments [1, 7].

## CONCLUDING REMARKS

Seasonal dynamics significantly impact the epidemiology of parasitic diseases in poultry, with fluctuations in temperature, humidity, and precipitation influencing parasite survival, development, and transmission. Warmer temperatures during spring and summer create favorable conditions for parasite proliferation, while colder temperatures in fall and winter may slow parasite development but promote environmental persistence. Changes in precipitation patterns affect parasite transmission rates, with increased rainfall facilitating breeding grounds for parasite vectors. Host-related factors like immune status and age also influence susceptibility to parasitic infections. Effective control of parasitic diseases requires a multifaceted approach, integrating sanitation, biosecurity, chemoprophylaxis, and vaccination strategies. Biosecurity measures, including strict hygiene protocols and controlled access to facilities, are essential for preventing parasite introduction and spread within poultry flocks. Chemoprophylaxis, using anthelmintic and acaricides, helps reduce parasite burdens, but judicious use is crucial to prevent drug resistance and environmental contamination. Vaccination programs stimulate the bird's immune system to produce protective antibodies against specific parasites, reducing infection risk and disease severity. Integrated pest management (IPM) strategies combine various control measures to minimize parasitic infections and mitigate their impact on poultry health and productivity. Overall, understanding seasonal dynamics and implementing targeted control measures are vital for optimizing poultry health and welfare in the face of parasitic challenges.

## REFERENCES

[1]   Ahmad R, Yu YH, Hua KF, *et al.* Management and control of coccidiosis in poultry — A review. Anim Biosci 2024; 37(1): 1-15.
[http://dx.doi.org/10.5713/ab.23.0189] [PMID: 37641827]

[2]   Barszcz M, Tuśnio A, Taciak M. Poultry nutrition. Phys Sci Rev 2024; 9(2): 611-50.
[http://dx.doi.org/10.1515/psr-2021-0122]

[3]   Chen L, Tang X, Sun P, *et al.* Comparative transcriptome profiling of *Eimeria tenella* in various developmental stages and functional analysis of an ApiAP2 transcription factor exclusively expressed during sporogony. Parasit Vectors 2023; 16(1): 241.
[http://dx.doi.org/10.1186/s13071-023-05828-8] [PMID: 37468981]

[4]   Coroian M, Fábián-Ravasz TZ, Dobrin PR, Györke A. Occurrence of *Eimeria* spp. and intestinal helminths in free-range chickens from northwest and central Romania. Animals (Basel) 2024; 14(4): 563.

[http://dx.doi.org/10.3390/ani14040563] [PMID: 38396531]

[5]     Hassoun A, Bekhit AED, Jambrak AR, *et al.* The fourth industrial revolution in the food industry—part II: Emerging food trends. Crit Rev Food Sci Nutr 2024; 64(2): 407-37.
[http://dx.doi.org/10.1080/10408398.2022.2106472] [PMID: 35930319]

[6]     Hauck R, Macklin KS. Vaccination against poultry parasites. Avian Dis 2024; 67(4): 441-9.
[PMID: 38300662]

[7]     Holubová N, Zikmundová V, Kicia M, *et al.* Genetic diversity of *Cryptosporidium* spp., *Encephalitozoon* spp. and *Enterocytozoon bieneusi* in feral and captive pigeons in Central Europe. Parasitol Res 2024; 123(3): 158.
[http://dx.doi.org/10.1007/s00436-024-08169-2] [PMID: 38460006]

[8]     Liana YA, Swai MC. Mathematical modeling of coccidiosis dynamics in chickens with some control strategies. Abstract and Applied Analysis. Hindawi 2024; 2024.

[9]     Lisovski S, Hoye BJ, Klaassen M. Geographic variation in seasonality and its influence on the dynamics of an infectious disease. Oikos 2017; 126(7): 931-6.
[http://dx.doi.org/10.1111/oik.03796]

[10]    Mesa-Pineda C, Navarro-Ruíz JL, López-Osorio S, Chaparro-Gutiérrez JJ, Gómez-Osorio LM. Chicken coccidiosis: From the parasite lifecycle to control of the disease. Front Vet Sci 2021; 8: 787653.
[http://dx.doi.org/10.3389/fvets.2021.787653] [PMID: 34993246]

[11]    Mir FH, Bharti P, Tanveer S, Para BA. Epidemiology and seasonal dynamics of gastrointestinal helminth infections of domestic fowl in Kashmir valley. India 2023.

[12]    Nagwa EA, El-Akabawy LM, El-Madawy RS, Toulan EI. Studies on intestinal protozoa of poultry in Gharbia Governorate. Benha Vet Med J 2013; 5(2): 78-83.

[13]    Paliy AP, Mashkey AM, Sumakova NV, Paliy AP. Distribution of poultry ectoparasites in industrial farms, farms, and private plots with different rearing technologies. Biosyst Divers 2018; 26(2): 153-9.
[http://dx.doi.org/10.15421/011824]

[14]    Rajesh C, Rao V D P, Gomez-Villamandos J C, Shukla S K, Banerjee P S. Diseases of poultry and their control. Diseases of poultry and their control 2001.

[15]    Shehata AA, Yalçın S, Latorre JD, *et al.* Probiotics, prebiotics, and phytogenic substances for optimizing gut health in poultry. Microorganisms 2022; 10(2): 395.
[http://dx.doi.org/10.3390/microorganisms10020395] [PMID: 35208851]

[16]    Shifaw A, Feyera T, Walkden-Brown SW, Sharpe B, Elliott T, Ruhnke I. Global and regional prevalence of helminth infection in chickens over time: a systematic review and meta-analysis. Poult Sci 2021; 100(5): 101082.
[http://dx.doi.org/10.1016/j.psj.2021.101082] [PMID: 33813325]

[17]    Sreedevi C, Jyothisree Ch, Rama Devi V, Annapurna P, Jeyabal L. Seasonal prevalence of gastrointestinal parasites in desi fowl (*Gallus gallus domesticus*) in and around Gannavaram, Andhra Pradesh. J Parasit Dis. 2016 Sep;40(3):656-61.
[http://dx.doi.org/10.1007/s12639-014-0553-0]

[18]    Soliman D, Adly E, Nasser M, Shehata M, Kamal M. Seasonal population dynamics of the common chewing lice *Columbicola columbae* infesting the domestic pigeon *Columba livia*. Orient Insects 2023; 57(3): 819-29.
[http://dx.doi.org/10.1080/00305316.2022.2136777]

[19]    Tirfie AM, Lulie MW. Economic impacts of coccidiosis on productivity and survivability of chicken in Ethiopia. Poult Fish Wildl Sci 2024; 12: 256.

# CHAPTER 3

# Principles of Parasitism in Parasitic Diseases

**Felix Uchenna Samuel[1,*], Clement Akotsen-Mensah[2] and Ibrahim Abdul Mohammed[3]**

*[1] Animal Science Program, Alabama Cooperative Extension System, Alabama A & M University, Normal, Alabama, USA*

*[2] Integrated Pest Control Program, Alabama Cooperative Extension System, Alabama A & M University, Normal, Alabama, USA*

*[3] Poultry Research Program, National Animal Production Research Institute, Shika-Zaria, Nigeria*

**Abstract:** "Principles of Parasitism in Parasitic Diseases of Poultry" discusses the fundamental aspects of parasitic diseases affecting poultry. It delves into the principles governing parasitism within this context, exploring the interactions between parasites and their avian hosts. The abstract highlights the significance of understanding these principles in the management and control of parasitic infections in poultry populations. By elucidating the mechanisms of parasite transmission, host-parasite interactions, and the impact of parasitic diseases on poultry health and productivity, the abstract underscores the importance of adopting comprehensive strategies for disease prevention and control. Furthermore, it emphasizes the role of integrated approaches involving parasite surveillance, biosecurity measures, and appropriate treatment protocols in mitigating the economic losses associated with parasitic infections in poultry farming. Overall, the abstract provides a concise overview of the central concepts and implications of parasitism in the context of poultry diseases, aiming to inform researchers, veterinarians, and poultry producers about the complexities of managing parasitic infections in avian populations.

**Keywords:** Biosecurity, Disease management, Host-parasite interactions, Parasitic diseases, Parasitism, Poultry.

## INTRODUCTION

Parasitic diseases pose significant challenges to poultry production worldwide, affecting bird health, welfare, and productivity [1]. The poultry industry has emerged as the primary provider of efficient and high-quality animal proteins on a global scale. Poultry meat and eggs offer numerous advantages over other sources of animal-based foods. Poultry meat stands out due to its favorable protein

---

*** Corresponding author Felix Uchenna Samuel:** Animal Science Program, Alabama Cooperative Extension System, Alabama A & M University, Normal, Alabama, USA; E-mail: felixsam75@yahoo.com

**Tanmoy Rana (Ed.)**

content, balanced amino acid profile, and rich supply of energy and micronutrients [2]. Moreover, when compared to mammalian meat, poultry meat, particularly when skinless, contains lower levels of fat, mainly attributed to the reduced presence of intramuscular fat in avian species, as highlighted [3]. Parasitism represents a type of ecological interaction wherein one organism, known as the parasite, derives benefits from utilizing resources obtained from another organism, referred to as the host. Over the course of evolution, species have coexisted alongside populations of parasites, which, along with various other ecological interactions, have played a role in regulating the sizes, population structures, and genetic compositions of these species. Parasites exert an influence on hosts akin to that of predators, competitors, and other natural adversaries. Indeed, the impact of a parasite on a host can extend to its response to competitors and mutualistic organisms, its reaction to environmental conditions, its overall health status, reproductive capabilities, resource acquisition abilities, and even its survival [4]. At the core of parasitism lies the intricate interaction between the parasite and its host. In essence, the crux of parasitism lies in the dynamics of the parasitic-host relationship, which constitutes a fundamental aspect of ecological studies examining the interplay between organisms and their surroundings. Yet, ecologically speaking, the relationship between parasite and host can be likened to a "double-edged sword". This is because the ecology of the host organism can concurrently influence the life cycle of a parasite, with the host effectively serving as a habitat for the parasite. Numerous biotic and abiotic factors contribute to shaping the ecology of hosts, thereby exerting a corresponding impact on the parasites they harbor [5].

In ecological terms, interactions between hosts and parasites are characterized by the relative fitness, encompassing factors like survival and reproduction, of each participating organism. Typically, parasitic interactions confer benefits to the parasite while imposing detrimental fitness outcomes on the host. However, the degree to which hosts are adversely affected by parasites can vary widely, with certain host-parasite relationships exhibiting characteristics akin to commensalism, where one organism benefits without causing significant harm to the other. The extent of fitness costs incurred by hosts is also heavily influenced by environmental factors, whereby ideal ecological conditions may render parasites relatively benign to hosts, whereas exposure to stressors like extreme weather or food scarcity can lead to noticeable survival or reproductive costs for hosts [6]. Moreover, host-parasite interactions can be examined from a physiological standpoint, focusing on the molecular and cellular interplay occurring when parasites come into contact with host tissues. In some instances, these interactions directly lead to host pathology, or negative fitness consequences, through mechanisms such as parasite-induced tissue damage, exploitation of host resources, or suppression of host immune responses by the parasite. Conversely, in other scenarios, the adverse fitness impacts of parasites on hosts predominantly stem from host-mediated responses to parasitism, such as immunopathology or alterations in host behavior that may impede reproductive success [7].

## BIOLOGY OF POULTRY PARASITES

Poultry parasites encompass a diverse array of organisms, including protozoa, helminths, arthropods, and other pathogens, that exploit birds as hosts to complete their life cycles. These parasites can affect various systems within the bird's body, including the gastrointestinal tract, respiratory system, integumentary system, and reproductive organs. Parasitic infections can lead to clinical signs such as diarrhea, weight loss, respiratory distress, decreased egg production, and increased mortality rates, posing significant challenges to poultry producers worldwide [8].

## CLASSIFICATION OF POULTRY PARASITES

Poultry parasites are classified into different taxonomic groups based on their evolutionary relationships, morphology, and life cycle characteristics. Protozoan parasites include species such as *Eimeria, Giardia,* and *Cryptosporidium*, which infect the gastrointestinal tract of poultry. Helminth parasites encompass nematodes (roundworms), cestodes (tapeworms), and trematodes (flukes), which can infect various organs and tissues in poultry. Arthropod parasites include mites, lice, fleas, and ticks, which infest the skin, feathers, and respiratory tract of birds [9].

## MORPHOLOGY AND LIFE CYCLES OF COMMON POULTRY PARASITES

Poultry parasites display a wide array of morphological adaptations that are tailored to their parasitic lifestyle. These adaptations enable them to effectively exploit their avian hosts and complete their life cycles [10].

### Protozoan Parasites

Protozoan parasites are single-celled organisms that can infect various tissues and organs of poultry. They exhibit complex life cycles that typically involve multiple developmental stages, each adapted to survive in different environmental conditions and host tissues. For example, the life cycle of *Eimeria spp.*, a common protozoan parasite in poultry, includes stages such as sporozoites, merozoites, gametocytes, and oocysts. Sporozoites are the infective stage of *Eimeria* parasites, released from sporulated oocysts upon ingestion by the host. These motile forms penetrate the intestinal epithelium and initiate infection. Inside the host cells, sporozoites undergo asexual reproduction, forming merozoites, which further multiply and cause tissue damage. Eventually, sexual stages develop, leading to the formation of gametocytes. These gametocytes undergo fertilization and produce oocysts, which are shed in the feces and serve as the source of infection for other birds (Fig. **1**).

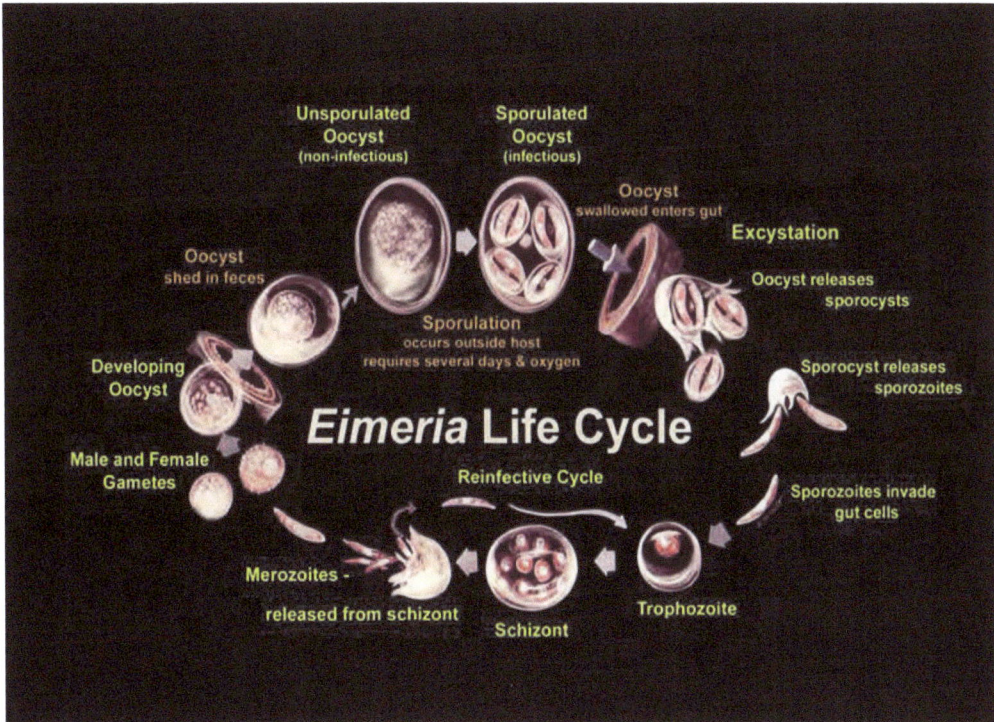

**Fig. (1).** Protozoan parasite life cycle (*Eimeria*) (Source: https://finevet.tumblr.com/post/142914665431/coccidiosis-is-a-parasitic-disease).

## Helminth Parasites

Helminth parasites are multicellular organisms that include nematodes (roundworms), cestodes (tapeworms), and trematodes (flukes). They vary in size, shape, and morphology, with some species possessing specialized structures for attachment and feeding. For example, *Ascaridia galli*, a common nematode parasite of poultry, has a cylindrical body with a tapered anterior end equipped with buccal capsules and teeth-like structures for attachment to the intestinal mucosa (Fig. **2**). The life cycles of helminth parasites often involve intermediate hosts, where larval development occurs before transmission to the definitive host. For instance, the life cycle of the tapeworm, *Hymenolepis* spp., includes a stage where eggs are ingested by intermediate hosts such as insects or earthworms. Inside the intermediate host, eggs hatch and release larvae, which develop into cysticercoids. When the definitive host consumes the infected intermediate host, the cysticercoids mature into adult tapeworms in the intestine, completing the life cycle [11].

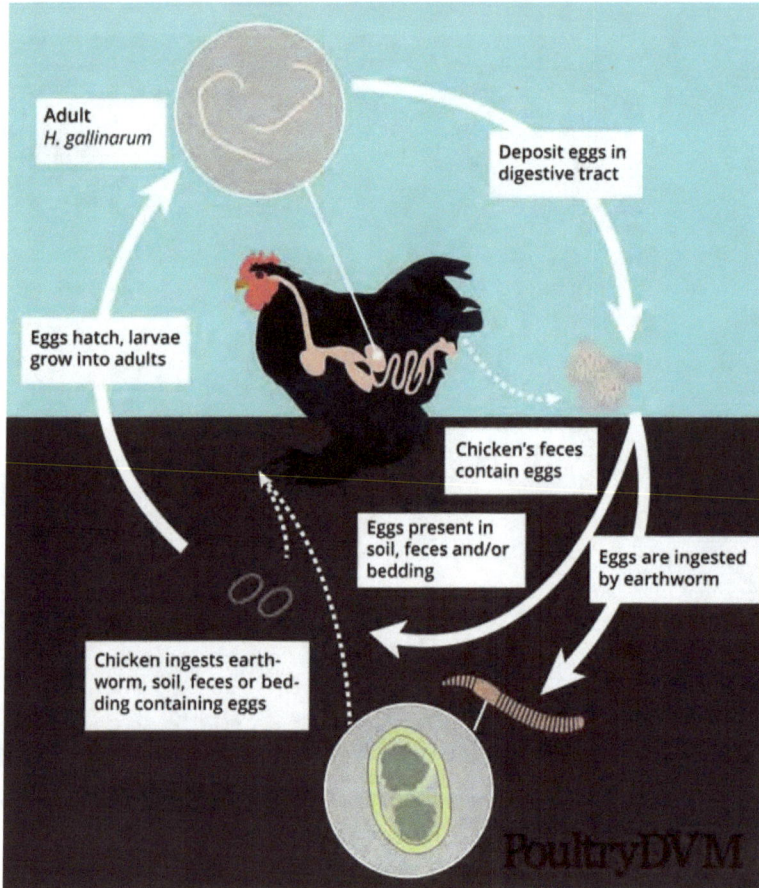

**Fig. (2).** Life cycle of helminth parasites of poultry. (https://i.pinimg.com/736x/66/7c/a1/667ca15ac40a-3ed06f76b5362adfcb43--life-cycles-poultry.jpg).

## Arthropod Parasites

Arthropod parasites, including mites, lice, fleas, and ticks, infest the skin, feathers, and respiratory tract of poultry. They possess distinct body segments, mouthparts, and appendages adapted for feeding, locomotion, and reproduction. For example, poultry mites like *Dermanyssus gallinae* have specialized mouthparts for piercing the skin and sucking blood from their avian hosts [12]. The life cycles of arthropod parasites often involve multiple stages, including eggs, nymphs, and adults, with each stage adapted to specific environmental conditions and host interactions (Fig. **3**). For instance, the life cycle of poultry lice begins with the deposition of eggs (nits) on the feathers or skin of the host. The eggs hatch into nymphs, which undergo several molts before reaching adulthood. Adult lice feed on the host's blood and reproduce, perpetuating the infestation.

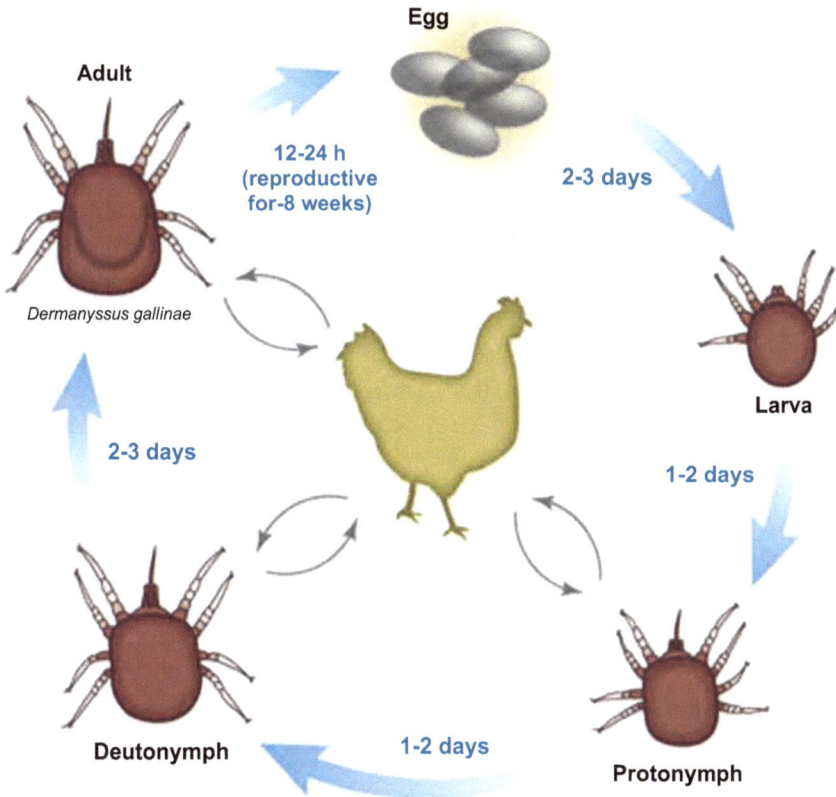

Sparagano OAE, et al. 2014.
Annu. Rev. Entomol. 59:447-66

**Fig. (3).** Life cycle of Arthropod parasite of poultry.

## TRANSMISSION ROUTES AND MODES OF INFECTION

The transmission of poultry parasites occurs through various routes, including ingestion of infective stages (*e.g.*, eggs, larvae, or cysts), direct contact with infected birds or vectors, and exposure to contaminated environments. Contaminated feed, water, bedding, and equipment can serve as sources of infection for poultry flocks [13]. Additionally, vectors such as mosquitoes, flies, and mites can transmit parasitic pathogens from one bird to another.

## Host Specificity and Tissue Tropism

Host specificity refers to the degree to which a parasite is adapted to infect a particular host species. In the context of poultry parasites, host specificity can vary widely, ranging from parasites capable of infecting multiple avian species to those that are highly specialized and restricted to specific hosts [14].

### *Factors Influencing Host Specificity*

Several factors contribute to the host specificity of poultry parasites, including genetic factors, host immune responses, and environmental conditions.

- **Genetic Factors**: Parasites possess genetic traits that determine their ability to infect and proliferate within specific host species. These traits may include surface antigens or receptors that facilitate host cell recognition and attachment. Genetic variability within parasite populations can influence host specificity, with certain strains or genotypes exhibiting greater affinity for particular hosts.
- **Host Immune Responses**: The immune system plays a critical role in determining the outcome of parasite infections, including host specificity. Hosts with robust immune responses may effectively resist or control parasite colonization, limiting the establishment of infection. Conversely, immunocompromised hosts may be more susceptible to parasitic diseases, allowing parasites to proliferate and cause pathology.
- **Environmental Conditions**: Environmental factors such as temperature, humidity, and habitat structure can also influence host specificity by affecting parasite survival, development, and transmission. Parasites adapted to specific environmental niches may exhibit preferences for certain host species that inhabit similar habitats [15].

## Tissue Tropism

In addition to host specificity, many poultry parasites exhibit tissue tropism, which refers to their preference for infecting specific organs or tissues within the host. Tissue tropism is influenced by a combination of parasite factors, host factors, and environmental conditions.

- **Parasite Factors**: The morphology, physiology, and life cycle of the parasite can influence tissue tropism. For example, parasites with specialized structures or adaptations for attachment and feeding may target specific host tissues where they can maximize nutrient acquisition and reproduction.
- **Host Factors**: The anatomy, physiology, and immune response of the host also play a crucial role in determining tissue tropism. Host tissues that provide suitable conditions for parasite survival and replication may be preferentially

targeted by parasitic invaders. Additionally, variations in host immune defenses across different tissues can influence parasite establishment and persistence [16].

- **Environmental Conditions**: Environmental factors such as oxygen availability, pH levels, and nutrient availability can impact tissue tropism by influencing parasite growth and development within specific host tissues. Parasites may exhibit adaptations to exploit environmental cues and colonize favorable microenvironments within the host.

## *Examples of Tissue Tropism in Poultry Parasites*

Many poultry parasites demonstrate tissue tropism, with distinct preferences for specific organs or tissues within the avian host. For example:

- **Gastrointestinal Parasites**: *Eimeria* species, which are protozoan parasites that cause coccidiosis in poultry, primarily infect the intestinal epithelium. These parasites invade the mucosal lining of the intestines, where they undergo a complex life cycle involving multiple developmental stages.
- **Respiratory Parasites**: Respiratory parasites such as *Ascaridia galli*, a nematode parasite, preferentially inhabit the trachea and bronchi of poultry. These parasites can cause respiratory symptoms such as coughing, wheezing, and dyspnea, leading to reduced respiratory function and compromised health [17].
- **Ectoparasites**: Ectoparasites like poultry mites and lice often target specific regions of the host's body, such as the skin, feathers, or respiratory tract. For example, *Dermanyssus gallinae*, commonly known as the red mite, feeds on the blood of poultry and typically infests roosting areas and nesting sites within the poultry house.

## Implications for Disease Management Host specificity and Tissue Tropism

The knowledge of host specificity and tissue tropism of poultry parasites is critical for developing targeted control strategies and implementing effective disease management practices. By identifying the specific hosts and tissues targeted by parasites, poultry producers can implement measures to reduce parasite exposure and minimize the risk of infection. This may include strategies such as improving biosecurity measures, implementing parasite surveillance programs, and using targeted treatments to control parasite populations in high-risk areas. Unravelling the tissue tropism can inform diagnostic approaches and help veterinarians and poultry producers identify the underlying cause of clinical signs and symptoms in affected birds. By understanding which organs or tissues are most likely to be affected by parasitic infections, practitioners can focus diagnostic efforts and tailor treatment regimens to address the specific needs of individual birds or flocks.

## ADAPTATIONS FOR PARASITISM IN POULTRY PARASITES

Poultry parasites have evolved a diverse array of adaptations to thrive within their avian hosts. These adaptations are crucial for their survival, reproduction, and transmission within the host environment [14].

### Evading Host Immune Responses

One of the key adaptations employed by poultry parasites is the ability to evade or modulate the host's immune response. Host immune defenses play a critical role in recognizing and eliminating invading parasites, but successful parasites have evolved strategies to evade or suppress these defenses. For example, protozoan parasites like *Eimeria spp.* can modulate host immune responses by secreting immunomodulatory molecules that interfere with the host's ability to mount an effective immune response. Similarly, helminth parasites like *Ascaridia galli* may secrete immunomodulatory proteins or molecules that down-regulate host immune defenses, allowing the parasite to establish and maintain infection within the host.

### Enhanced Attachment to Host Tissues

Another important adaptation exhibited by poultry parasites is the ability to attach securely to host tissues, facilitating nutrient acquisition and preventing expulsion from the host. Many parasites possess specialized structures or organs for attachment, such as suckers, hooks, or specialized mouthparts. For example, the coccidian parasite *Eimeria spp.* produces specialized structures called sporocysts and oocysts, which contain protective walls that enable them to survive outside the host and resist environmental stresses. Once ingested by the host, these structures release infective sporozoites that attach to and invade host intestinal cells, where they undergo replication and development. Similarly, helminth parasites like *Heterakis gallinarum* possess specialized structures such as buccal capsules and stylets that facilitate attachment to the intestinal mucosa, allowing the parasite to feed on host blood or tissue fluids [10].

### Optimizing Nutrient Acquisition

Poultry parasites have also evolved mechanisms to optimize nutrient acquisition from the host environment. Parasites rely on host resources for energy, growth, and reproduction, and have developed adaptations to maximize their nutrient uptake. For example, coccidian parasites like *Eimeria* spp. absorb nutrients directly from host intestinal cells, exploiting host cell metabolism for their own benefit. These parasites may also induce changes in host cell physiology to enhance nutrient availability or suppress host immune responses, creating a favorable environment for parasite survival and reproduction. Similarly, helminth parasites like *Ascaridia galli* possess specialized structures such as a well-developed digestive system and body cavity filled with nutrient-rich fluid, allowing them to absorb nutrients from host blood or tissue fluids [9].

## Evolution of Resistance Mechanisms

In response to the selective pressure exerted by parasitic infections, poultry hosts have evolved a variety of resistance mechanisms to limit parasite establishment and replication. These resistance mechanisms may involve both innate and adaptive immune responses, as well as behavioral or physiological adaptations that reduce parasite exposure or susceptibility. For example, poultry hosts may exhibit increased mucosal antibody production, enhanced cellular immune responses, or changes in gut microbiota composition that confer resistance to parasitic infections. Additionally, hosts may exhibit behavioral adaptations such as preening or grooming behaviors that remove ectoparasites from the body surface, reducing parasite burdens and transmission rates [8].

## Interactions with Host Microbiota

Recent research has highlighted the importance of interactions between poultry parasites and the host microbiota in shaping parasite-host interactions and disease outcomes. The host microbiota, consisting of diverse communities of bacteria, fungi, and other microorganisms inhabiting the gastrointestinal tract, plays a crucial role in modulating host immune responses, nutrient metabolism, and overall health. Poultry parasites may interact with the host microbiota in several ways, including modulating microbial composition, altering microbial metabolism, or exploiting microbial products for their own benefit. Conversely, the host microbiota may exert protective effects against parasitic infections by competing for resources, producing antimicrobial compounds, or stimulating host immune responses. Understanding these interactions is essential for elucidating the mechanisms underlying parasite-host interactions and developing novel strategies for parasite control in poultry populations [7].

## Implications for Disease Management

Adaptations employed by poultry parasites are crucial for developing effective strategies for disease management and control. By targeting key parasite adaptations, such as mechanisms for evading host immune responses or optimizing nutrient acquisition, researchers and veterinarians can develop novel therapeutics, vaccines, or control measures to disrupt parasite life cycles, reduce transmission rates, and minimize the impact of parasitic diseases in poultry populations. Additionally, understanding the role of the host microbiota in modulating parasite-host interactions provides new opportunities for the development of probiotics or microbiome-based interventions to enhance host resistance to parasitic infections. Overall, a comprehensive understanding of parasite adaptations is essential for developing integrated, sustainable approaches to poultry parasite control that mitigate the impact of parasitic diseases on poultry health and welfare [6].

## TRANSMISSION ROUTES AND MODES OF INFECTION IN POULTRY PARASITES

Poultry parasites employ diverse strategies for transmission, utilizing various routes to infect susceptible hosts and perpetuate their life cycles [4, 5].

### Direct Transmission

Direct transmission involves the transfer of parasites between infected and susceptible hosts through direct contact or close proximity. In poultry, direct transmission commonly occurs through contact with contaminated feces, respiratory secretions, or skin lesions of infected birds. For example, coccidian parasites like *Eimeria* spp. shed infective oocysts in the feces of infected birds, which can contaminate the environment and serve as a source of infection for susceptible individuals within the flock. Similarly, ectoparasites such as poultry lice or mites can spread directly from bird to bird through close contact, leading to infestations within the flock.

### Indirect Transmission

Indirect transmission involves the transfer of parasites *via* intermediate hosts, contaminated environments, or vectors. In poultry, indirect transmission routes are common for parasites with complex life cycles that require intermediate hosts or environmental stages for development and transmission. For example, helminth parasites like *Ascaridia galli* have indirect life cycles that involve earthworms as intermediate hosts. Poultry ingests earthworms containing infective larvae, allowing the parasites to complete their life cycle within the avian host. Similarly, coccidian parasites like *Eimeria* spp. have indirect life cycles involving environmental stages (oocysts) that must sporulate in the external environment before becoming infective to poultry hosts [3].

### Horizontal Transmission

Horizontal transmission refers to the spread of parasites between individuals within the same generation. In poultry, horizontal transmission is common in flock settings, where parasites can be transmitted through direct or indirect contact between birds. Horizontal transmission may occur through shared feeding and drinking sources, communal nesting areas, or close social interactions between flock members. For example, respiratory parasites like gapeworms (*Syngamus trachea*) can be transmitted horizontally between birds through shared airspace or contaminated respiratory secretions, leading to respiratory infections within the flock [12].

## Vertical Transmission

Vertical transmission involves the transfer of parasites from parent birds to offspring, typically through the egg or embryo. In poultry, vertical transmission may occur transovarially, where parasites infect the reproductive organs of the parent bird and are subsequently passed on to the developing eggs. Alternatively, parasites may infect developing embryos within the egg, leading to the hatching of infected chicks. Vertical transmission can play a significant role in perpetuating parasitic infections within poultry populations, particularly in breeding or parent stock flocks. For example, coccidian parasites like *Eimeria spp.* can be transmitted vertically from parent birds to chicks through infected eggs, resulting in an early onset of infection in the offspring.

## Environmental Transmission

Environmental transmission involves the transfer of parasites through contaminated environments, including soil, water, bedding, and feed sources. In poultry, environmental transmission is common for parasites with robust environmental stages, such as coccidian oocysts or helminth eggs. These environmental stages can persist in the external environment for extended periods, serving as a reservoir of infection for susceptible birds. For example, poultry may ingest infective coccidian oocysts or helminth eggs present in contaminated soil, water, or feed, leading to the establishment of infection within the host. Additionally, vectors such as arthropods (*e.g.*, mosquitoes, and flies) can serve as mechanical or biological vectors for parasite transmission, carrying infective stages between birds or introducing parasites directly into the host environment [9].

## MODES OF INFECTION

The modes of infection describe the specific mechanisms by which parasites enter and establish infection within the host. In poultry, modes of infection vary depending on the parasite species and its life cycle requirements. Common modes of infection include ingestion of infective stages (*e.g.*, eggs, larvae, cysts) *via* contaminated food, water, or soil, or exposure to infective stages through direct contact with infected birds or vectors. For example, coccidian parasites like *Eimeria spp.* are typically ingested by poultry through contaminated feed or water sources, allowing the parasites to establish infection within the intestinal tract [10]. Similarly, helminth parasites like *Ascaridia galli* may be ingested by poultry through the consumption of contaminated feed or soil, while ectoparasites like poultry lice or mites may infest birds through direct contact or exposure to contaminated environments [8].

## FACTORS INFLUENCING PARASITE DEVELOPMENT AND SURVIVAL IN POULTRY

Parasitic diseases pose significant challenges to poultry production worldwide, affecting bird health, welfare, and productivity. The development and survival of parasites within poultry hosts are influenced by a myriad of factors, including environmental conditions, host factors, and management practices [11].

### Environmental Conditions

#### *Temperature*

Temperature plays a crucial role in the development and survival of poultry parasites. Different parasites have varying temperature requirements for optimal development, with some species thriving in warm conditions while others prefer cooler temperatures. For example, coccidian parasites like *Eimeria spp.* typically exhibit optimal development at temperatures ranging from 20°C to 30°C, making the summer months conducive to parasite proliferation. Conversely, certain helminth parasites may have lower temperature thresholds for larval development, allowing them to persist in the environment during colder seasons [2].

#### *Humidity*

Humidity levels also influence the survival of poultry parasites, particularly those with environmental stages such as oocysts or eggs. Higher humidity levels can enhance the viability and sporulation of parasite stages outside the host, increasing the risk of infection for susceptible birds. In contrast, arid conditions may limit parasite survival and transmission, reducing the overall prevalence of parasitic diseases in poultry flocks [6].

#### *Moisture*

Moisture levels in the environment can impact the development and transmission of poultry parasites, especially those with aquatic or soil-based life stages. Excessive moisture can create favorable breeding grounds for parasite vectors such as mosquitoes or flies, increasing the risk of transmission to poultry hosts. Proper drainage and ventilation in poultry housing facilities are essential for minimizing moisture buildup and reducing the proliferation of parasitic organisms.

## Host Factors

### Age

The age of poultry hosts can influence their susceptibility to parasitic infections. Young birds, particularly chicks or poults, may be more vulnerable to certain parasites due to their immature immune systems and physiological development. In contrast, older birds may have acquired immunity to certain parasites through previous exposure or vaccination, reducing their susceptibility to reinfection.

### Immune Status

The immune status of poultry hosts plays a critical role in determining their ability to resist parasitic infections. Birds with compromised immune systems, either due to genetic factors, stress, or concurrent diseases, may be more susceptible to parasitic diseases. Conversely, birds with robust immune responses may be able to control parasite replication and limit the severity of infection [5].

### Genetic Resistance

Genetic factors also contribute to the susceptibility of poultry hosts to parasitic infections. Some bird breeds or genetic lines may exhibit inherent resistance or tolerance to specific parasites, reducing the overall prevalence of infection within the population. Selective breeding programs may target genetic traits associated with resistance to parasitic diseases to improve overall flock health and productivity.

## HOST-PARASITE INTERACTIONS

### Immune Responses to Parasitic Infections in Poultry

The immune response to parasitic infections in poultry is a complex and coordinated process involving both innate and adaptive components. Upon exposure to parasitic organisms, the host's immune system recognizes and responds to the invading pathogens, aiming to eliminate the parasites and prevent further infection. The innate immune system acts as the first line of defense, providing immediate, nonspecific protection against a wide range of pathogens. This includes physical barriers such as the skin and mucous membranes, as well as cellular components such as phagocytes (*e.g.*, macrophages, neutrophils) and natural killer (NK) cells. In addition to the innate immune response, poultry possesses an adaptive immune system that provides more specific and long-lasting protection against parasites. The adaptive immune response involves the activation of T and B lymphocytes, which work together to recognize and eliminate parasite-infected cells and produce specific antibodies against parasitic antigens. T cells play a central role in orchestrating the immune response, with different subsets of T cells (*e.g.*, T helper cells, cytotoxic T cells) performing distinct functions in combating parasitic infections. B cells produce antibodies that bind to parasite antigens, marking them for destruction by other immune cells or neutralizing their harmful effects. The immune response to parasitic infections in poultry is influenced by various factors, including the type of parasite, the route of infection, and the host's genetic background. Different parasites have evolved diverse strategies to evade or suppress host immune responses, allowing them to establish chronic infections and persist within the host [4].

## PATHOGENESIS OF PARASITIC DISEASES IN POULTRY

The pathogenesis of parasitic diseases in poultry involves a complex interplay between the parasite, the host immune system, and environmental factors. Parasitic organisms can cause tissue damage directly through their feeding activities, migration through host tissues, or the release of toxic metabolites. For example, helminth parasites like *Ascaridia galli* can disrupt the integrity of the intestinal mucosa, leading to hemorrhage, inflammation, and impaired nutrient absorption. Protozoan parasites such as *Eimeria* spp. invade and replicate within host cells, causing cell lysis and tissue destruction. In addition to direct tissue damage, parasitic infections can induce immune-mediated pathology, where the host immune response contributes to tissue injury and inflammation. Excessive activation of immune cells and the release of inflammatory mediators can lead to collateral damage to host tissues, exacerbating the severity of parasitic diseases. Chronic inflammation associated with persistent parasitic infections can also impair host organ function and promote the development of secondary infections. The pathogenesis of parasitic diseases in poultry is influenced by various factors, including the virulence of the parasite, the host's immune status, and environmental conditions such as temperature, humidity, and hygiene practices [5].

### Host Resistance and Susceptibility in Poultry

Host resistance and susceptibility to parasitic infections in poultry are influenced by a combination of genetic, immunological, and environmental factors. Some poultry breeds or genetic lines may exhibit inherent resistance or susceptibility to specific parasites, reflecting differences in immune responsiveness or physiological traits. For example, certain chicken breeds may produce higher levels of antibodies against specific parasitic antigens, conferring protection against infection. Additionally, host age, nutritional status, and stress levels can affect susceptibility to parasitic diseases, with young or immunocompromised birds being more vulnerable to infection. Host resistance to parasitic infections can also be influenced by previous exposure to parasites, leading to the development of acquired immunity. Upon initial infection, the host immune system generates memory T and B cells that provide rapid and specific protection upon re-exposure to the same parasite. Vaccination programs can also induce protective immunity against specific parasites, reducing the overall prevalence of infection within poultry populations [6].

## Immunomodulation by Parasites in Poultry

Parasites have evolved sophisticated mechanisms to evade or modulate host immune responses, allowing them to establish chronic infections and persist within the host environment. Immunomodulation by parasites can take various forms, including the inhibition of host immune cell activation, the induction of regulatory T cells, and the production of immunosuppressive molecules. For example, certain helminth parasites release excretory-secretory products that interfere with host cytokine signaling pathways, dampening pro-inflammatory responses and promoting parasite survival. Additionally, some parasites can manipulate host immune responses to their advantage, promoting a tolerogenic environment that facilitates their persistence within the host. This may involve the induction of regulatory T cells or the production of anti-inflammatory cytokines that suppress effector immune responses and promote parasite survival [7]. By subverting host immune defenses, parasites can establish long-term infections and evade host immune surveillance [8].

## Host Behavioral Changes Induced by Parasites in Poultry

Parasitic infections can induce behavioral changes in poultry hosts, altering their feeding, grooming, and social interactions in ways that facilitate parasite transmission and survival. These behavioral changes are often driven by the parasite's need to complete its life cycle or enhance its chances of transmission to new hosts. For example, certain avian malaria parasites manipulate the behavior of their mosquito vectors, increasing their propensity to feed on infected birds and transmit the parasite to uninfected individuals. In addition to vector manipulation, parasites can also directly influence the behavior of their avian hosts, altering their foraging behavior, activity levels, and reproductive strategies. For example, *Toxoplasma gondii*, a protozoan parasite that infects birds and mammals, has been shown to alter the behavior of infected rodents, making them more susceptible to predation by cats, the parasite's definitive host. Similarly, parasitic nematodes like *Heterakis gallinarum* can induce changes in the feeding behavior of infected poultry, leading to increased exposure to infective parasite stages [9].

## IMPACT OF PARASITIC INFECTIONS ON POULTRY PERFORMANCE

Parasitic infections can have significant impacts on poultry performance, including growth rates, feed efficiency, egg production, and overall profitability. Chronic parasitic diseases can impair nutrient absorption and utilization, leading to reduced growth rates and poor feed conversion efficiency in infected birds. Additionally, the inflammatory responses elicited by parasitic infections can divert energy away from productive processes, further compromising performance. In laying hens, parasitic infections can lead to declines in egg production, egg quality, and hatchability, resulting in economic losses for producers. Parasite-induced pathology, such as intestinal damage or reproductive tract inflammation, can disrupt normal physiological processes and impair reproductive performance in infected birds. Moreover, parasitic infections may increase susceptibility to secondary bacterial or viral infections, exacerbating the severity of disease and further impacting poultry performance [4].

## EPIDEMIOLOGY OF PARASITIC DISEASES IN POULTRY

### Factors Influencing Disease Transmission in Poultry

The transmission of parasitic diseases in poultry is influenced by a multitude of factors, including the presence of infected birds, the density of the poultry population, environmental conditions, and management practices. Direct contact between infected and susceptible birds is a common route of transmission for many parasitic organisms, especially those that reside in the gastrointestinal tract or respiratory system. Close confinement of birds in poultry houses or on farms can facilitate the spread of parasites through direct contact, increasing the likelihood of disease transmission within flocks. In addition to direct contact, parasitic diseases can also be transmitted indirectly through contaminated feed, water, or bedding materials. Parasite eggs, larvae, or cysts shed in the feces of infected birds can contaminate the environment, leading to subsequent infection of susceptible individuals through ingestion or inhalation of infectious stages. Poor sanitation practices, overcrowding, and inadequate biosecurity measures can exacerbate the risk of environmental contamination and transmission of parasitic diseases in poultry flocks. Environmental conditions play a crucial role in the survival and transmission of parasitic organisms in the poultry environment. Factors such as temperature, humidity, and the presence of intermediate hosts or vectors can influence the viability and infectivity of parasite stages outside the host. Warm and humid conditions are often conducive to the development and transmission of parasites, particularly those with external life stages or intermediate hosts that thrive in such environments. Conversely, extreme temperatures or drought conditions may inhibit parasite survival and transmission, reducing the risk of disease outbreaks in poultry populations. Management practices, including flock density, stocking density, and the use of preventive measures such as vaccination or deworming programs, can also impact disease transmission dynamics in poultry. High stocking densities and overcrowding can promote the rapid spread of parasitic diseases within flocks, increasing the likelihood of disease outbreaks and reducing overall flock health and productivity. Implementing biosecurity protocols, such as restricting access to poultry facilities, disinfecting equipment, and monitoring bird health, can help mitigate the risk of disease transmission and prevent the introduction of parasites into poultry populations [11].

## Seasonal Dynamics of Parasitic Diseases in Poultry

Seasonal variations in environmental conditions can influence the prevalence and transmission dynamics of parasitic diseases in poultry. Factors such as temperature, humidity, and precipitation can impact the survival, development, and transmission of parasitic organisms, leading to fluctuations in disease incidence and severity throughout the year.

Warmer temperatures during the spring and summer months create favorable conditions for the survival and proliferation of many parasites, leading to increased disease prevalence in poultry flocks. Higher temperatures accelerate the development and maturation of parasite stages outside the host, increasing the likelihood of environmental contamination and transmission. Additionally, warmer weather may favor the growth and reproduction of intermediate hosts or vectors, amplifying the risk of parasite transmission within poultry populations.

Conversely, colder temperatures during the fall and winter months may slow down parasite development but can also promote their persistence in the environment or within host organisms. Some parasites have evolved strategies to survive harsh environmental conditions or overwinter within host tissues, allowing them to persist through the colder months and reemerge when conditions become more favorable. Additionally, fluctuations in humidity levels can affect the viability of parasite stages outside the host, with higher humidity favoring survival and transmission.

Seasonal changes in precipitation patterns also play a role in the epidemiology of parasitic diseases in poultry. Increased rainfall can create conducive breeding grounds for parasite vectors, such as mosquitoes and flies, leading to higher transmission rates. On the other hand, drought conditions may reduce environmental moisture levels, limiting parasite survival and transmission. Understanding the seasonal patterns of parasitic diseases can inform the timing of control measures and help poultry producers mitigate the risk of disease outbreaks in their flocks.

## Host Population Dynamics and Density Dependence in Poultry

The dynamics of host populations, including fluctuations in population size, density, and composition, can influence the transmission and spread of parasitic diseases in poultry. Changes in population density, resulting from factors such as birth rates, mortality rates, or migration, can impact the intensity and frequency of contact between infected and susceptible individuals, affecting the transmission dynamics of parasitic organisms within poultry flocks. High-density poultry production systems, characterized by large numbers of birds confined in limited spaces, can facilitate the rapid spread of parasitic diseases within flocks. Overcrowding and high stocking densities increase the likelihood of direct contact between infected and susceptible birds, promoting the transmission of parasites and leading to higher disease prevalence. Additionally, increased population density can create stressful conditions for poultry, compromising their immune function and making them more susceptible to parasitic infections. Density-dependent processes, where the rate of disease transmission depends on the density of susceptible hosts within a population, can further exacerbate the spread of parasitic diseases in poultry. As the density of susceptible hosts increases, so does the likelihood of disease transmission, leading to higher infection rates and greater disease burden within poultry populations [15].

Population demographics, including the age structure and reproductive status of poultry flocks, can also influence disease transmission dynamics. Young or immunocompromised birds may be more susceptible to parasitic infections, as their immune systems are still developing or compromised by other factors. Additionally, changes in the composition of poultry populations, such as the introduction of new birds or the removal of infected individuals, can impact the spread of parasitic diseases and the overall health of poultry flocks [11].

## Geographic Distribution and Spread of Parasitic Infections in Poultry

The geographic distribution of parasitic diseases in poultry is influenced by a combination of factors, including climate, host availability, environmental conditions, and human activities. Different parasites have distinct geographic ranges, reflecting differences in their life cycles, transmission dynamics, and ecological requirements. Climate plays a significant role in shaping the geographic distribution of parasitic diseases, with temperature, humidity, and precipitation influencing the survival, development, and transmission of parasitic organisms. Parasites with temperature-dependent life cycles may be restricted to certain geographical regions with suitable climatic conditions for their development and transmission. Additionally, environmental factors such as soil type, vegetation cover, and water availability can impact the distribution of intermediate hosts or vectors, further influencing the spread of parasitic infections in poultry. Host availability and population density also influence the geographic distribution of parasitic diseases in poultry. Areas with dense poultry populations or high levels of commercial poultry production may experience higher rates of disease transmission and greater disease burden compared to regions with lower poultry densities. The movement of infected birds, contaminated equipment, or vehicles can facilitate the spread of parasitic infections between farms or regions, contributing to the geographic distribution of parasitic diseases. Human activities, including trade, travel, and migration, can play a significant role in the spread of parasitic infections in poultry. International trade in live birds, poultry products, or equipment can introduce parasites into new regions or countries, leading to the emergence of novel disease outbreaks. Similarly, the movement of migratory birds or wild animals can introduce parasites into domestic poultry populations, increasing the risk of disease transmission and spread. Understanding the role of human activities in the geographic distribution of parasitic diseases is crucial for implementing biosecurity measures and preventing the introduction of parasites into poultry populations.

## Risk Factors for Disease Outbreaks in Poultry

Several risk factors contribute to the occurrence and spread of parasitic diseases in poultry, including management practices, environmental conditions, host susceptibility, and the presence of vectors or intermediate hosts. Identifying and

mitigating these risk factors is essential for preventing disease outbreaks and maintaining the health and productivity of poultry flocks.

Poor biosecurity practices, including inadequate sanitation, overcrowding, and insufficient pest control, can increase the risk of disease outbreaks in poultry. Contaminated feed, water, or bedding materials can serve as sources of infection, introducing parasites into poultry facilities and facilitating disease transmission within flocks. Additionally, the introduction of infected birds or equipment from other farms or regions can introduce parasites into naïve poultry populations, leading to the emergence of new disease outbreaks [10].

Environmental conditions, such as temperature, humidity, and precipitation, can influence the survival and transmission of parasitic organisms, impacting the likelihood of disease outbreaks in poultry. Warm and humid conditions are often conducive to the development and proliferation of parasites, increasing the risk of disease transmission within poultry flocks. Similarly, areas with poor drainage or standing water may provide breeding grounds for parasite vectors, amplifying the risk of disease transmission and spread.

Host susceptibility and immunity play a critical role in determining the likelihood of disease outbreaks in poultry. Young or immunocompromised birds may be more susceptible to parasitic infections, as their immune systems are still developing or compromised by other factors. Additionally, changes in the composition of poultry populations, such as the introduction of new birds or the removal of infected individuals, can impact the spread of parasitic diseases and the overall health of poultry flocks [8].

The presence of vectors or intermediate hosts can also increase the risk of disease outbreaks in poultry. Parasite vectors, such as mosquitoes, flies, or ticks, can transmit parasitic organisms between birds, amplifying the spread of infections within poultry populations. Similarly, intermediate hosts, such as earthworms or snails, can serve as reservoirs for parasitic organisms, contributing to the persistence and transmission of diseases in poultry flocks. Implementing integrated pest management strategies, including vector control and habitat modification, can help reduce the risk of disease outbreaks and minimize the impact of parasitic infections on poultry health and productivity.

## SURVEILLANCE AND MONITORING STRATEGIES

Surveillance and monitoring of parasitic diseases are essential components of effective disease control programs in poultry. By detecting and identifying disease outbreaks early, poultry producers can implement timely interventions to prevent the spread of parasites and minimize the impact of infections on flock health and productivity. Several surveillance and monitoring strategies are employed in poultry production systems to assess disease prevalence, monitor trends, and identify risk factors for disease outbreaks. Active surveillance involves routine sampling and testing of poultry populations for the presence of parasitic infections, using diagnostic tests such as fecal examinations, serological assays, or molecular techniques. Sampling may be conducted at regular intervals, targeting specific age groups, production stages, or geographical regions, to assess disease prevalence and monitor changes over time. Passive surveillance relies on the voluntary reporting of suspected cases of parasitic diseases by poultry producers, veterinarians, or diagnostic laboratories. Reported cases are investigated further through laboratory testing and epidemiological analysis to confirm the presence of parasites and determine the extent of disease spread. Sentinel surveillance involves the systematic monitoring of specific sentinel flocks or sites within poultry production systems to detect the presence of parasitic infections and assess disease risk. Sentinel flocks are typically selected based on factors such as location, age, production type, or health status, and are regularly monitored for clinical signs of parasitic diseases or evidence of infection. Surveillance data collected from sentinel flocks can provide early warning of disease outbreaks and help inform targeted control measures to prevent further spread. In addition to surveillance, monitoring of environmental conditions and risk factors for disease transmission is essential for identifying and addressing potential sources of infection in poultry populations. Environmental monitoring may involve regular assessment of water quality, feed hygiene, pest populations, and other factors that can impact the transmission and spread of parasitic diseases. Risk factor analysis aims to identify management practices, biosecurity lapses, or other factors that increase the likelihood of disease outbreaks in poultry flocks, allowing producers to implement corrective actions and mitigate disease risk. Integration of surveillance and monitoring data into decision-making processes is essential for effective disease control and management in poultry production systems. By combining information on disease prevalence, environmental conditions, and risk factors, poultry producers can develop targeted control measures, such as vaccination programs, biosecurity improvements, or treatment protocols, to minimize the impact of parasitic diseases on flock health and productivity. Regular review and evaluation of surveillance data are critical for identifying emerging threats, adapting control strategies, and optimizing disease prevention efforts in poultry populations [7, 9].

## DIAGNOSIS OF PARASITIC DISEASES

### Clinical Signs and Symptoms in Poultry

Parasitic diseases in poultry can manifest with a wide range of clinical signs and symptoms, which can vary depending on the specific parasite involved, the severity of the infection, and the affected organ systems. Clinical observations play a crucial role in the diagnosis of parasitic diseases in poultry, as they provide valuable information about the nature and progression of the infection [12].

### *Gastrointestinal Parasites*

Gastrointestinal parasites are among the most common parasites affecting poultry worldwide. These parasites, including coccidia, roundworms (nematodes), and tapeworms (cestodes), primarily infect the digestive tract and can cause a variety of clinical signs in affected birds.

## Coccidiosis

Coccidiosis, caused by protozoan parasites of the genus *Eimeria*, is one of the most economically significant parasitic diseases in poultry. Clinical signs of coccidiosis vary depending on the *Eimeria* species involved and the severity of the infection but commonly include diarrhea (often bloody), dehydration, reduced feed intake, weight loss, lethargy, and decreased egg production in laying hens. Severe cases of coccidiosis can result in high mortality rates, particularly in young or immunocompromised birds.

## Roundworm Infections

Roundworm infections, caused by nematodes such as *Ascaridia* spp., *Heterakis* spp., and *Capillaria* spp., can also lead to a range of clinical signs in poultry. Common symptoms include reduced growth rates, poor feed conversion, emaciation, anemia (pale comb and wattles), and occasionally, diarrhea. Severe infections may result in intestinal obstruction, leading to a condition known as "gape" or "gaping" where affected birds stretch their necks and gasp for air due to the presence of large numbers of worms in the trachea [9].

## Tapeworm Infections

Tapeworm infections in poultry, caused by cestodes such as *Raillietina* spp. and *Choanotaenia* spp., are less common but can still cause significant morbidity and mortality. Clinical signs may include weight loss, poor growth, reduced egg production, and occasionally, intestinal obstruction. In severe cases, tapeworm segments may be visible in the feces or around the cloaca of affected birds.

## Respiratory Parasites

Respiratory parasites affect the respiratory tract of poultry and can cause a range of respiratory signs and symptoms. Common respiratory parasites in poultry include gapeworms (*Syngamus trachea*) and nasal mites (*e.g., Ornithonyssus* spp.).

## Gapeworm Infections

Gapeworm infections are characterized by respiratory distress, gasping, coughing, and sneezing in affected birds. Severe infections can lead to asphyxiation and death, particularly in young or susceptible birds. Post-mortem examination may reveal the presence of adult worms in the trachea and bronchi of infected birds [11].

## Nasal Mite Infestations

Nasal mite infestations can cause irritation, inflammation, and obstruction of the nasal passages, leading to nasal discharge, sneezing, head shaking, and respiratory distress in affected birds. In severe cases, nasal mites may cause deformities of the nasal passages and sinuses, impairing breathing and feeding.

## Cutaneous Parasites

Cutaneous parasites infest the skin and feathers of poultry and can cause a range of dermatological signs and lesions. Common cutaneous parasites in poultry include poultry lice (*Mallophaga* and *Anoplura* spp.) and poultry mites (*Dermanyssus* spp. and *Ornithonyssus* spp.).

## Poultry Lice Infestations

Poultry lice infestations can cause irritation, feather damage, anemia, and reduced egg production in affected birds. Clinical signs may include feather loss, feather pecking, skin irritation, and restlessness. Lice and their eggs (nits) may be visible on the skin and feathers of affected birds, particularly around the vent, neck, and under the wings [14].

## Poultry Mite Infestations

Poultry mite infestations can cause similar clinical signs to lice infestations, including feather damage, skin irritation, and reduced egg production. In severe cases, poultry mites can lead to anemia, weight loss, and increased susceptibility to secondary infections. Mites and their eggs may be visible on the skin, feathers, and in the housing environment of affected birds.

## General Clinical Signs

In addition to specific clinical signs associated with particular types of parasites, poultry affected by parasitic infections may exhibit general signs of illness, including lethargy, reduced activity, fluffed feathers, decreased feed and water intake, weight loss, pale combs and wattles, and decreased egg production in laying hens. Post-mortem examination and laboratory diagnostics are often necessary to confirm the presence of parasitic infections and identify the causative agents in affected poultry flocks (Figs. **4** and **5**).

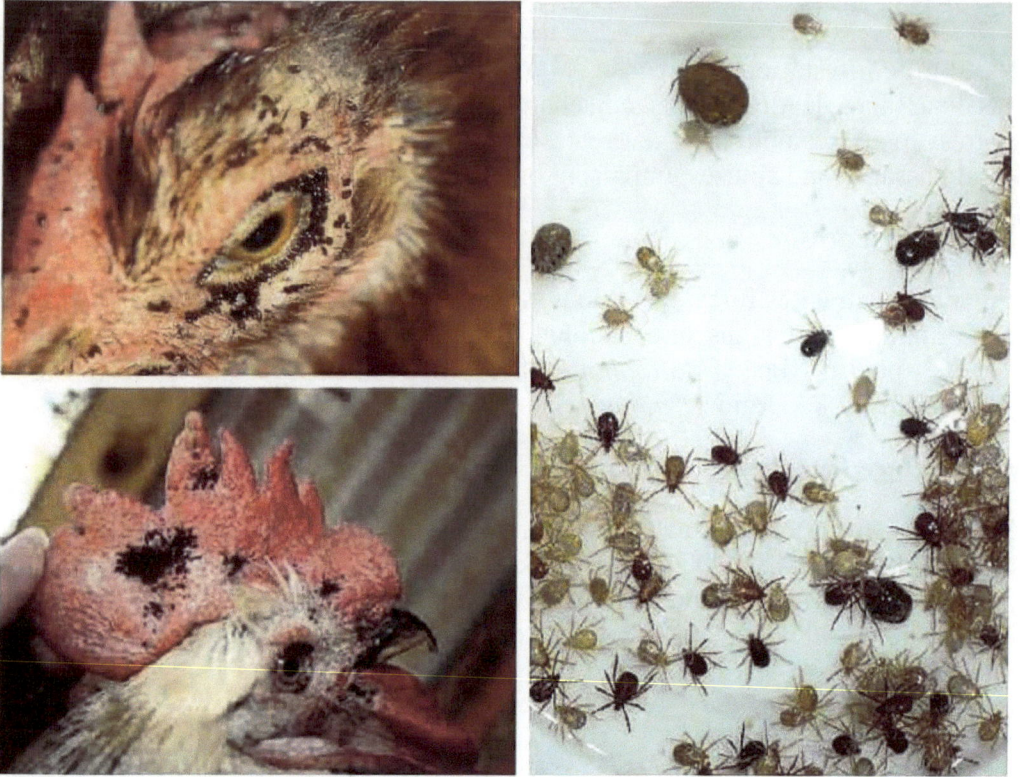

**Fig. (4).** Parasitic disease of poultry (https://cs-tf.com/wp-content/uploads/2020/03/chicken-parasite.jpg).

## PREVENTION AND CONTROL STRATEGIES

Parasitic diseases pose significant challenges to poultry health and productivity worldwide. Effective prevention and control strategies are essential for minimizing the impact of parasitic infections on poultry flocks and ensuring sustainable production.

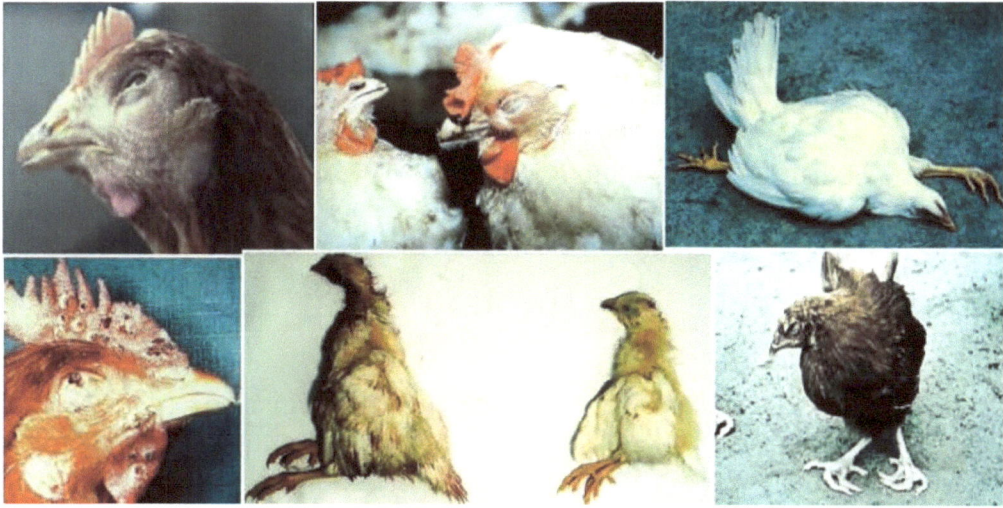

**Fig. (5).**    Clinical signs of poultry parasitic diseases (https://www.hightoppoultry.com/wp-content/uploads/poultry-disease-control-and-prevention-800x389.jpg).

## Biosecurity Measures for Parasite Prevention in Poultry

Biosecurity measures are fundamental for preventing the introduction and spread of parasitic diseases in poultry flocks. Biosecurity protocols should be implemented at all stages of poultry production, including breeding, hatching, rearing, and laying. Key biosecurity measures include:

**Restricted Access:** Limiting access to poultry facilities to essential personnel only helps reduce the risk of introducing parasites from external sources.

**Footwear and Equipment Disinfection:** Disinfecting footwear, equipment, vehicles, and other items before entering and leaving poultry premises helps prevent the transmission of parasites.

**Quarantine and Testing:** Implementing quarantine measures for newly acquired birds and conducting diagnostic testing for parasites before introducing them to existing flocks can help prevent the spread of infection [10].

**Wildlife and Pest Control:** Implementing measures to control wildlife, rodents, and insects that may act as vectors for parasites helps reduce the risk of transmission to poultry.

**Manure Management**: Proper disposal of manure and regular cleaning and disinfection of poultry housing facilities help reduce environmental contamination and parasite buildup.

## SANITATION AND HYGIENE PRACTICES IN POULTRY

Maintaining clean and hygienic poultry facilities is essential for minimizing the risk of parasitic diseases. Regular cleaning and disinfection of housing facilities, equipment, feeders, and waterers help reduce the environmental contamination of parasites and their transmission to poultry. Proper waste management, including the removal and disposal of litter, bedding, and manure, helps prevent the buildup of parasite eggs, larvae, or cysts in the poultry environment.

## INTEGRATED PEST MANAGEMENT (IPM) APPROACHES IN POULTRY

Integrated Pest Management (IPM) involves the coordinated use of multiple control strategies to manage pests, including parasites, in poultry flocks. IPM approaches may include:

**Biological Control**: Introducing natural predators or parasitoids to control parasite populations.

**Cultural Control**: Implementing management practices such as rotational grazing, pasture management, and habitat modification to reduce parasite exposure.

**Mechanical Control**: Using physical barriers, traps, or mechanical removal methods to control parasite populations.

**Chemical Control**: Applying pesticides, acaricides, or parasiticides to control parasite populations. However, the judicious use of chemical control methods is essential to prevent the development of resistance and minimize environmental contamination [11].

**Chemoprophylaxis**: Anthelmintics, Acaricides in Poultry. Chemoprophylaxis involves the use of chemotherapeutic agents, such as anthelmintics (for helminth parasites) and acaricides (for arthropod parasites), to prevent parasitic infections in poultry flocks. Anthelmintics are commonly used to control nematode infections in poultry, while acaricides are used to control mite and tick infestations. However, the overuse or misuse of anthelmintics and acaricides can lead to the development of drug resistance in parasite populations, highlighting the importance of proper dosage, rotation, and management practices.

## VACCINATION PROGRAMS FOR PARASITIC DISEASES IN POULTRY

Vaccination is an effective strategy for preventing parasitic diseases in poultry. Vaccines stimulate the bird's immune system to produce protective antibodies against specific parasites, reducing the risk of infection and minimizing the severity of disease. Live attenuated or recombinant vaccines are commonly used for diseases such as coccidiosis and Marek's disease, providing long-term protection and reducing the reliance on chemoprophylaxis. However, the development of effective vaccines for certain parasitic diseases, such as helminth infections, remains challenging due to the complex nature of host-parasite interactions [17, 18].

## GENETIC SELECTION FOR RESISTANCE IN POULTRY

Genetic selection for resistance to parasitic diseases is an important component of disease control strategies in poultry. Breeding programs aimed at selecting birds with inherent resistance or tolerance to parasitic infections can help reduce the prevalence and impact of diseases in poultry flocks. Genetic markers associated with resistance to specific parasites can be identified through genome-wide association studies and used to selectively breed resistant poultry lines. However, genetic selection should be combined with other control measures, such as biosecurity, sanitation, and vaccination, for optimal disease management outcomes [8].

## NUTRITIONAL STRATEGIES TO ENHANCE HOST IMMUNITY IN POULTRY

Nutritional strategies aimed at enhancing host immunity can help improve the resistance of poultry to parasitic infections. Providing balanced diets with adequate levels of essential nutrients, vitamins, and minerals supports the development and function of the immune system. Additionally, the inclusion of immunomodulatory feed additives such as probiotics, prebiotics, organic acids, and plant extracts can help stimulate immune responses and improve overall health and resilience in poultry flocks. However, nutritional interventions should be tailored to the specific requirements of poultry species and production systems to achieve optimal outcomes.

## EMERGING CHALLENGES AND FUTURE DIRECTIONS IN POULTRY

Parasitic diseases continue to pose significant challenges to poultry production worldwide. As the poultry industry evolves and adapts to changing environmental, socioeconomic, and technological factors, new challenges and opportunities emerge in the field of parasitology. In this chapter, we will explore emerging challenges and future directions in poultry parasitology, focusing on areas such as emerging parasitic diseases, antimicrobial resistance, climate change, advances in parasite control technologies, the One Health approach, and research needs and opportunities [10, 18].

## Emerging Parasitic Diseases in Poultry

As poultry production systems evolve and intensify, the emergence of new parasitic diseases poses a significant threat to poultry health and productivity. Emerging parasitic diseases may arise due to factors such as changes in host populations, environmental conditions, and the introduction of exotic parasites through global trade and travel. Surveillance and monitoring programs are essential for detecting and responding to emerging parasitic diseases in poultry, allowing for the timely implementation of control measures to prevent further spread and minimize economic losses [5].

## Antimicrobial Resistance in Poultry Parasites

Antimicrobial resistance (AMR) is a growing concern in the field of poultry parasitology. Overuse and misuse of antimicrobial agents in poultry production have led to the development of resistance among parasitic organisms, rendering commonly used drugs ineffective for disease control. AMR not only compromises the efficacy of treatment but also poses risks to public health through the transmission of resistant pathogens to humans *via* the food chain. Strategies to combat AMR in poultry parasites include the prudent use of antimicrobial agents, the development of alternative treatment options, and the implementation of biosecurity and hygiene measures to prevent disease transmission.

## Climate Change and Parasitic Diseases in Poultry

Climate change is expected to have profound effects on the epidemiology and distribution of parasitic diseases in poultry. Changes in temperature, precipitation patterns, and humidity levels can alter the survival, development, and transmission of parasitic organisms, leading to shifts in disease prevalence and distribution. Climate change may also influence the distribution and abundance of vector species, such as mosquitoes and ticks, which play a crucial role in the transmission of certain parasitic diseases. Adaptation strategies, such as the development of climate-resilient poultry breeds and the implementation of vector control measures, are needed to mitigate the impact of climate change on poultry parasitology [9].

# ADVANCES IN PARASITE CONTROL TECHNOLOGIES IN POULTRY

Advances in parasite control technologies offer promising solutions for managing parasitic diseases in poultry. Innovations in diagnostics, therapeutics, vaccines, and genetic approaches provide new opportunities for disease prevention and control. Molecular diagnostic techniques, such as polymerase chain reaction (PCR) and next-generation sequencing (NGS), allow for rapid and accurate identification of parasitic pathogens, facilitating targeted treatment and control measures. Novel therapeutics, including alternative chemotherapeutic agents and biopesticides, offer alternative treatment options for controlling parasitic infections while minimizing environmental impact. Vaccines and genetic selection for disease resistance provide long-term solutions for preventing parasitic diseases in poultry populations [13].

## One Health Approach to Parasitic Disease Management in Poultry

The One Health approach emphasizes the interconnectedness of human, animal, and environmental health and recognizes the importance of collaboration between different sectors to address complex health challenges, including parasitic diseases. Adopting a One Health approach to poultry parasitology involves integrating expertise from multiple disciplines, including veterinary medicine, public health, environmental science, and social sciences, to develop holistic and sustainable solutions for disease management. One Health initiatives focus on identifying shared risks and implementing coordinated strategies to prevent and control parasitic diseases in both poultry and human populations, ultimately improving health outcomes for all stakeholders [14, 18].

## CONCLUDING REMARKS

In conclusion, understanding the principles of parasitism is essential for the effective management and control of parasitic diseases in poultry. By exploring the biology of poultry parasites, host-parasite interactions, epidemiology, diagnosis, prevention, and control strategies, poultry producers can implement comprehensive approaches to minimize the impact of parasitic diseases and ensure the health and welfare of their flocks. Continued research, surveillance, and collaboration are essential for addressing emerging challenges and advancing our understanding of parasitic diseases in poultry.

## REFERENCES

[1]    Belete A, Addis M, Ayele M. Review on major gastrointestinal parasites that affect chickens. J Biol Agric Healthc 2016; 6(11): 11-21.

[2]    BN A. Clinical signs and pathological changes and differential diagnosis Of Marek's disease of poultry. Excellencia: Int Multi-disc J Educ 2024; 2(2): 145-50.

[http://dx.doi.org/10.5281/]

[3]    Bohrer BM. Review: Nutrient density and nutritional value of meat products and non-meat foods high in protein. Trends Food Sci Technol 2017; 65: 103-12.
[http://dx.doi.org/10.1016/j.tifs.2017.04.016]

[4]    Gadde U, Chapman HD, Rathinam T, Erf GF. Cellular immune responses, chemokine, and cytokine profiles in Turkey poults following infection with the intestinal parasite *Eimeria adenoeides*. Poult Sci 2011; 90(10): 2243-50.
[http://dx.doi.org/10.3382/ps.2011-01558] [PMID: 21934006]

[5]    Hoste H. Adaptive physiological processes in the host during gastrointestinal parasitism. Int J Parasitol 2001; 31(3): 231-44.
[http://dx.doi.org/10.1016/S0020-7519(00)00167-3] [PMID: 11226449]

[6]    Kumari P, Bhattacharyya S, Chattopadhyay S, Raj A, Banik A. Parasites in poultry faeces: should we be concerned?. Eur J Biomed Res 2024; 11(4): 181-6.

[7]    López-Osorio S, Chaparro-Gutiérrez JJ, Gómez-Osorio LM. Overview of poultry *Eimeria* life cycle and host-parasite interactions. Front Vet Sci 2020; 7: 384.
[http://dx.doi.org/10.3389/fvets.2020.00384] [PMID: 32714951]

[8]    Maqsood R, Khan A, Mushtaq MH, *et al.* Risk factors for outbreaks caused by variant strain of Newcastle disease on environmentally controlled broiler chicken farms in Lahore, Pakistan Pol J Vet Sci 2021; 24(4): 497-503.
[http://dx.doi.org/10.24425/pjvs.2021.139974] [PMID: 35179843]

[9]    Mohsin M, Abbas RZ, Yin G, *et al.* Probiotics as therapeutic, antioxidant and immunomodulatory agents against poultry coccidiosis. Worlds Poult Sci J 2021; 77(2): 331-45.
[http://dx.doi.org/10.1080/00439339.2021.1883412]

[10]   Muzaffar SB. 2007.Diseases and parasites of birds: ecology and epidemiology in a changing world. Doctoral (PhD) thesis, Memorial University of Newfoundland. https://research.library.mun.ca/9125/

[11]   Olano J P, Weller P F, Guerrant R L, Walker D H. Principles of parasitism: host–parasite interactions. Tropical Infectious Diseases: Principles, Pathogens and Practice 2011; 1-7.

[12]   Ravindran V, Abdollahi M R. Advances and future directions in poultry feeding: an overview. Achieving Sustainable Production of Poultry Meat 2017; 2: 113-30.

[13]   Trees A J. Parasitic diseases. In: Pattison M, Mc-Mullin P, Bradbury J M, Alexander D, Eds. Poultry Diseases. 2001; 6: pp. 444-56.

[14]   Mohammed Adnan AB, Shamal Abdullah AM. Phylogenetic analysis of lice infested chicken (*Gallus gallus domisticus*) with new records in Kurdistan of Iraq. Ann Parasitol. 2021; 67: pp. (2)161-8.
[http://dx.doi.org/10.17420/ap6702.325] [PMID: 34331852]

[15]   Tůmová E. Teimouri Fat deposition in the broiler chicken: a review. Sci Agric Bohem 2010; 41(2): 121-8.

[16]   Wells K, Clark NJ. Host specificity in variable environments. Trends Parasitol 2019; 35(6): 452-65.
[http://dx.doi.org/10.1016/j.pt.2019.04.001] [PMID: 31047808]

[17]   Yegani M, Korver DR. Factors affecting intestinal health in poultry. Poult Sci 2008; 87(10): 2052-63.
[http://dx.doi.org/10.3382/ps.2008-00091] [PMID: 18809868]

[18]   Abdulla NR, Loh TC, Foo HL, Alshelmani MI, Akit H. Influence of dietary ratios of n-6: n-3 fatty acid on gene expression, fatty acid profile in liver and breast muscle tissues, serum lipid profile, and immunoglobulin in broiler chickens. J Appl Poult Res 2019; 28(2): 454-69.
[http://dx.doi.org/10.3382/japr/pfz008]

CHAPTER 4

# Pathological Significance of Parasitic Diseases

**P.N. Bashetti**[1] and **Debolina Dattaray**[2,*]

[1] *Divisison of Veterinary Pathology, IVRI, Izatnagr, Uttar Pradesh, India*

[2] *Department of Veterinary Pharmacology and Toxicology, Institute of Veterinary Science and Animal Husbandry, Siksha 'O' Anusandhan University, Bhubaneswar, Odisha, India*

**Abstract:** Parasitic diseases in poultry pose substantial pathological and economic challenges, affecting both commercial and backyard flocks. This chapter comprehensively overviews the most common parasitic infections, including coccidiosis, nematodiasis, cestodiasis, and ectoparasitic infestations like mites and lice. It explores the pathological changes caused by these parasites, such as tissue damage, immunosuppression, reduced feed conversion, and impaired growth rates. Special attention is given to the interaction between parasites and the host's immune system, leading to secondary infections and exacerbating other health conditions. The chapter also discusses the economic losses associated with reduced egg production, increased mortality, and the cost of treatment and prevention. Current strategies for diagnosis, treatment, and control, as well as emerging trends in parasite management, are also addressed, emphasizing the need for integrated approaches to safeguard poultry health.

**Keywords:** Cestodes, Ectoparasite, Nematodes, Pathological significance, Protozoal infection.

## INTRODUCTION

The poultry industry in India is growing tremendously. It is one of the fastest growing industries in the world. India ranks third in egg production and sixth in meat production in the world. Human protein needs can be fulfilled by both poultry eggs and meat so this industry contributes to both the economic status of the country as well as the nutritional status of the health. Nonetheless, the economics of poultry farming are frequently marred by outbreaks due to poor management practices, which resulted in various infectious diseases such as bacterial, viral, and parasitic diseases [1]. Among these, parasitic diseases are a major concern in poultry production worldwide. These diseases can significantly impact the health, productivity, and economic viability of the poultry industry.

[*] **Corresponding author Debolina Dattaray:** Department of Veterinary Pharmacology and Toxicology, Institute of Veterinary Science and Animal Husbandry, Siksha 'O' Anusandhan University, Bhubaneswar, Odisha, India; E-mail: debolinadattaray10@gmail.com

**Tanmoy Rana (Ed.)**

Parasites in poultry can be broadly categorized into ectoparasites and endoparasites. Again ectoparasites contain various types of fleas, mites, lice, and ticks. Endoparasites can be classified as nematodes, cestodes, and protozoa. Each type has unique challenges and various pathological consequences [2]. This chapter explores the pathological significance of various parasitic diseases in poultry, including their effects on the health and productivity of affected birds, as well as the economic implications for the poultry industry (Table **1**).

Table 1. Classification of different poultry parasites with their common names.

| Class of Parasite | Scientific Name | Common Name | Description |
|---|---|---|---|
| Ectoparasite: A) Mites | 1. Dermanyssus *gallinae* | Red Mite | Red in color when fed, mostly fed at night. |
| | 2.Ornithonyssus *sylvarum* | Northern Fowl Mite | Causes irritation, blood loss, and decreased egg production. |
| | 3. *Ornithonyssus bursa* | Tropical fowl mite | Colonize the vent feathers, and feed on blood. |
| | 4. *Cnemidocoptes mutans* | Scaly leg mite | Burrows under the scales of legs and feet, causing thickening and crusting. |
| | 5. *Cnemidocoptes gallinae* | Depluming mite | Causing severe itching and feather plucking. |
| B) Lice | 1. *Menacanthus stramineus* | Chicken body louse | Feeds on skin scales, feathers, and blood, leading to irritation and decreased productivity. |
| | 2. *Menopon gallinae* | Shaft louse | Lives on feathers causing feather damage and irritation. |
| C) Fleas | 1. *Echidnophaga gallinacea* | Sticktight flea | Attaches firmly to the skin, particularly around the eyes and comb, causing irritation and anemia. |
| D) Ticks | 1. *Argas persicus* | Fowl tick (blue bug) | Feeds on blood at night and hides in cracks during the day, causing weakness and disease transmission. |
| Endoparasites which affect the Gastrointesinal portion A) Nematodes | 1. *Ascaridia galli* | Large roundworm | Found in the small intestine, causing weight loss and intestinal blockage. |
| | 2. *Heterakis gallinarum* | Cecal worm | Found in the ceca, can transmit *Histomonas meleagridis* (blackhead disease). |
| | 3. *Capillaria spp.* | Hairworm or threadworm | Affects the crop and intestine, leading to weight loss and diarrhea. |
| B) Cestodes | 1. *Raillietina spp.* | Tapeworm | Causes weight loss, diarrhea, and intestinal damage. |
| | 2. *Davainea proglottina* | Tapeworm | Causes nodular lesions in the intestine. |

(Table 1) cont.....

| Class of Parasite | Scientific Name | Common Name | Description |
|---|---|---|---|
| C) Protozoa | 1. *Eimeria spp.* | Coccidia | Causes coccidiosis, characterized by diarrhea, weight loss, and sometimes death. Different species affect different parts of the intestine (*e.g.*, *Eimeria tenella* in the ceca, *Eimeria maxima* in the mid-gut). |
| | 2. *Histomonas meleagridis* | Blackhead disease agent | Causes blackhead disease, primarily affecting turkeys but can also affect chickens, leading to liver and cecal lesions. |
| | 3. *Trichomonas gallinae* | Avian trichomoniasis agent | Causes lesions in the upper digestive tract. |
| Other parasites | | | |
| Helminths | *Syngamus trachea* | Gapeworm | Resides in the trachea, causing respiratory distress and gaping in affected birds. |

## PROTOZOAL INFECTION

There are three major groups of protozoa in the birds which include phylum Apicomplexa, phylum Parabasalia, and the less important Microspora group. The first phyla Apicomplexa (coccidia) are mostly intracellular parasites. In this group, the major parasites include *Eimeria, Isospora, Plasmodium*, and *Cryptosporidium*. Phylum Parabasalia has mostly flagellates and amoebas like *Histomonas, Entamoeba, Trypanosoma, and Cochlosoma*. The third group contains *Encephalitozoon cuniculi*, which has lesser importance in the poultry industry. The parasites that have shorter and more direct life cycles can affect modern and commercial poultry through diseases like coccidiosis. The only exception to this is the Blackhead Disease (histomoniasis) which spreads easily in turkeys despite having a complex lifecycle [3].

## *EIMERIA* SPP.

There are almost 1700 species of the genus *Eimeria,* which are monoxenous parasites that affect specific domestic mammals and birds. The *Eimeria* has seven species that infect the poultry industry, each having a different pathogenicity. All these *Eimeria* species have different invasion sites within the intestine. Along with this, they also produce different lesions and severity. *E. acervulina, E. maxima, and E. tenella* are responsible for having a major impact on gut health in both young and older birds. Whereas *E. mitis and E. praecox* cause subclinical coccidiosis, which leads to reduced broiler growth. *E. brunetti and E. necatrix* primarily affect long-living birds, such as laying-hens and breeders, causing severe injuries and high mortality. Broilers are typically unaffected by these due to their short lifespan [4].

## Life Cycle

All *Eimeria* species exhibit a direct life cycle characterized by high tissue and host specificity. It involves stages of asexual and sexual multiplication, with three development phases. The first is the formation of schizogony (agamogony/merogony). The second is the phase of gametogony, where gamete formation takes place for sexual production and sporogony.

Transmissions of the disease can occur through the fecal-oral route, which includes the ingestion of sporulated oocysts containing eight sporozoites. Sporozoites are the infective stage of this species. In the digestive tract, enzymes and mechanical action break down the oocyst wall and these sporozoites are released. The process of the release of sporozoites from the oocyst is called excystation. Released sporozoites enter into the intestinal lumen and infect intestinal cells [5]. Sporozoites penetrate directly into the host's intestinal epithelial cells in the gut lining in various regions depending on the species of *Eimeria*. After entering into the intestinal cells, sporozoites transform into trophozoites. A trophozoite is the growing stage that absorbs nutrients from the host and enters a feeding period that lasts for 12–48 hours. Inside the parasitophorous vacuole, these trophozoites enlarge and undergo multiple asexual divisions to form schizonts. These schizonts are filled with multiple merozoites. This phase is the asexual phase and is called merogony. The Merozoites lyse out of the original infected host intestinal epithelial cell to infect new intestinal epithelial cells, completing a second cycle of merogony. This asexual reproduction phase increases the number of merozoites in preparation for sexual reproduction. Each species of *Eimeria* has a predetermined number of cycles of merogony which range between 2 and 4, leading to a characteristic prepatent period [6].

In the gametogony stage, the merozoites develop into gametocytes, which then differentiate into microgametes and macrogametes. The number of microgametes varies by species. The *E. acervulina* produce 20-30 microgametes and the *E. maxima* produce over 100 oocysts with resistant double wall forms, which protects the undifferentiated zygote. Then the zygotes undergo meiosis and mitosis to form infectious sporozoites [7]. The parasite's internal phase duration is determined by the time needed to complete both asexual and sexual reproduction, which leads to oocyst formation. Then, this oocyst can excrete from the feces and enter into the sporulation phase. The sporulation process begins with the zygote's nucleus dividing twice, resulting in four nuclei within the oocyst. The cytoplasm reorganizes, forming sporoblasts that transform into oval-shaped sporocysts. Within each sporocyst, two sporozoites are formed through a final nuclear division [8]. These sporozoites have a specialized Stieda body, which aids in their release when they infect a new host. This process is important for the parasite as it makes the parasite infectious. It depends on various environmental conditions like oxygen, temperature, and humidity. Sporulation times can vary depending on the *Eimeria* species and environmental conditions. For instance, the sporulation rate of *E. maxima* is more efficient under dry conditions, while higher moisture levels can negatively impact this process [9].

## Pathogenesis

The *Eimeria* infection can be initiated through the ingestion of the sporulated oocyst. The route of infection is mostly fecal-oral which can occur through ingestion of contaminated feed and water. After ingestion, the infectious excystation of oocyst takes place resulting in the release of an infective form *i.e.* sporozoite. These sporozoites then infect epithelial cells in the intestine. Intraepithelial lymphocytes play an important role in the transmission of the sporozoites to the site's primary lesion. Then these sporozoites invade the lining of the intestinal epithelial cells through specific receptors and surface molecules present in the host cells. This invasion leads to tissue damage, which results in specific clinical signs like reduced feed intake, poor absorption of nutrients, dehydration, blood loss, and poor growth [10]. This tissue damage can also predispose the bird to bacterial infections such as *Clostridium* and *Salmonella*. All such diseases can suppress the bird's immune system and result in the exacerbation of the severity of coccidiosis. Though the pathogenesis for all *Eimeria* species is the same the presence of concurrent disease and, the nutritional status of the bird can influence the disease severity. Among all the *Eimeria* species , *Eimeria necatrix* and *Eimeria tenella* are highly pathogenic in chickens because schizogony occurs in the lamina propria and crypts of the epithelium of the small intestine and cecum, respectively, causing extensive hemorrhage. Whereas the development of other species takes place in the lining villi of intestinal epithelial cells [11].

## Pathogenicity and Clinical Signs

There are two forms of coccidiosis that include clinical and subclinical. Clinical coccidiosis is characterized by symptoms like diarrhea, bloody feces, dehydration, reduced feed intake, and finally mortality. Affected chickens often appear tired, with drooping wings and closed eyes, and may die within days. The severity of this disease can be affected by many factors such as ingested oocysts, the pathogenicity of the *Eimeria* species, the age of the bird, and management practices. The other more subtle form is subclinical coccidiosis. However, this form can cause poor weight gain and a decreased feed conversion ratio in economic losses. The other aspect of coccidial infection is the secondary bacterial infection, particularly *Clostridium* species. Birds surviving severe infections may recover but often with permanent growth and production setbacks [12].

As the severity depends on the type of the species affected, the different species of *Eimeria* have different pathogenicity. The highly pathogenic *Eimeria* species is *Eimeria tenella,* which primarily affects the ceca. It causes severe cecal coccidiosis characterized by bloody diarrhea, high mortality, and the formation of cecal cores, which are clotted blood and tissue debris. This species often results in significant losses, especially in young birds. Along with this, *Eimeria necatrix* is also highly pathogenic and targets the mid-small intestine and ceca. It is known for causing a distinctive "salt and pepper" appearance on the intestinal serosa and can lead to severe symptoms including thickened intestinal walls, bloody mucus, and dehydration. This species can cause extensive damage that can affect both the health and productivity of birds [13].

The other common species that affects the upper small intestine is *Eimeria acervulina.* It is less severe but can cause moderate disease, which can be characterized by whitish patches on the intestinal surface. This species often results in a poor growth of the birds, which causes an increase in culling and contributes to economic losses through reduced feed conversion efficiency. An *Eimeria maximum* has moderate pathogenicity and affects the mid-small intestine. It is known for causing the thickening of the intestinal wall, petechial hemorrhages, and the presence of reddish-orange fluid. Although its impact is less severe than that of *E. tenella* or *E. necatrix*, it can still lead to significant production losses. The major intestinal part can be targeted by the *Eimeria brunetti,* which affects the lower small intestine, rectum, ceca, and cloaca. It causes mucosal disruption and coagulative necrosis, with severe infections leading to sloughing of the mucosa. This species can cause notable damage and affect bird growth and health. The less pathogenic species are *Eimeria mitis* and *Eimeria praecox. E. mitis* affects the distal small intestine and generally causes milder lesions similar to *E. brunetti, E. praecox* impacts the proximal small intestine and is considered less economically important which only causes mild growth impairment. However, *Eimeria hagani* and *Eimeria mivati* develop in the proximal small intestine. *E. mivati* can cause severe lesions similar to those of *E. acervulina,* while *E. hagani* causes less distinct lesions. These species' effects can vary, making their impact on poultry health and production somewhat variable [14].

In turkeys, species like *Eimeria adenoides* and *Eimeria meleagrimitis* can be more lethal, mostly in younger birds. Game birds and waterfowl, including ducks and geese, are also susceptible, with certain *Eimeria* species causing high mortality in young flocks. The impact of coccidiosis can be severe across various bird species, requiring careful management and treatment to prevent outbreaks and economic losses [15].

## Necropsy Findings

There are distinct characteristics of lesions caused by various *Eimeria* species in poultry based on the specific species involved.

*Eimeria tenella,* which is known to cause the cecal coccidiosis is responsible for severe inflammation and necrotic lesions in the ceca. Macroscopically, this results in the accumulation of blood clots, tissue debris, and oocysts in the cecal lumen, which is known as the cecal core. Postmortem examination reveals a markedly swollen cecum filled with bloody masses. Microscopically, the lesions reveal extensive necrosis of the cecal mucosa, hemorrhages, and the presence of numerous oocysts within the damaged tissue. The infection often results in severe diarrhea, high mortality, and significant economic losses [16].

*Eimeria necatrix* produces distinctive macroscopic lesions in the proximal and mid-small intestine. There is a ballooning of the mid-small intestine, the mucosa is thickened and the limen is filled with blood and tissue debris. The serosal surface shows a characteristic "salt and pepper" appearance due to the presence of small haemorrhagic and necrotic foci of white or black plaques. Microscopic examination shows numerous clusters of large schizonts and oocysts. These are the characteristics of this species that distinguish it from other species. Along with this, there is severe mucosal damage, including thickened walls and hemorrhagic lesions. This species can lead to marked dehydration and significant health impacts [17].

*Eimeria acervulina* usually affects the upper part of the small intestine involving the duodenum. Macroscopically, the mucosal surface is covered by white plaques which are arranged in a manner that gives it a ladder-like appearance. The intestine is pale and contains fluid. Microscopically, there is localized epithelial damage and the presence of oocysts in the mucosa, which results in reduced feed efficiency and poor growth.

*Eimeria maxima* affects the mid-small intestine. Gross lesions include thickening of the intestinal wall, petechial hemorrhages, and reddish-orange fluid exudate. Whereas the microscopic lesions include fine pinpoint hemorrhages on the serosal surface of the middle portion of the intestine and may contain large size of oocysts and gametocytes. This species can cause moderate to severe damage, affecting growth and production.

*Eimeria brunetti* targets the lower small intestine, rectum, ceca, and cloaca. Macroscopically it causes severe mucosal disruption, coagulative necrosis, and sloughing of the mucosa. This results in bloody diarrhea. Severe infections can lead to extensive damage across the intestinal tract, affecting overall bird health and productivity.

*Eimeria mitis* affects the distal small intestine and typically causes less severe lesions. The lesions are often similar to moderate infections caused by *E. brunetti*, with small, round oocysts found in association with the lesions. This species generally results in milder disease [18].

*Eimeria praecox* infects the proximal small intestine and is characterized by indistinct lesions. It may cause some impairment in growth, but its impact is generally less severe compared to other species. Oocysts of *E. praecox* are larger and more numerous than those of *E. acervulina*.

*Eimeria hagani* and *Eimeria mivati* both infect the proximal small intestine. *E. mivati* can cause severe lesions similar to those of *E. acervulina*, while *E. hagani* presents with less distinct lesions. The impact of these species can vary, affecting the overall health and productivity of affected flocks.

**Diagnosis**

This disease can be diagnosed based on clinical observations, post-mortem fecal examination, and advanced molecular techniques. Signs like bloody fecal material, dysentery, and diarrhea are indicative of coccidiosis. Oocysts can be detected by using fecal examination with the flotation method. Actual identification of *Eimeria* species depends on measuring oocysts under a microscope and noting their size, shape, and sporulation characteristics [19].

Based on macroscopic and microscopic lesions and their location, appearance, and severity we can diagnose the infection. Gross lesions observed during post-mortem examination, including their location, appearance, and severity, provide crucial diagnostic information. The more recent advancement in molecular diagnostics techniques is that it has become easier to diagnose the coccidiosis species. These techniques involve Polymerase Chain Reaction (PCR) assays and offer precise identification by targeting specific genomic sequences of *Eimeria* species. Differential diagnosis is important as intestinal coccidiosis can be mistaken for necrotic enteritis, hemorrhagic enteritis, or other enteric diseases.

Cecal coccidiosis may also be confused with histomoniasis or salmonellosis due to similar lesions.

## Treatment

Treatment for coccidiosis involves various anticoccidial drugs, including amprolium, clopidol, diclazuril, ethopabate, halofuginone, and ionophores (*e.g.*, monensin, lasalocid). Amprolium inhibits thiamine, crucial for coccidian growth, while ionophores disrupt cell membranes and have antibacterial properties, aiding in secondary disease prevention. Effective treatment aims to address both affected and unaffected birds to build immunity. Anticoccidials are often withdrawn from broilers 3-7 days before the bird is slaughtered to comply with regulations and lower costs. However, continuous use can lead to drug resistance, reducing effectiveness over time.

## Control and Prevention

Effective prevention of coccidiosis relies on good management practices and the use of anticoccidial drugs. Key strategies include maintaining dry litter, proper ventilation, and regular cleaning of feeders and drinkers. Prophylactic measures involve using coccidiostats like amprolium, ionophores, and sulphaquinoxaline, which inhibit parasite development and promote immunity. Vaccination with either attenuated or virulent strains of *Eimeria* provides an alternative to drug use, though costs and effectiveness vary. Genetic selection for resistance and natural feed additives, such as oregano extract and Moringa leaf powder, also offer promising approaches. The integration of these methods helps manage and prevent coccidiosis outbreaks, effectively [20].

## *HISTOMONAS MELEAGRIDIS*

*Histomonas meleagridis,* the flagellate protozoan, causes the disease histomonosis also known as the blackhead disease or infectious enterohepatitis. It was first described in turkeys by Cushman in 1893. It is mostly found in turkeys and is characterized by severe lesions in the caeca and liver. Along with this, an important sign of this disease is the high mortality. The chickens are less affected and lesions are mostly confined to the caeca. It is a unicellular parasite in the Parabasalia. It can change its morphology between flagellated and amoeboid forms depending on its location within the ceca or liver. It measures 10-14 μm. In the cecal lumen, it usually has a single flagellum. This flagellum sheds when it invades the mucosal tissue and instead of a flagellum, it develops pseudopods. The species reproduces by binary fission and lacks mitochondria. For energy metabolism, these parasites depend on hydrogenosomes. A related species,

*Histomonas wenrichi* or *Parahistomonas wenrich*, is non-pathogenic and appears as a 4-flagellated or amoeboid form, with a larger size of 20–30 μm.

## Life Cycle

The life cycle of *Histomonas meleagridis* has several distinct stages. In the early stages, the parasites are in amoebic size, which is about 8 to 17 micrometers in diameter. These stage parasites are mostly found in the liver and caeca of infected turkeys. These forms are believed to be the invasive stage of the parasite. They actively spread through the host's tissues. There is a transformation of this stage into the flagellar form as the disease progresses inside the host tissue. This can cause a severe inflammatory response leading to the severe swelling of the host tissue. The later stage of infection is characterized by the formation of smaller, rounded cells with dense surface membranes. Although early studies did not identify flagella in these cells, later research confirmed that *H. meleagridis* has a single flagellum per cell so it can be classified into the flagellate group. This results in the amoeboid or rhythmic pulsating movements of the parasite. The full life cycle of *H. meleagridis* is not completely understood, specifically how it spreads among poultry flocks. However, it is confirmed that this parasite uses the nematode *Heterakis gallinarum* as an intermediate host. Inside this intermediate host, the parasite can be found in the intestinal wall as well as in the nematode's eggs and larvae. The special feature of this parasite is that it shrinks in size as it moves through the nematode's reproductive system. It cannot survive outside the host for more than a few minutes unless protected by the *Heterakis* egg or earthworm. Earthworms serve as transport hosts in which *Heterakis* eggs can hatch and young worms survive in tissues in an infective stage. Recent studies have also found cyst-like stages of *H. meleagridis* in lab cultures. These cysts might form for the survival of the parasite outside the host, which helps the parasite in its persistence outside the host and possibly aids in the spread of the disease among the poultry. These findings suggest that *H. meleagridis* can take on different forms depending on its environment, but more research is needed to fully understand how these forms contribute to the transmission of the disease [21].

## Pathogenesis

The target organ for the *Histomonas meleagridis* is the cecum. The parasites invade the caecal mucosa and spread through the blood to the liver. Their migration to the liver *via* hepatic portal blood causes characteristic lesions in the liver and caseous cores in the ceca. These lesions are characteristic of the disease and are often used for diagnosis. However, the primary sites of infection are the ceca and liver but the parasite can spread to other organs such as the brain, pancreas, heart, lungs, kidneys, and spleen. In some cases, the parasites can be found in the bursa of Fabricius, mostly in younger chickens. This suggests that the intra-cloacal route may be the natural pathway for infection [22]. As discussed earlier, Turkeys are most susceptible to histomonosis and show high mortality rates in affected flocks sometimes reaching as high as 80-100%. In chickens, there is less severity but they can act as reservoirs for the occasionally developing clinical symptoms. The major route of transmission in turkeys is cloacal drink and the bird's behavioral tendencies like huddling and having high litter moisture provide a favorable environment for the survival of the parasite and spread even in the absence of vectors like *Heterakis gallinarum*. Horizontal transmission of the disease in chickens is less common unless vectors are present. Factors like age, the genetic makeup of the birds, and strain-specific virulence of *H. meleagridis* could influence the severity of infection and mortality rates among the different poultry species. Recent studies indicate that while chickens might often be asymptomatic, they are not entirely resistant to infection and can still carry and spread the parasite under certain conditions.

## Clinical Signs

Histomoniasis mostly affects the caeca and liver of the poultry leading to significant morbidity and mortality mostly in turkeys. Turkeys show a very severe form of the disease often leading to acute outbreaks with high mortality rates. Infected birds show symptoms like depression, reduced appetite, ruffled feathers, and sulfur-yellow droppings. As the disease progresses, birds may develop cyanosis of the head, which suggests the name "blackhead" disease. In chickens, this disease is less severe but still shows clinical signs like diarrhea and lethargy. In both turkeys and chickens, younger birds are more susceptible to the disease.

## Lesions

The most characteristic lesions are found in the ceca and liver, which include thickening of the caecal wall due to severe inflammatory response caused by parasites. The lumen of the ceca is filled with caseous core. Along with this, ulceration of the caecal wall may lead to the perforation of the organ and generalized peritonitis. In the liver, circular depressed necrotic foci are present, which are mostly yellow to greenish lesions. These lesions are pathognomic of this disease. Microscopically early changes in the caecal wall include hyperemia and heterophil infiltration whereas in the later phase, there is infiltration of the lymphocytes and macrophages in the affected tissue. The caseous core of the caecal lumen is composed of the sloughed epithelium, fibrin, erythrocytes, and leukocytes along with the trapped ingesta. The microscopic lesions seen in the liver include the infiltration of inflammatory cells near the portal area and necrotic foci [23].

## Diagnosis

It can be made mostly on the gross lesions and microscopic lesions of the affected organs like the ceca and liver, which can show the presence of amoeboid forms of the parasite in the tissue while flagellated forms are found in the lumen of the ceca. Molecular techniques like PCR can be used to detect *H. meleagridis* DNA in tissue samples, providing a highly specific diagnosis.

## Prevention and Control

The major prevention and controlling factor in the poultry industry is biosecurity, which involves the isolation of the birds, cleanliness, and managing intermediate hosts like cecal worms and earthworms. Along with this regular deworming, control of the *Heterakis gallinarum* is also important. Proper management practices, such as keeping litter dry and avoiding contact with contaminated soil, are important. It is also advisable to keep the chickens and turkeys separate as chickens can carry the parasite without showing the symptoms. Stress can be minimized through good ventilation, nutrition, and by avoiding overcrowding, which help reduce the susceptibility to the disease. Additionally, prophylactic measures like specific feed additives or medications as advised by a veterinarian can further help in preventing outbreaks [24].

## TRICHOMONAS GALLINAE

*Trichomonas gallinae* is a protozoan parasite that has a distinctive morphology and is a causative agent of trichomoniasis. This disease is mostly found in birds like pigeons, doves, and chickens. The morphology of this parasite is somewhat different. It has a pear-shaped body measuring 7-11 μm, with four anterior flagella and undulating membranes that extend along the body. This undulating membrane helps in the motility and adherence to the host tissue. The nucleus is ovoid and placed centrally. They lack mitochondria but instead, they have hydrosomes for energy metabolism. Also, these parasites have a special structure called an axostyle used for rigid support. This is an extended structure from apical-basal bodies to the posterior end. This parasite thrives in warm, moist environments and is commonly transmitted through direct contact, contaminated water, or feeding regurgitated food to an offspring [25].

## Life Cycle

The life cycle of *Trichomonas gallinae* is simple and direct and involves only the trophozoite stage. The cyst form of this parasite is absent so this leads to the desiccation of the parasite very easily outside the host tissue. In the infective trophozoite stage, it can be transmitted between the birds through contaminated feed and water or during the courtship and feeding of the younger birds. After ingestion of the trophozoite, the parasite colonizes in the upper digestive tract, mostly in the oropharynx, esophagus, and crop. They replicate in the upper respiratory tract by binary fission.

## Pathogenesis

As discussed earlier, parasites colonize and multiply in the upper respiratory tract of the bird and can cause damage mostly to the upper respiratory tract. These parasites can adhere to the mucosal surface of the upper digestive tract and enter into the epithelial cells where multiplication takes place inside the epithelial cells by binary fission. This leads to severe tissue damage and an inflammatory response. As a result of the inflammatory response, there is the formation of the caseous plug, which can obstruct the esophagus and crop. This hinders the bird's ability to eat or drink. There are various strains of these parasites, and the severity depends on the strain type and the bird's immunity status [26].

## Clinical Signs

Affected birds may show signs such as difficulty in swallowing, regurgitation, and drooling. As there is formation of the caseous plug in the esophagus, this results in the bird losing weight being unable to ingest the food properly. Along with this, the bird may appear lethargic, with ruffled feathers, and impaired health.

## Lesions

Grossly, we can see a characteristic yellowish to white caseous plug in the esophagus or the masses in the oral cavity, pharynx, and crop. These lesions can coalesce to form larger masses, leading to the obstruction of the digestive tract. Microscopically affected tissue reveals the infiltration of various inflammatory cells like heterophils and macrophages. Parasites can be seen in the necrotic area. Chronic cases may show fibrosis and granulomatous inflammation.

## Diagnosis

We can diagnose this disease based on the clinical signs and post-mortem lesions. Wet mount preparations from the lesions can show that motile trophozoites can also be helpful. Molecular techniques such as PCR can be used for specific identification, and culture methods can isolate the organism for further study.

## GASTROINTESTINAL HELMINTHS

Gastrointestinal helminthiasis in poultry is caused by roundworms (nematodes), tapeworms (cestodes), and flukes (trematodes) [27]. Among these, nematodes are the most important helminths in poultry as they can have a great economic impact on the poultry industry. Nematodes can cause reduced feed conversion ratio, weight loss, and decreased egg quality and production. Along with this, they can damage the intestinal tissue, which may result in the weakening of the intestinal barrier and make birds susceptible to secondary bacterial infection due to reduced immunity. Helminth infection is most prevalent in chickens that are kept in the backyard or in free-range systems. The infection can be influenced by various factors such as climate, agroecological zones, the accumulation of infective larvae or eggs in the environment, the presence of an intermediate host, and the susceptibility of the host. The transmission and survival of the infective stage of the parasites can be determined by two important factors *i.e.*, temperature and humidity.

## NEMATODES

These parasites belong to the phylum Nemathelminthes and class Nematoda. They are unsegmented worms that are cylindrical and elongated in shape. They have cuticles, which are smooth or have various types of ornamentation. These parasites have complete alimentary tracts and both sexes are different, which makes them different from other parasites. The life cycle of all nematodes is mostly direct but may involve one or two indirect intermediate hosts. In the poultry industry, the most common and important nematodes are *Ascaridia galli,* which infect the jejunum of the small intestine [28]. *Heterakis gallinarum,* also called caecal worm, and various *Capillaria* species, are found in the crop. All these worms are mostly long and spindle-shaped. The color is mostly creamy to yellow. All poultry nematodes have a direct life cycle, and the primary mode of infection is the fecal-oral route. This route of infection is more common in free-range and floor poultry production systems where birds are in close contact with their excreta and soil.

## ASCARIDIA GALLI

In chickens, there are more than 30 helminthic parasites that have been identified. But among these, *Ascaridia galli* is the most common, which is then followed by the cecal nematode *Heterakis gallinarum*. In tropical regions, the most prevalent infection in poultry is *Ascaridia galli* in domestic fowls. This parasite resides in the intestine of the host, causing damage to the intestinal tissue. It is a large, white, or cream-colored parasite with a cylindrical and elongated body that tapers at both ends. These worms can grow up to 7-12 cm in length. The anterior end has three prominent lips, and there is a smooth cuticle on the entire body surface. The eggs of these parasites are oval with thick, smooth shells. These eggs are often excreted in the fecal material of the infected birds. Its most important characteristic is that it can be seen with the naked eye during the post-mortem examination. *Ascaridia galli* affects the small intestine of chickens, pigeons, and wild birds, particularly the duodenum, leading to anemia, emaciation, and reduced production efficiency [29].

## Life Cycle

As discussed earlier, the life cycle of all nematodes is direct, which involves a single host, mostly chickens. As the eggs are excreted in the feces of the infected host, their life cycle begins with this step. Under a suitable environment, the eggs are embryonated in the litter or soil and become infective. When chickens ingest such contaminated feed and water, the infection is initiated. The embryonated eggs contain the larvae, which are at either the second (L2) stage or (L3) stage of development. After ingestion of such embryonated eggs, the eggs hatch inside the proventriculus or duodenum and release the young larvae, which live free in the lumen of the duodenum for at least 9-10 days. After this period, these larvae penetrate the mucosal lining of the intestine again, which causes severe hemorrhages and bleeding, which leads to anemia in birds. This phase of the interaction of larvae with the intestinal mucosa is called the Tissue Phase. Sometimes, a few larvae can penetrate the deep tissue but most of the larvae have a very brief association with the intestinal mucosa [30]. Then these larvae undergo developmental stages in the intestinal wall and return to the lumen of the intestine, where they mature into adult worms. The adult worms then reside in the small intestine, where they feed on the intestinal feed material of the host. The adult worms reproduce inside the lumen of the host's intestine and complete the life cycle by laying eggs; these eggs pass out through the feces of the infected host. The transmission of the *Ascaridia galli* can be influenced by the age, sex, diet, and genetics of the host and so the young birds are more susceptible to the infection as compared to the adult birds. All these factors can play a role in the susceptibility of the host. Along with this, the age of the infective eggs and the dose of the ingested eggs also affect the infection [31].

## Pathogenesis

As discussed earlier, when chickens ingest the embryonated eggs through contaminated feed and water, the infection begins and these ingested eggs hatch inside the duodenal lumen and release the larvae inside it, which later invade the mucosa, resulting in severe hemorrhages. For one week these larvae reside inside the anterior parts of the intestine, then move slowly to the posterior part of the intestine as the infection progresses. Most of the hatched larvae develop inside the lumen, but some may remain stunted and can be associated with the mucosa. In the histotrophic phase or tissue phase, which is around 3 to 54 days, they penetrate the crypts of Lieberkühn, resulting in necrosis of these crypts and a significant inflammatory response characterized by the infiltration of eosinophils, lymphocytes, and macrophages. After the development of the larvae into the adult worm, the adult worm returns to the lumen of the intestine and can create a blockage of the intestinal lumen, leading to the malabsorption of nutrients. This can cause deficiencies and impaired growth of the affected host. Again it can cause intestinal obstruction or intussusception due to hypermobility. Additionally, adult worms may travel *via* the lamina propria of the large intestine and cloaca to the oviduct, where they can become incorporated within the eggs [32].

More recently it has been found that *A. galli* can interfere with the host's immune system. In the tissue phase, where larvae are in contact with the intestinal wall, they can secrete excretory and secretory (E/S) products that modulate and inhibit the immune system of the host, which help the larvae to grow and mature within the intestinal tissue. This results in chronic infection. Along with this, it is observed that larvae can move strategically within the tissue to avoid detection by the host's immune system, which helps the parasite evade the host's immune system, survive and develop [33].

## Clinical Signs and Symptoms

The parasite causes direct losses by damaging the intestinal tract, leading to malabsorption, malnutrition, and immunosuppression. Clinical signs related to the *Ascaridia galli* infection include loss of appetite, weight loss, ruffled feathers, drooped wings, delayed muscular and skeletal development, hormonal imbalances, anorexia, depression, and increased mortality. *A. galli* can also act as a vector for other pathogens like *Salmonella enterica* and impair immune responses following vaccinations, such as those against the Newcastle disease virus. Co-infections with *A. galli* and bacteria like *E. coli* or *Pasteurella multocida* can significantly impact weight gain and egg production. Due to its direct life cycle, *A. galli* transmits rapidly, especially in deep litter systems, with earthworms serving as transport hosts in rural settings. However, experimental infection-laying hens often show no clinical signs even after multiple inoculations. But when hens are co-infected with other pathogens like *Pasteurella multocida,* they can result in more severe symptoms such as depression, anorexia, ruffled feathers, and mortality. Mostly there is mixed infection of all the helminthic parasites like *A. galli, Heterakis gallinarum,* and *Raillietina spp.* All these infections can impact the poultry in the same way by reducing the feed intake, body weight gain, egg production, and overall health. Infected hens also show behavioral changes like no movement, increased nest time, and severe feather pecking. Along with these changes, the infection with this parasite can cause reduced nutrient absorption which can result in a lower lipid reserve. This impacts the health and productivity of the infected birds. Both humoral and cellular immune systems get activated in response to the *A. galli* infection with a specific antibody response, which suggests the complex interaction between the parasite and the host's immune system [34].

## Lesions

There are significant macroscopic and microscopic lesions in the host. Grossly, due to the invasion of the larvae to the intestinal wall, there is a severe inflammatory response that can cause the thickening of the intestinal wall, severe hemorrhagic patches, and edema. Microscopically we can see an abundant infiltration of the inflammatory cells in the affected tissue, which include lymphoid cells and eosinophils. As the larvae penetrate the intestinal wall, there occurs hemorrhagic enteritis that can also damage the glandular epithelium of the intestine leading to the proliferation of mucus-secreting goblet cells. This causes the fusion of mucosal villi. Mature worms exert pressure on the villi, leading to mucosal necrosis, while larvae up to 7 mm long can be found within the mucosa. The ulcerative proventriculus is another change that can be noticed in some cases, which results in the epithelial desquamation frequently observed in the duodenal villi, acting as a barrier to L3 larval penetration. To overcome the cell damage and cell loss, there is hyperplasia of the intestinal villi. In high parasitic loads, there is degeneration and necrosis of epithelial cells in the small intestine, which reduces the surface area for absorption and results in an increased number of goblet cells, inflammatory cells, and mast cells preventing further larval penetration into the mucosa. There are more recent findings of the presence of live calcified parasites in the egg albumin, which confirms that parasites can migrate through the oviduct [35].

## Diagnosis

There are various ways of detecting the *A. galli* infection in poultry. One of the most basic methods involves detection of the specific antibodies by enzyme-linked immunosorbent assay (ELISA). Both serum and egg yolk samples can be used for this method. However, the egg yolk provides the most suitable and easy method as it can be collected non-invasively. ELISA measures the host's immune response indirectly but it can't detect the intensity of the infection directly. Along with this, antibody levels can remain high even after the infection has been cleared out which complicates the results. When there is co-infection with other helminthic infections, more accurate results can be provided by ELISA, which targets the antigen called coproantigen ELISA. This test detects the antigen in the excreta and provides improved sensitivity and specificity. Indirect methods like the evaluation of inflammatory markers, including acute phase proteins can serve as indicators of health. These markers, which are part of the innate immune response to infection, stress, or inflammation, can potentially indicate the early stages of infection before clinical signs become visible. There are various recent advancements in diagnostic tests, which include the detection of *A. galli* eggs in fecal samples using a LAMP-LFD test that visually identifies the eggs by targeting specific genetic markers. Another method called duplex digital droplet PCR (ddPCR) can detect *A. galli* DNA and distinguish it from *Heterakis gallinarum*. This method is more accurate and effective compared to the traditional flotation technique [36].

**Prevention and Control**

It involves strict hygiene maintenance in poultry mostly in deep litter systems where moisture can increase the risk of infection among the birds. To avoid excessive moisture in the litter, it should be changed regularly. Along with this, good ventilation is also a key factor in avoiding any kind of infection. Young birds should be separated from the older ones to avoid infection in younger ones as they are more susceptible. In the poultry industry, disinfection is a major factor to avoid any type of outbreak but the effectiveness of disinfection is limited. Along with this, managing mental practices such as nutritional management including diets low in non-starch polysaccharides (NSP) and selective breeding for disease-resistant poultry breeds, regular deworming with anthelmintics, biosecurity measures, such as proper disposal of dead birds and preventing wild animals from accessing poultry areas, is crucial.

## *HETERAKIS GALLINARUM*

*Heterakis gallinarum* is a small, white cecal worm with three equal-sized lips and lateral membranes extending almost the entire length of its body. The male worm is 7-13 mm long, featuring a pre-anal sucker, long alae, and unequal spicules. The female, measuring 10-15 mm, has a prominent vulva and a long, narrow tail. Eggs are thick-shelled, ellipsoid, and unsegmented when deposited, measuring around 63-75 x 36-50 μm. Recent research has focused on the worm's role in transmitting *Histomonas meleagridis*, a protozoan that causes blackhead disease in poultry, highlighting its significance in poultry health [37].

**Life Cycle**

The life cycle of this parasite is similar to the *A. galli* which is direct but the only difference is that it is present in the caecal part of the large intestine. All the development and maturation phases take place in the caecal tissue causing pathological changes in the caecum of the host. Along with this *Heterakis gallinarum* is the vector for the protozoan *Histomonas meleagridis*, which causes blackhead disease, adding to its impact on poultry health.

## Pathogenicity and Necropsy Findings

The pathogenic effect of *Heterakis gallinarum* in poultry includes damage to the cecum because the maturation and development of the parasite take place in the mucosal layer of the cecum. There is a marked inflammatory response to the cecal tissue as it causes irritation which mostly leads to mucosal damage resulting in impaired nutrient absorption and poor growth in the affected host. As discussed earlier this parasite acts as a vector for the protozoal disease histomoniasis caused by *Histomonas meleagridis*. This association complicates the infection, resulting in more severe cecal and liver damage. Macroscopically the cecal wall is swollen due to severe inflammation and necrotic areas are also found due to the severe damage caused by the parasites. The affected area may show the presence of both the eggs and the adult worm of the parasites. Along with that when the bird is infected with the blackhead disease there are distinct necrotic lesions in the liver and cecum that can be noticed [38].

## *CAPILLARIA* SPECIES

These parasites have a small hair-like structure and affect various parts of the gastrointestinal tract of the poultry. There are six species that most commonly affect both the wild and domesticated chickens. These include *Capillaria annulata* and *Capillaria contorta,* which affect the crop and esophagus. *Capillaria caudinflata,* C*apillaria bursata* and *Capillaria obsignata* mostly affect the small intestine of the host. Whereas *Capillaria anatis* has the cecum as a predilection site. Due to their smaller size, these worms pose great challenges for their detection. Male worms measure approximately 6-25 mm in length but females are longer than males. They have characteristics of eggs with bipolar plugs. These parasites are cosmopolitan and affect poultry worldwide.

## Life Cycle

The life cycle of this parasite is mostly specie-specific and involves direct or indirect routes of transmission. *C. annulata* and *C. contorta* are mostly found in the crop and esophagus of the affected host. The life cycle of these species is direct and involves the shedding of eggs in the fecal material of the infected birds. Healthy birds can catch the infection by ingesting infected eggs through contaminated feed and water. Then these eggs are hatched inside the host's intestinal tract. Their further development and maturation take place in the host and they mature into adult worms.

*C. caudinflata, C. bursata,* and *C. obsignata* are found in the small intestine. All these parasites can have an indirect life cycle, which involves one intermediate host such as earthworms. The eggs are ingested by the earthworms and here inside the earthworms, these eggs hatch and develop into the infective larvae. When a bird ingests such infected intermediate hosts, the infective larvae are released inside the intestine of the bird. The development and maturation will take place inside the intestine of the final host where adult worms would be formed. The cycle is completed when adult worms lay eggs and these eggs pass through the feces of the infected host. These eggs can be ingested by the new healthy birds that would acquire the infection. This cycle continues, which leads to the reinfection of poultry flocks especially in poor hygienic farms where birds have access to contaminated feed and water [5].

## Pathogenicity and Clinical Signs

Both the birds kept in free-ranging and deep litter systems can be affected by *Capillaria* species. *Capillaria contorta* and *C. annulata* can cause mild infection in birds, leading to the inflammation and thickening of the crop and esophagus but sometimes, they may cause heavy infection leading to severe thickening and catarrhal and croupous inflammation in these areas. *C. caudinflata, C. bursata, C. obsignata,* or *C. anatis* affects the small intestine or caeca and causes hemorrhagic enteritis. This results in bloody diarrhea and severe anemia. In pigeons, *C. obsignata* is particularly pathogenic and can lead to high mortality rates.

The clinical signs and pathogenicity depend on the species and the part of the intestine involved in the disease. When crop and esophagus are involved, there is a severe inflammation of these organs, which causes obstruction leading to reduced nutrient intake and weight loss. Whereas in the small intestine and caeca, the damage to the intestinal tissue results in impaired absorption of nutrients, which causes emaciation and hemorrhagic enteritis and contributes to anemia [7].

## Necropsy Findings

In infections caused by *Capillaria contorta* and *Capillaria annulata,* the crop and the esophageal wall are the target organs and there is severe inflammation of both of these organs resulting in marked thickening of the crop and esophageal walls. The mucosal lining of the crop and esophageal wall shows catarrhal and croupous inflammation leading to mucus accumulation and the presence of diphtheritic membranes. The mucosal surface may be severely ulcerated and thickened which gives it a rough appearance in the very highly infected host. When the small intestine and caeca are infected with *C. caudinflata, C. bursata, C. obsignata,* or *C. anatis,* there is severe inflammation resulting in the thickening of the intestinal wall. The most characteristic lesion of this infection is the presence of hemorrhagic enteritis that is characterized by the presence of blood in the intestinal contents and darkened, congested areas of the intestinal lining. The mucosal layer of the intestine becomes necrotic and may be ulcerated in severe cases. In the cecum of the affected bird, the presence of necrotic debris mixed with blood indicates this infection. In pigeons, infected with *C. obsignata* that is highly pathogenic, there is extensive hemorrhagic enteritis with significant thinning of the intestinal walls due to chronic blood loss, and severe anemia, evidenced by pale mucous membranes and reduced fat deposits [9].

## CESTODES

These are called tapeworms, which belong to the phylum Platyhelminthes and the class *Cestoda*. They are hermaphrodites having both male and female reproductive systems inside them. They have very flat and segmented body structures and they don't have a digestive tract, which makes them tape-like structures; the so-called tapeworms. Poultry tapeworms measure about 30-50 cm in length. The body is divided into 3 parts, which include the head part called scolex, the neck, and the strobila. Scolex helps in the attachment of the parasite to the intimal wall of the host whereas strobila has a series of segments called proglottids that develop from the neck. Each proglottid has a complete set of sex organs. These proglottids become mature when they move away from the neck and finally detach from the body. The detached segments can be called gravid proglottids as they are filled with eggs. These eggs can be released in the environment when they are excreted through the affected host. The normal healthy bird can acquire infection by ingesting such contaminated material and the life cycle of the parasite continues. The most commonly found poultry tapeworms are *Davainea proglottina, Choanotaenia infundibulum, Raillietina tetragona,* and *Raillietina echinobothrida*. The smallest tapeworm is *Davainea proglottina,* which measures about 4 mm in length and is found in the duodenum. The *Choanotaenia infundibulum* can reach up to a size of 25 cm and is mostly found in the distal duodenum and jejunum. *Raillietina tetragona* also measures around 25 cm and is located in the distal jejunum. Among all these tapeworms, the *Raillietina echinobothrida* measures 30 cm, which makes it the largest cestode. It can be found in the jejunum and is responsible for nodular granulomas and catarrhal enteritis [11].

## *RAILLIETINA*

This genus was named in 1920 after Louis-Joseph Alcide Railliet who was a French veterinarian and helminthologist. There are almost 37 species of this genus with the more commonly found parasites being *Raillietina echinobothrida, Raillietina tetragona,* and *Raillietina cesticillus*. All these mentioned parasites have a very significant pathogenic impact with a high prevalence rate in the poultry industry. The adult worms have elongated ribbon-like structures. Their Scolex is bulbous and has suckers and rostellum, which helps the parasite attach to the host cells. The proglottids are covered with fine hair-like structures called microtriches, which are specialised structures for the absorption of nutrients.

## Life Cycle

The life cycle of this parasite can start with the ingestion of the gravid proglottids, which contain numerous eggs. Such gravid proglottids are excreted in the fecal material of the infected host. These eggs can be ingested by the intermediate host like ants of genera *Pheidole* and *Tetramorium*, beetles of genera *Calathus* and *Amara*, and other insects. Inside the intermediate host, the eggs hatch in the intestine and release the embryo called the oncosphere. The embryo can penetrate the wall of the intestine and develop in the next developmental stage, which is the cysticercoid larva in the intermediate host. This cysticercoid stage remains dormant in the intermediate host until it has been ingested by the final host. After the ingestion of such an intermediate host with the cysticercoid stage of the larvae inside them, the larva gets activated by the bile juice from the intestine of the final host. This activated larva gets attached to the intestinal wall through its scolex and develops into an adult tapeworm. The gravid segments are formed as the tapeworm matures and they are excreted again through the fecal material of the final host. This cycle again continues when such mature proglottids are ingested by the intermediate host [13].

## Pathogenicity and Clinical Signs

Among the all species, *Raillietina echinobothrida* are important as they can cause chronic infection in the bird leading to a significant effect on the birds. The disease can be initiated when the parasite attaches to the intestinal wall through their hooks and sucker. This results in severe irritation and damage to the intestinal wall leading to the formation of nodules and results in the hyperplasia of the intestinal cell. In these cases, there is extensive hyperplasia of the intestinal cells and severe inflammatory response of the host tissue, which gives it a nodular appearance. Thus, this infection can be called "Nodular tapeworm disease," which is noticed only in heavily infected cases and can severely impair the absorption process of the host.

Clinical signs include reduced growth, emaciation, and general weakness. Infected birds may exhibit signs of poor feed conversion, lethargy, and weight loss as a result of the inability of the bird to absorb the nutrients from the intestine. Along with this, the affected bird may show immune suppression, which makes the bird susceptible to other bacterial infections. In chronic infection with

*Raillietina echinobothrida,* there is persistent emaciation and reduced productivity. The combination of nutrient malabsorption and the body's response to the infection can also lead to anemia and a compromised immune system, making the birds more susceptible to other diseases [18].

## Necropsy Findings

The presence of nodules in the intestinal wall is a characteristic lesion of this disease. These nodules can be formed due to the local inflammatory reaction caused by the attachment of the tapeworms with their hooks and suckers. Nodules are typically firm and raised areas that are found at the site where parasite scolex attaches to the wall of the intestine. The size of the nodule depends on the parasitic load present in that area. Along with this, the intestine shows hyperplastic lesions and there is the presence of a thickened and hyperplastic mucosal lining of the intestine caused due to chronic inflammation. The Lumen of the intestine may contain numerous numbers of the proglottids and adult worms, which can be seen by the naked eyes.

## *DAVAINEA PROGLOTTINA*

These are minute or small tapeworms of poultry, which particularly affect the gallinaceous worms like chickens, turkeys, guinea fowl, and grouse. They have very small sizes ranging from 0.5 to 3 mm in length, with only 4 to 9 segments, or proglottids. They are mostly found in the mucosal layer of the duodenum. Their invasion into the mucosal layer can cause severe damage to the intestinal wall [19].

They also have an indirect life cycle, which involves snails as an intermediate host. The intermediate host ingests the eggs from the contaminated environment and its development takes place inside the host. Birds can get infected when they eat such infected snails. *Davainea proglottina* can cause significant pathology in the host, including inflammation and lesions in the duodenum. The infestation can lead to weight loss, decreased egg production, and in severe cases, death, particularly in young or immunocompromised birds. Diagnosis is often made by identifying the proglottids or eggs in the host's feces.

## Pathogenicity and Clinical Signs

Young birds are most susceptible to this infection. As they also attach to the intestinal mucosa through their sucker causing trauma to the mucosal lining, resulting in severe inflammatory response and local damage. Their attachment can lead to thickening, inflammation, and hemorrhages, which can lead to anemia in the infected host. There is secretion of the fetid mucus and necrosis of the affected tissue in the small intestine.

The affected birds are dull and depressed and they show reduced body weight emaciation due to the inability to absorb nutrients. Along with this, some birds may show dyspnoea, slow movements, and lethargy as the systemic effects of the infection caused by this parasite. In severe cases, leg paralysis can occur, and if the infection is left untreated, it can lead to death, particularly in young or immunocompromised birds.

## TREATMENT OF TAPEWORM INFECTION IN POULTRY

Tapeworm infection in poultry can be treated by Praziquantel, which is highly effective against tapeworms, and Niclosamide these drugs can be added to the feed and given to the affected flocks. Butynorate is another anthelmintic drug that can treat tapeworm infection effectively. All these treatments require a starvation period before administration to the bird. When there occur a complication with coccidiosis, sulphonamide drugs like sulphaquinoxaline can be used in combination with diaveridine or sulphadimidine, which can be given through drinking water. Along with these supplements, Vitamin A and K enhance the immune system of the birds by supporting the healing process of the damaged intestinal mucosa [22].

## CONTROL AND PREVENTION OF TAPEWORM

For the effective control of the tapeworm, it is important to disrupt the life cycle of the parasite, which can be achieved by targeting intermediate hosts like snails and slugs. The most effective method for this is the application of the snail bait containing the metaldehyde around the poultry house. Along with this, biosecurity is the most important factor in the poultry industry to control and prevent, not only parasitic disease but all infective diseases.

## NEMATODES CAUSING RESPIRATORY DISEASE

### *SYNGAMUS TRACHEA*

The parasite is Y-shaped and is called "tracheal worm" of the poultry as it is responsible for causing respiratory disease in poultry. These parasites are mostly found in the trachea, bronchi, and bronchioles of chickens, turkeys, geese, and many other birds. It affects the respiratory tract and causes the condition called "gapes" which causes difficulty in breathing, hence these worms can also be called "gapeworms of the poultry". It can also be called as "red worm of the poultry" because it is red. The adult worms are large and they have anteriorly directed buckle capsules. They use this buckle capsule for their attachment to the tracheal lining. Both males and females are permanently paired forming the characteristic "Y shape" and can also be called a "forked worm". Males measure around 5.8 mm and females measure 10-15 mm. The eggs of these parasites are oval and have a thick shell that measures approximately 70-85 μm by 50-60 μm [25].

## Life Cycle

The life cycle of *Syngamus trachea* is direct or indirect, involving earthworms as intermediate hosts. Eggs of these parasites are shed into the environment through the feces of the infected host and these eggs become infective after their development into larvae (L3) in the environment only. These embryonated eggs can be directly ingested by the birds and acquire infection which comprises the direct life cycle. But sometimes birds acquire the infection through ingestion of earthworms, which contain the free larvae or encysted larvae that they obtain by feeding on contaminated soil. Female worms deposit the eggs through the vulvar opening and the eggs that reach the mouth cavity are swallowed by the birds and pass through the fecal material. In suitable environmental conditions, the released eggs get embryonated. They hatch and release the larvae free in the soil. Earthworms feed on such contaminated soil and they become infected. Within the earthworm, the larvae penetrate the intestinal wall and enter the body cavity. Then from there, they invade the musculature of the earthworm. These larvae of *Syngamus trachea* can remain infective for 4 years. Poultry become infected by ingesting larvae-containing earthworms. These larvae penetrate the intestinal wall in birds as well. Some larvae can penetrate the wall of the crop and esophagus and penetrate the lungs directly. However, most of the larvae can penetrate the duodenum and they are carried to the respiratory system through the portal. These larvae can break the capillaries and come out. These released larvae migrate to the heart and trachea. In the trachea, they mature into adults, where they attach and feed. The adults lay eggs that are expelled through the trachea into the esophagus and then out through the feces, perpetuating the cycle [27].

## Pathogenicity and Clinical Signs

We discussed earlier that the larvae penetrate the mucosal surface of the trachea and that this causes severe irritation, resulting in an inflammatory response. This damage obstructs airflow and respiratory distress. Chronic irritation from worms can make birds susceptible to secondary bacterial infection.

## Clinical Signs

Birds affected with this disease show respiratory distress, which is characterized by labored breathing, gasping, and coughing. Infected birds with this parasite have heavy worm load in the trachea leading to the blockage of the lumen of the trachea and so the birds commonly exhibit respiratory distress, characterized by labored breathing, gasping, and coughing. This symptom is due to the obstruction of the trachea by the worms. Birds may display a characteristic "gape" behavior, where they open their mouths widely as if gasping for air. Other signs include emaciation and weakness resulting from impaired respiration and reduced feed intake. Additionally, changes in vocalizations, often becoming more hoarse or raspy, may be observed [29].

## Lesions

Grossly the trachea of the infected bird shows a severe inflammatory response and there is attachment of the parasite to the mucosal lining of the trachea throughout the life of the parasites. The trachea can be swollen and petechial hemorrhages can be seen. Some necrotic patches can be seen on the tracheal wall. In severe cases, there may be mucus accumulation and evidence of secondary bacterial infections. Microscopically, there is marked hyperplasia of the epithelial lining of the trachea and infiltration of the inflammatory cells in the affected tissue. The ulceration and hemorrhages can be seen at the place where the parasite attaches to the trachea.

## Diagnosis

Diagnosis of *Syngamus trachea* infections typically involves clinical examination, where signs such as respiratory distress and gape behavior are noted. The fecal examination can confirm the presence of eggs, though they may be difficult to find. Direct examination of the trachea during necropsy or endoscopic procedures can reveal the characteristic presence of adult worms.

## Prevention and Control

Maintain hygiene in poultry housing by regular cleaning, disinfection, and removal of contaminated litter. Control the environment to reduce infection risks and intermediate hosts. Treat flocks with anthelmintics like fenbendazole or ivermectin for *Syngamus trachea* control. Implement biosecurity to prevent parasite introduction from wild birds [35].

## ECTOPARASITES OF THE POULTRY

External parasitism is responsible for the greatest economic losses to the poultry industry followed by viral diseases. This is more common in the villages where the backyard raring system is predominant. Along with this, the tropical areas are also prone because of the favorable climatic conditions for their development.

These parasites compete for feed or cause distress to the birds as they live their whole life on the body surface of the bird this may lead to anemia, reduced growth, egg production, and death. This class of parasites includes mites, lice, ticks, and fleas.

## MITES

Poultry mites may spend their entire life on the body of a bird but when their infestation reaches certain levels, they can cause severe dermatitis. Certain mites have blood-sucking habits that lead to anemia and may even lead to death. The most significant mites that cause serious impact on health care are *Dermanyssus gallinae* (red mite of poultry) and *Ornithonyssus sylviarum* (northern fowl mite) as both of them are bloodsuckers and can damage both skin and feathers. Among these two, *Dermanyssus gallinae* is widely distributed throughout the world and imposes a major threat to the layers.

## *DERMANYSSUS GALLINAE*

This is also called as "red mite of the chicken" or "roost mite" which is a small ectoparasite. It measures approximately 1.5 mm in length. It is grey to brown-red in color depending on the feeding status. This parasite does not reside on the host's body surface permanently. They are mostly nocturnal and feed on the host at night. They hide during the day in cracks and crevices. This mite has a genetic structure that allows it to rapidly adapt to its host, contributing to its host specificity.

### Life Cycle

*D. gallinae* mostly hides in secluded areas like cracks in wooden joints. The life cycle of this parasite occurs off the host bird. It can find the host by using specific signals like suitable temperature, chemical signals, and level of carbon dioxide. It feeds on the host during the night for a short period. The life cycle can be completed in 14 days and requires a suitable climatic condition. The eggs are smooth, white, and oval in shape, measuring approximately 400 x 270 µ in size. These eggs can hatch at suitable temperatures mostly between 28°C and 30°C within 2 to 3 days. Larvae that are six-legged and white coloured emerge from the eggs. In this stage larva cannot feed on the host. In the next developmental stage, which occurs in one day, these larvae molt into the next stage which is protonymph. Protonymph stage larvae have eight legs and they can feed on the host's blood. After feeding the proto-nymphal stage again molts into the next stage *i.e.* deutonymph. After feeding, it gets converted into the adult mite. These adult mites begin mating and females start laying the eggs [26].

Adult mites, either male or female, begin mating shortly after molting. Within 12 hours of mating, females start feeding and laying eggs. This cycle can be repeated for the full life span of the parasite. One female can lay at least 30 eggs in her total life span. Around 1.2 weeks are required to complete one life cycle and this depends on suitable environmental conditions such as temperature and humidity. This mite has very great potential in reproduction with a capacity of tripling in just 10 days. Along with this they are very sturdy and can live without feeding for even 12 months.

## Pathogenicity

This parasite is the primary ectoparasite of the laying hens. These mites are haematopagus meaning they feed on the blood of the host. Their constant feeding on the host may result in anemia and reduce egg production, fertility, and feed conversion efficiency. In severe cases, mite feeding can lead to increased mortality mostly in younger birds. Along with this, these mites have the potential to transmit various diseases as they can act as a vectors for various viruses and bacteria. They can transmit both animal as well as human pathogens which include *Borrelia anserine*, fowl poxvirus, Eastern equine encephalitis virus, and *Salmonella*. The ability of *D. gallinae* to transmit *Salmonella* to its offspring poses a potential risk for zoonotic salmonellosis.

## *ORNITHONYSSUS* SPP.

It is also called a Northern fowl mite which is small and oval-shaped and measures about 0.7 to 1.1 mm long. The color of this parasite is dark and the body is covered with short bristles. They have eight legs and the mouth parts are adapted for the feeding of blood. The body of the mite is flexible for navigation through feathers. Along with this, they have a dorsal shield which protects the mite. The eggs are small, oval, and white. They are laid in clusters. These mites also feed on the blood and can be found in the vent area of poultry. In the vent area, their infestation can cause skin inflammation, irritation, and scabbing. They can appear in large numbers, reaching tens of thousands per bird, resulting in feather discoloration from the accumulation of live and dead mites, eggs, and feces [29].

## Life Cycle

The Northern fowl mite completes its life cycle on the host with all stages including egg, larva, protonymph, deutonymph, and adult. The time taken by the mite to complete the life cycle is very short mostly one week. The protonymph stage feeds once or twice before molting into the deutonymph. This stage does not feed on the blood and develops into the adult. Mite populations can rapidly explode, particularly in young birds with immature immune systems.

## Pathogenicity

Northern fowl mites are also blood feeders that can cause significant harm to infested poultry. They induce blood loss, scabbing, and pruritus, leading to anemia and reduced egg production. Infestations also divert energy from growth and egg production as the bird's immune system attempts to control the mites. In breeder flocks, the irritation can lower rooster libido and egg fertility. Mites can also affect egg-processing workers, causing pruritus and irritation, and potentially leading to refusal to work.

## *KNEMIDOCOPTES MUTANS*

These mites are the scaly leg mites of poultry. These are tiny in size and can infest the shanks and feet of birds, including both wild and domesticated fowl. They are burrowing mites and can burrow deep inside the host tissue. These mites cause significant damage by burrowing into the skin, leading to tissue swelling, enlarged and protruding scales, and leakage of lymphatic fluid. The burrowing behavior of these mites results in the characteristic scaly appearance of the affected limbs which gives them the name the "scaly leg" mite.

## Life Cycle

The entire life cycle of *Knemidocoptes mutans* occurs on the host bird. The mites are transmitted through direct contact between infected and healthy birds. The mites live under the scales of the bird's legs and feet where they feed on keratin. The continuous feeding on the keratin of the leg can cause severe damage and scaling of the leg. As the mites reproduce, the infestation worsens leading to more extensive scale lifting and tissue damage.

## Pathogenicity

As they are burrowing mites and their activity can lead to severe skin irritation, inflammation. The tissue damage may result in secondary bacterial infection. It requires immediate treatment to avoid the secondary bacterial complication and if not treated, the infestation can cause significant deformities in the legs and claws, which may result in the legs deformities and finally lameness in the birds. In severe cases, the bird's overall health may deteriorate due to the stress and discomfort caused by the mites [31].

## *KNEMIDOCOPTES LAEVIS*

They are called "depluming mites" of the poultry. These mites are also burrowing mites, which burrow deep into the skin at the base of the feathers. They are smaller in size and difficult to see by the naked eye. The burrowing activity of the mites causes severe irritation to the bird, leading to feather-pulling and significant discomfort.

### Pathogenicity

They are harmful due to their burrowing habit and they feed on the host tissue which leads to intense irritation and itching, prompting birds to pull out their feathers. This behavior results in feather loss, which can cause stress and further health issues for the affected bird. If left untreated, the infestation can lead to more extensive feather damage, skin infections, and a decline in the bird's overall health.

## *NEOSCHOENGASTIA AMERICANA*

These are the larval chiggers and are also very small. They are often found on turkeys in large numbers, typically around 100 per bird. These mites are visible during the larval stage which is the infective stage, where they cluster together and feed on the bird's skin. At the larval stage, they attach to the host for 4-6 days and feed on the host to develop into their next stage and finally become adults in the environment. The subsequent life stages of chiggers are nonparasitic and do not pose a direct threat to birds.

### Pathogenicity

Chiggers are mostly harmful to the turkeys. Their feeding habit on the skin results in skin inflammation which can lead to carcass downgrading and financial loss. The irritation and stress caused by chigger infestations can also impact the overall health and productivity of the birds.

### CONTROL AND PREVENTION OF MITES IN POULTRY

As mites can impact the poultry industry their control is very important. The most important approach to prevent and control the mite population is the Integrated Pest Management (IPM) approach. Quarantine of the new bird is also the key factor for the control of ectoparasite infestation in poultry flocks. Regular monitoring of the flock is essential for early detection and timely action against mite infestations, which can help prevent their spread and escalation. Maintenance of a clean and well-managed area with the help of a proper use of disinfectant and controlling access to wild birds and other potential mite carriers, reduces the risk of infestations. When infestations do occur, a combination of IPM strategies should be employed. Topical treatments with pesticides are crucial, although ensuring adequate coverage and penetration through feathers can be challenging. Dusting with acaricidal powders, while a labor-intensive approaches, can be effective if applied correctly to the infestation sites. Systemic treatments, such as off-label use of ivermectin under veterinary supervision, may also be employed to treat infestations internally. By integrating these approaches, poultry producers can manage mite infestations more effectively, minimizing their impact on bird health and productivity [12].

## FLEAS

*Echidnophaga gallinacean,* which is also called a sticktight flea, is the most important flea pest affecting poultry primarily in backyard flocks. These are small and measure around 2mm in length. They can also infest other animals including dogs, cats, and swine when they come across the infested birds. Adult female sticktight fleas attach themselves deeply to the skin of their hosts. The sight of attachment is around the head in large clusters whereas the male mite can move through the entire body of the host and mate with the female. This behavior distinguishes them from other flea species that only intermittently feed on birds and mammals. Infestations, particularly around the eyes, can cause swelling and vision problems in poultry.

The life cycle of the sticktight flea begins when females lay eggs that fall off the host and develop in the surrounding environment, such as litter. The larvae feed on organic debris and eventually pupate in the same area. Adult fleas can emerge within a week, but if hosts are unavailable, they can remain dormant for extended periods. This highlights the importance of cleaning bedding to prevent flea population resurgence. Small infestations can be managed by manually removing the fleas with tweezers.

To prevent re-infestation, treating the birds with a pyrethroid insecticide and altering the flea larval habitat is crucial. Regularly cleaning and replacing bedding, along with spraying insect growth regulators like methoprene or pyriproxyfen, helps disrupt the flea life cycle. Continued monitoring of the birds ensures that any subsequent infestations are caught and treated promptly.

## POULTRY LICE

Lice present in the poultry industry are small and wingless. They can infest chickens, turkeys, and other birds too. These lice feed on the bird's skin feathers. Sometimes they can feed on the blood of the host causing irritation, reduced egg production, and overall stress to the birds. The most common types of lice found in poultry include *Menacanthus stramineus, Menopon gallinae, Cuclotogaster heterographus, Lipeurus caponis,* and *Goniocotes gallinae.*

Mallophaga order contains chewing-lice which are primary parasites that infest birds. They feed on the feathers, skin scales, feather debris, and dermal materials. They also chew through feather shafts and ingest fresh blood but they do not depend on the blood as a primary food source. More than 40 species of lice have been identified in domestic birds, though most are rare in commercial flocks. Chickens typically host seven louse species, while turkeys have three common species. Although the economic impact of louse infestations is not well-documented, they can significantly affect young birds, leading to stunted growth and reduced feed efficiency [17].

**Common Poultry Lice**

The *Menacanthus stramineus* can be called a chicken body louse. It is the most common species found in adult chickens. It primarily feeds on the skin in lightly dense feather area, which is present around the vent but can spread the entire body of the chicken. These are straw-colored lice and they can move very fast on the skin. The chicken body louse feeds on skin debris and at the base of feathers, causing skin irritation, scabbing, and reduced weight gain due to the constant discomfort.

The shaft louse or small body louse is the *Menopon gallinae*. It is similar in appearance to the chicken body louse but is smaller in size. It primarily infests the feathers of the breast and thighs. When feathers are parted, these lice can be seen scurrying down the feather shafts, trying to hide. Shaft lice feed on feathers, which can lead to significant feather damage. Heavily infested birds often become restless, which can impact their overall health and productivity.

The chicken head louse *i.e. Cuclotogaster heterographa* is greyish, approximately 1 mm in length, and is typically found around the head and neck of birds. It positions itself near the host's skin at the base of feathers, particularly on the top and back of the head and under the beak. Female head lice attach their pearly white eggs to small head feathers, with the eggs hatching within five days. Although head lice do not feed on blood, they can cause significant irritation, especially in young birds. In severe infestations, young chickens and turkeys may suffer from decline and die before they reach one month of age.

## Life Cycle of the Lice

The life cycle starts with the laying of eggs which are small, and white in colour. These eggs are called nits. They are firmly attached to the base of the feather near the skin. Depending on the temperature and humidity, these eggs are hatched in the nymphal stage within 4-7 days. This stage is crucial for the infestation to continue, as each egg hatches into a young louse ready to begin feeding on the bird. This nymph stage looks similar to the louse but its size is smaller and cannot reproduce. They can undergo further stages of development which can be called instars. Each stage of development lasts approximately 3-7 days. During the development process, they can molt and grow faster and larger. They require a permanent food source that can be provided by the host. After the final molt, the lice become adults, fully capable of reproducing and continuing the cycle. Adult lice are larger and have fully developed reproductive organs. They typically start laying eggs within a day or two after reaching maturity. A single female louse can lay between 50 to 100 eggs throughout her lifetime. Adult lice continue to feed on the host and can live for several weeks on the bird. However, if they are separated from their host, they typically die within a few days due to a lack of sustenance. The entire life cycle, from egg to adult, usually spans about 3 to 4 weeks, making lice infestations difficult to control without consistent management efforts [23].

## Pathology of Lice Infestation

Lice infestations can lead to skin irritation because of their movement on the body of the chicken. As lice feed on the skin debris and base of the feathers, they cause constant discomfort to the host. This continuous irritation can cause scabbing of the skin. The heavy infestation may lead to severe feather damage and some lice also chew feathers, which impacts the quality of feathers and the appearance of the bird. Birds affected by lice may experience reduced weight gain due to the continuous irritation and stress caused by the parasites. Additionally, some lice can feed on the blood which can cause anemia and can decrease feed conversion efficiency, which means that birds are not able to properly convert feed into body mass, which can lead to economic losses in poultry production. In severe cases, especially with head lice, heavy infestations can be fatal to young birds, with deaths occurring before the birds reach one month of age.

## Control of the Lice

Lice can be controlled by a combination of regular monitoring, environmental management, and treatment. Another way of controlling lice is regular inspection under the wings and around the vent which is the most favourable site of the infestation. Keeping the poultry environment clean and dry is essential, with frequent cleaning of coops, nesting boxes, and perches to reduce the risk of lice.

Providing dust baths, supplemented with diatomaceous earth or wood ash, allows birds to naturally remove parasites. Chemical treatments like permethrin or pyrethrins can be used to treat lice, applied as sprays, dusts, or dips. It is crucial to treat all birds in the flock at once to prevent re-infestation, and re-treatment may be necessary after 7 to 10 days to eliminate newly hatched lice [31].

## FOWL TICK (*ARGAS PERSICUS*)

The most important soft tick in the bird is *Argas persicus* that is commonly called a fowl tick or blue bug. It is known to have originated in Central Asia but now can be found in many countries. The most common host for this tick is the domestic chicken but it can also be found in birds like pigeons, and other fowl. In the absence of chickens, the tick may latch on to humans. These ticks can bite the host and cause severe irritation. This tick can act as a vector for many diseases like *Borrelia anserine*, which causes avian spirochetosis. It may play a role in the transmission of *Mycobacterium avium*, the bacterium responsible for fowl tuberculosis. Along with this, it can cause fowl paralysis. These ticks are hidden in the cracks and crevices in the natural environment away from the host. They are nocturnal and feed in the night on the blood of the host. The female can lay up to 500 eggs in secluded areas. The eggs can take anywhere from a few weeks to several months to hatch, depending on environmental conditions, adding to the challenge of controlling infestations.

## Life Cycle

After the laying of the eggs by the female, they hatch in the environment and the larvae are released. The released larvae crawl to the host, feed on the bird, and take their first blood meal. After feeding, they detach from the host and hide to molt into the nymphal stage. These ticks undergo multiple nymphal stages and every developmental stage feeds on the blood of the host. Repeated feeding by large populations of fowl ticks can lead to significant blood loss in the host, resulting in emaciation and, in severe cases, fatal anemia. Adult ticks are sturdy and can survive over a year without feeding which complicates eradication efforts [35].

## Pathogenicity

As they feed on the blood of the host, anemia is the most prominent pathological intervention caused by these ticks. In addition to physical weakening, *Argas persicus* is known to transmit various pathogens that can lead to serious diseases in poultry, such as spirochetes, rickettsias, and bacteria, which can be particularly problematic in regions where these diseases are prevalent. The nocturnal feeding habits of these ticks mean they may go unnoticed unless birds are examined at night, allowing infestations to progress undetected.

## Control of the ticks

*Argus persicus* spends most of its life off the host so controlling the population of such a tick is difficult. All cracks and crevices where ticks may hide must be treated with an appropriate acaricide to eliminate the infestation. While fowl ticks are more common in backyard flocks, typical commercial poultry operations have rarely provided the environmental conditions conducive to their populations [32]. However, changes in caging and husbandry practices may alter this dynamic, making it increasingly important to monitor and control tick infestations in various poultry settings.

## CONCLUDING REMARKS

Parasites can cause a wide range of pathophysiological effects on the host. Internal parasites cause anemia involving various mechanisms associated with the destruction of red cells as well as possible defects in red cell production. Parasites are responsible for causing the disturbance of heart function, and the nervous, immune as well as urinary systems. The major groups of parasitic diseases are proximately associated with the gastrointestinal tract of poultry. Gastrointestinal nematode parasites can cause alteration in feed intake, disturbed gastrointestinal function, and protein and energy metabolism by raising pathophysiological responses by the host to parasitic infections.

## REFRENCES

[1]    Abebe E, Gugsa G. A review on poultry coccidiosis. Abyssinia J Sci Technol 2018; 3(1): 1-12.

[2]    Al-Badrani MA, Al-Muffti SA. Poultry farming: New perspectives and applications chapter–parasitic diseases of chickens In: Téllez-Isaías G, Poultry Farming-New Perspectives and Applications. IntechOpen. 2023.

[3]    Amin A, Bilic I, Liebhart D, Hess M. Trichomonads in birds – a review. Parasitology 2014; 141(6): 733-47.
       [http://dx.doi.org/10.1017/S0031182013002096] [PMID: 24476968]

[4]    Arabkhazaeli F, Nabian S, Modirsanei M, Madani S A. The efficacy of a poultry commercial anticoccidial vaccine in experimental challenge with *Eimeria* field isolates. Iranian J Vet Med. 2014.

[5]    Arce SI, Manzoli DE, Saravia-Pietropaolo MJ, *et al.* The tropical fowl mite, *Ornithonyssus bursa* (Acari: Macronyssidae): environmental and host factors associated with its occurrence in Argentine passerine communities. Parasitol Res 2018; 117(10): 3257-67.
       [http://dx.doi.org/10.1007/s00436-018-6025-1] [PMID: 30069828]

[6]    Hauck R, Macklin KS. Vaccination against poultry parasites. Avian Dis. 2024 Jan;67(4):441-449.
       [http://dx.doi.org/10.1637/aviandiseases-D-23-99989]

[7]    Bedford GAH. The external parasites of poultry with measures for their control. J Dep Agric 1924; 9(2): 123-40.

[8]     Khayatnouri . The effect of ivermectin pour-on administration against natural *Heterakis gallinarum* infestation and its prevalence in native poultry. Am J Anim Vet Sci 2011; 6(1): 55-8. [http://dx.doi.org/10.3844/ajavsp.2011.55.58]

[9]     De Gussem M. Coccidiosis in poultry: review on diagnosis, control, prevention and interaction with overall gut health. Proceedings of the 16th European Symposium on Poultry Nutrition. 253-61.

[10]    Bilic I, Leberl M, Hess M. Identification and molecular characterization of numerous *Histomonas meleagridis* proteins using a cDNA library. Parasitology. 2009 Apr;136(4):379-91. [http://dx.doi.org/10.1017/S0031182008005477]

[11]    Fatoba AJ, Adeleke MA. Diagnosis and control of chicken coccidiosis: a recent update. J Parasit Dis 2018; 42(4): 483-93. [http://dx.doi.org/10.1007/s12639-018-1048-1] [PMID: 30538344]

[12]    Hafez HM. Poultry coccidiosis: prevention and control approaches. Arch Geflugelkd 2008; 72(1): 2-7. [http://dx.doi.org/10.1016/S0003-9098(25)00872-0]

[13]    Alves LFA, Johann L, Oliveira DGP. Challenges in the biological control of pests in poultry production: a critical review of advances in Brazil. Neotrop Entomol. 2023 Apr;52(2):292-301. [http://dx.doi.org/10.1007/s13744-022-01021-1]

[14]    Hess M, Liebhart D, Bilic I, Ganas P. *Histomonas meleagridis*—New insights into an old pathogen. Vet Parasitol 2015; 208(1-2): 67-76. [http://dx.doi.org/10.1016/j.vetpar.2014.12.018] [PMID: 25576442]

[15]    Hinkle N C, Corrigan R M. External parasites and poultry pests In: Swayne DE, Boulianne M, Logue CM, McDougald LR, Nair V, Suarez DL, de Wit S, Grimes T, Johnson D, Kromm M, Prajitno TY, Rubinoff I, Zavala G, Eds, Diseases of Poultry, 2020; 1135-56. [http://dx.doi.org/10.1002/9781119371199.ch26]

[16]    Jahantigh M, Esmailzade Dizaji R, Teymoori Y. Prevalence of external parasites of pigeon in Zabol, southeast of Iran. J Parasit Dis. 2016 Dec;40(4):1548-1551. [http://dx.doi.org/10.1007/s12639-015-0725-6]

[17]    Höglund J, Daş G, Tarbiat B, Geldhof P, Jansson DS, Gauly M. *Ascaridia galli* - An old problem that requires new solutions. Int J Parasitol Drugs Drug Resist 2023; 23: 1-9. [http://dx.doi.org/10.1016/j.ijpddr.2023.07.003] [PMID: 37516026]

[18]    Kebede A, Abebe B, Zewdie T. Study on prevalence of ectoparasites of poultry in and around Jimma town. Eur J Biol Sci 2017; 9(1): 18-26.

[19]    Knežević S, Pajić M, Petrović A, *et al*. *Dermanyssus gallinae*-overview: life cycle, morphology, prevalence and control measures in poultry farms. Arh Vet Med 2017; 10(2): 53-62. [http://dx.doi.org/10.46784/e-avm.v10i2.73]

[20]    Ladds P. Helminth Diseases in Birds. In: Pathology of Australian Native Wildlife. CSIRO Publishing. 2009; pp. 323-45.

[21]    Lilić S, Ilić T, Dimitrijević S. Coccidiosis in poultry industry. Met Technol 2009; 50(1-2): 90-8.

[22]    López-Osorio S, Chaparro-Gutiérrez JJ, Gómez-Osorio LM. Overview of poultry *Eimeria* life cycle and host-parasite interactions. Front Vet Sci 2020; 7: 384. [http://dx.doi.org/10.3389/fvets.2020.00384] [PMID: 32714951]

[23]    McBurney S, Kelly-Clark WK, Forzán MJ, Vanderstichel R, Teather K, Greenwood SJ. Persistence of *Trichomonas gallinae* in Birdseed. Avian Dis 2017; 61(3): 311-5. [http://dx.doi.org/10.1637/11545-113016-RegR1] [PMID: 28956991]

[24]    Montasser AA. The fowl tick, *Argas (Persicargas) persicus* (Ixodoidea: Argasidae): Description of the egg and redescription of the larva by Scanning Electron Microscopy. Exp Appl Acarol 2010; 52(4): 343-61. [http://dx.doi.org/10.1007/s10493-010-9377-5] [PMID: 20607364]

[25] Munsch M, Gräfner G, Popp J, Henning M. Development of *Histomonas meleagridis* under *in vitro* conditions. Parasitol Res 2009; 105(4): 887-95.

[26] Pritchard J, Kuster T, Sparagano O, Tomley F. Understanding the biology and control of the poultry red mite *Dermanyssus gallinae* : a review. Avian Pathol 2015; 44(3): 143-53.
[http://dx.doi.org/10.1080/03079457.2015.1030589] [PMID: 25895578]

[27] Saikia M, Bhattacharjee K, Sarmah PC, Deka DK, Upadhyaya TN, Konch P. Prevalence and pathology of *Trichomonas gallinae* in domestic pigeon (*Columba livia domestica*) of Assam, India. Indian J Anim Res 2021; 55(1): 84-9.

[28] Scholtyseck E, Mehlhorn H, Hammond DM. Electron microscope studies of microgametogenesis in coccidia and related groups. Z Parasitenkd 1972; 38(2): 95-131.
[http://dx.doi.org/10.1007/BF00329023] [PMID: 4622927]

[29] Schuster M. Electron microscopic demonstration of flagella in *Histomonas meleagridis*. J Parasitol 1968; 54(4): 809-10.

[30] Sharma N, Hunt PW, Hine BC, Ruhnke I. The impacts of *Ascaridia galli* on performance, health, and immune responses of laying hens: new insights into an old problem. Poult Sci 2019; 98(12): 6517-26.
[http://dx.doi.org/10.3382/ps/pez422] [PMID: 31504894]

[31] Shifaw A, Feyera T, Walkden-Brown SW, Sharpe B, Elliott T, Ruhnke I. Global and regional prevalence of helminth infection in chickens over time: a systematic review and meta-analysis. Poult Sci 2021; 100(5): 101082.
[http://dx.doi.org/10.1016/j.psj.2021.101082] [PMID: 33813325]

[32] Singh R, Gupta I, Patil R D. 2023.Ascariasis in poultry: A comprehensive review
[http://dx.doi.org/10.22271/tpi.2023.v12.i11Sj.24021]

[33] Sparagano OAE, George DR, Harrington DWJ, Giangaspero A. Significance and control of the poultry red mite, *Dermanyssus gallinae*. Annu Rev Entomol 2014; 59(1): 447-66.
[http://dx.doi.org/10.1146/annurev-ento-011613-162101] [PMID: 24397522]

[34] Sparagano OAE, Ho J. Parasitic mite fauna in Asian poultry farming systems. Front Vet Sci 2020; 7: 400.
[http://dx.doi.org/10.3389/fvets.2020.00400] [PMID: 32733926]

[35] Sparagano O, Di Domenico D, Venturelli C, Papadopoulos E, Smallegange RC, Giangaspero A. Arthropod pests in the poultry industry. Pests and vector-borne diseases in the livestock industry. Wageningen Academic Publishers 2018; p. 109.
[http://dx.doi.org/10.3920/978-90-8686-863-6_2]

[36] Yim D, Kang SS, Kim DW, Kim SH, Lillehoj HS, Min W. Protective effects of *Aloe vera*-based diets in *Eimeria maxima*-infected broiler chickens. Exp Parasitol 2011; 127(1): 322-5.
[http://dx.doi.org/10.1016/j.exppara.2010.08.010] [PMID: 20723543]

[37] Zaragatzki E, Munsch M, Henning M. Observation of cyst-like stages in *Histomonas meleagridis* and their survival in the host. Vet Parasitol 2010; 170(1-2): 25-33.

[38] Beer LC, Petrone-Garcia VM, Graham BD, Hargis BM, Tellez-Isaias G, Vuong CN. Histomonosis in poultry: A comprehensive review. Front Vet Sci. 2022 May 6;9:880738.
[http://dx.doi.org/10.3389/fvets.2022.880738]

# CHAPTER 5

# Immuno-pathological Purview of Parasitic Infection

## Felix Uchenna Samuel[1,*]

[1] *Animal Science Program, Alabama Cooperative Extension System, Alabama A & M University, Normal , Alabama, USA*

**Abstract:** Parasitic infections pose a major challenge in poultry farming, affecting both the health and productivity of birds. Immunopathology plays a key role in determining the severity of these infections and the host's ability to resist them. The immunopathological processes in poultry parasitic infections involve a complex interplay between the host's immune response and the parasite's tactics to evade or alter immunity. Parasites stimulate immune responses, leading to the activation of immune cells, the release of cytokines, and the recruitment of inflammatory mediators to the infection site. However, if these responses become dysregulated, they can cause tissue damage, inflammation, and pathological changes in the affected organs. An overactive immune response can result in immunopathology marked by excessive inflammation and tissue damage. On the other hand, parasites may suppress the host's immune response, allowing them to survive and spread within the host.

**Keywords:** Disease management, Host-parasite interactions, Immune response, Parasitic infections, Poultry, Immunopathology.

## INTRODUCTION

Immunopathology refers to the study of abnormal immune responses that result in tissue damage, inflammation, and disease. Immunopathology represents a medical discipline concerned with immune responses linked to various diseases. Immunopathology encompasses a spectrum of pathological conditions arising from dysregulated or aberrant immune responses. These responses may be triggered by infectious agents, environmental factors, genetic predispositions, or autoimmune processes, leading to tissue damage, inflammation, and disease. Within biology, it denotes harm inflicted upon an organism due to its immune system's response, often occurring as a consequence of infection [1]. Parasitic infections present substantial challenges to poultry health and production globally,

---

* **Corresponding author Felix Uchenna Samuel:** Animal Science Program, Alabama Cooperative Extension System, Alabama A & M University, Normal, Alabama, USA; E-mail: felix.samuel@aamu.edu

**Tanmoy Rana (Ed.)**

causing economic losses and raising welfare concerns. Understanding the immunopathology of these infections is crucial for developing effective control and management strategies. Poultry have a complex immune system, consisting of diverse organs, cells, and molecules that work together to protect against pathogens, including parasites. While their immune system shares core features with that of mammals, poultry also displays unique immune adaptations suited to their distinct physiological and ecological needs [1].

## Mechanisms

Immunopathological mechanisms involve a complex interaction among various immune system components, including immune cells like lymphocytes, macrophages, and neutrophils, along with signaling molecules such as cytokines, chemokines, and other inflammatory mediators. Together, these elements coordinate to generate immune responses against invading pathogens or foreign substances. When immune responses become dysregulated, however, this can lead to abnormal outcomes. Overactivation of the immune system may result in excessive inflammation and tissue damage, whereas immunodeficiency arises when the immune system cannot adequately respond to pathogens, leaving the host susceptible to infections. Autoimmunity, another consequence of immune dysregulation, occurs when the immune system mistakenly attacks the body's own cells and tissues, potentially leading to chronic inflammation and tissue damage. Hypersensitivity reactions, characterized by exaggerated immune responses to harmless substances, trigger inflammatory responses that can damage surrounding tissues. These reactions are classified into four types (Type I to Type IV) based on their immunological mechanisms [2].

## INNATE IMMUNITY

**Poultry Innate Immune Mechanisms:** The First Line of Defense

In the complex fight between poultry and pathogens, innate immune mechanisms serve as the first line of defense, rapidly activating to combat invading microorganisms. This section explores the key components of the innate immune system in poultry, emphasizing their roles in detecting and eliminating pathogens [3, 4].

**Physical Barriers**

*Skin*

The skin acts as the primary defense against external pathogens in poultry, forming a formidable barrier that prevents microbial invasion and protects the body from infections.

## Structure of the Avian Skin

The avian skin is a multifunctional organ composed of several layers, each with distinct structural and functional characteristics. The anatomy of the skin of the birds is crucial for appreciating its role as a physical barrier against pathogens (Fig. **1**).

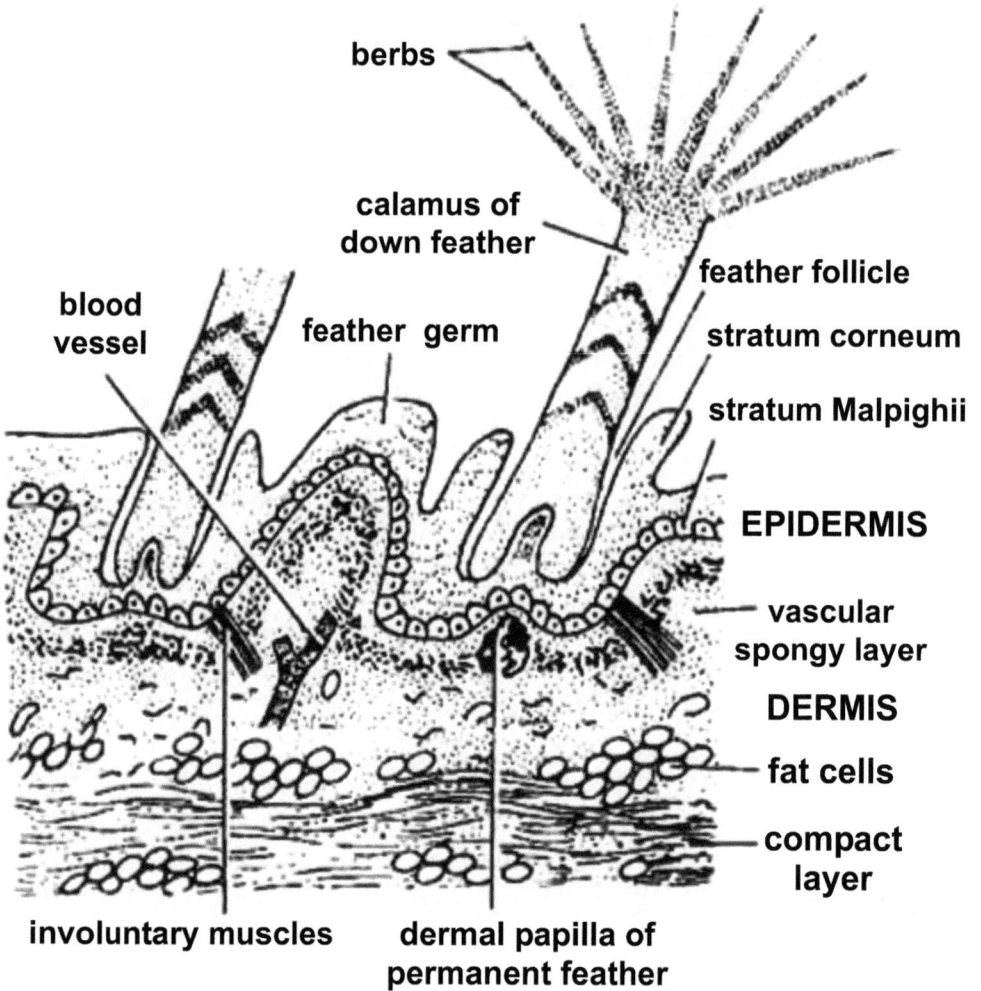

**Fig. (1).** Structure of the Avian skin.

## Epidermis

The epidermis is the outermost layer of the skin, consisting primarily of epithelial cells called keratinocytes. Keratinocytes form a stratified epithelium, providing mechanical strength and protection against physical and chemical insults. Tight junctions between keratinocytes contribute to the impermeability of the epidermis, preventing the entry of pathogens and toxins.

## Dermis

Beneath the epidermis lies the dermis, a connective tissue layer rich in blood vessels, nerves, and immune cells. Fibroblasts in the dermis produce collagen and elastin fibers, imparting elasticity and resilience to the skin. Blood vessels in the dermis regulate temperature and nutrient supply to the skin, supporting its metabolic functions.

## Adnexal Structures

Adnexal structures, including feathers, follicles, and glands, are embedded within the dermis and extend into the epidermis.

Feathers are specialized epidermal appendages that provide insulation, protection, and visual communication in birds.

Feather follicles house the developing feathers and serve as sites for feather growth and regeneration.

Glands, such as sebaceous glands and uropygial glands, secrete oils and other substances that lubricate the skin and feathers, enhancing their waterproofing and antimicrobial properties.

## Feather Covering: A Protective Shield Against Pathogens

Feathers play a crucial role in protecting poultry from environmental hazards, including microbial pathogens. The arrangement and structure of feathers contribute to their effectiveness as a barrier against pathogen entry.

## Feather Structure

Feathers are composed of a central shaft (rachis) with numerous branches (barbs) extending from either side. Interlocking barbules and barbicels form a cohesive structure, creating a tight barrier that prevents the penetration of pathogens and other foreign particles (Fig. 2).

**Main tail or wing feather**

**Soft body feather**

Quill

Web

Fluff

Staff

Quill

Web

Fluff

Staff

**Downy hairs**

Hooks on barb

Barb

Quill

**Enlarged detail of web**

Barb

Quill

**Enlarged detail of down or fluff**

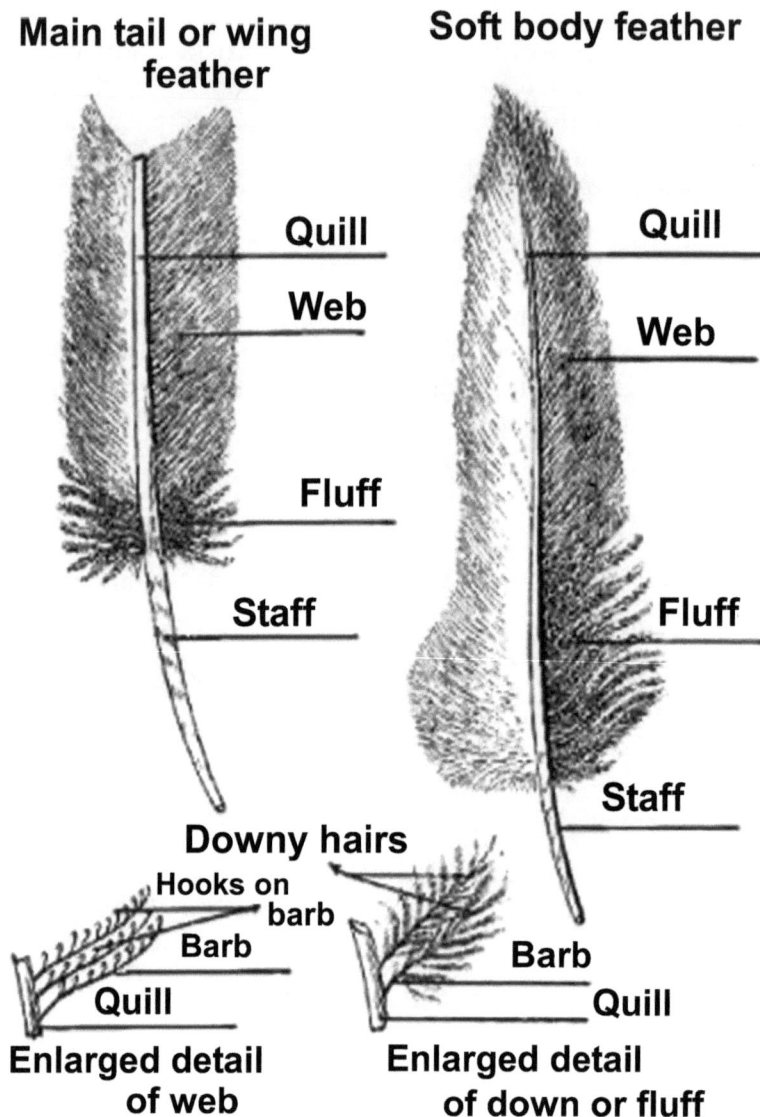

**Fig. (2).** Feather structure.

## *Waterproofing and Contaminant Repellence*

The outermost layer of feathers, the vaned region, is coated with a waterproofing agent produced by the uropygial gland. This lipid-rich substance, known as preen oil, helps repel water and contaminants, reducing the risk of pathogen adherence and colonization on the feather surface.

## Thermal Insulation and Thermoregulation

Feathers provide thermal insulation, helping birds maintain optimal body temperature in various environmental conditions. By trapping air between the feathers and the skin, insulation is enhanced, reducing heat loss and conserving metabolic energy. Additionally, feathers can fluff up or lie flat, allowing birds to adjust their insulation properties and regulate body temperature as needed.

## Antimicrobial Properties of the Epidermis

In addition to physical barriers provided by feathers, the epidermis of poultry skin possesses innate antimicrobial properties, further enhancing its defense against microbial pathogens.

## Keratinocytes and Antimicrobial Peptides

Keratinocytes in the epidermis produce a variety of antimicrobial peptides (AMPs), small cationic molecules that exhibit broad-spectrum antimicrobial activity. AMPs, such as β-defensins and cathelicidins, disrupt microbial cell membranes, inhibit protein synthesis, and modulate immune responses. These peptides serve as natural antibiotics, contributing to the maintenance of skin health and integrity.

## Maintenance of Skin Microbiota

The avian skin harbors a diverse microbial community, including commensal bacteria that play a role in protecting against pathogen colonization. Commensal bacteria compete with potential pathogens for nutrients and space, limiting their growth and colonization on the skin surface. Furthermore, the skin microbiota can produce antimicrobial substances that inhibit the growth of pathogenic microorganisms, contributing to skin homeostasis and defense.

## Mucosal Surfaces

Mucosal surfaces, lining the respiratory, gastrointestinal, and reproductive tracts, play a crucial role in protecting poultry against pathogens. The basic method of mucosal surface defense system is the secretion of mucus and antimicrobial peptides to prevent pathogen adherence and combat infections (Fig. **3**) [6, 7].

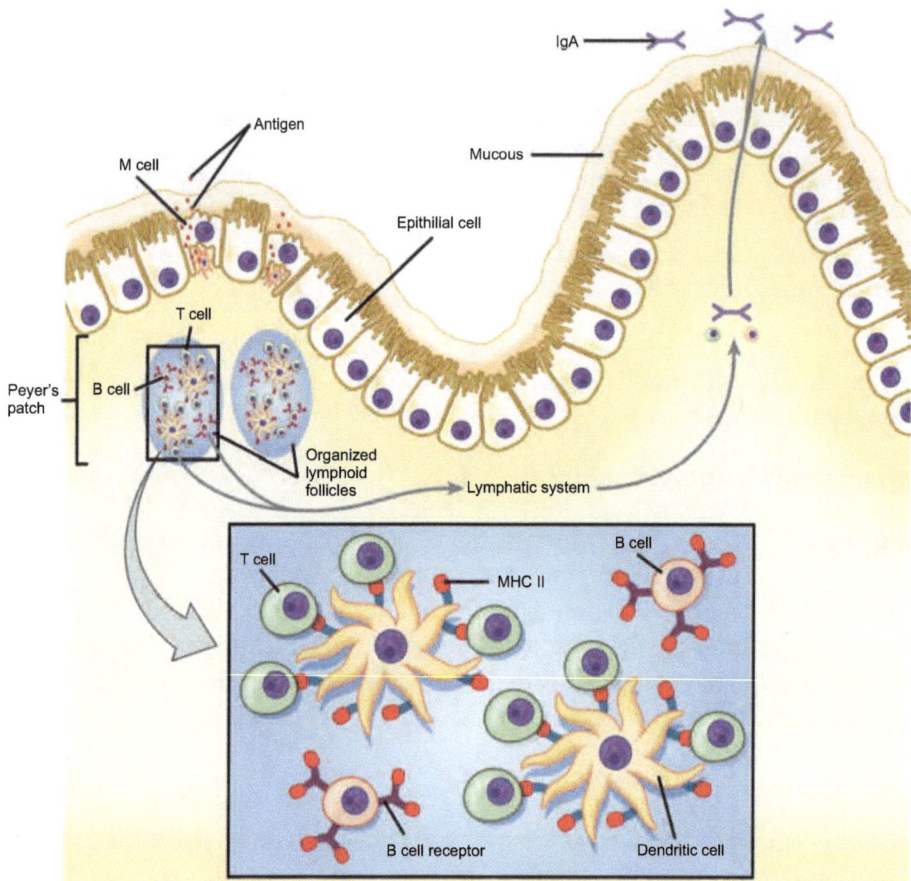

**Fig. (3).** Mucosal surfaces.

## *Importance of Mucosal Surfaces*

### *Respiratory Tract*

The respiratory tract serves as the primary route of entry for airborne pathogens, including bacteria, viruses, and fungi. Mucosal surfaces lining the nasal passages, trachea, and bronchi act as a barrier against inhaled pathogens, preventing their penetration into the lower respiratory tract.

### *Gastrointestinal Tract*

The gastrointestinal tract is constantly exposed to a wide range of pathogens present in feed, water, and the environment. Mucosal surfaces of the stomach, intestines, and ceca play a critical role in nutrient absorption and immune surveillance, while also serving as a barrier against ingested pathogens.

## Reproductive Tract

The reproductive tract in poultry comprises the oviduct and cloaca, which are susceptible to microbial colonization and infection. Mucosal surfaces lining the oviduct provide an environment conducive to fertilization and embryo development, while also defending against ascending infections.

## Mucus Secretion: Trapping and Immobilizing Pathogens

### Composition and Function of Mucus

Mucus is a viscous fluid secreted by specialized goblet cells and mucous glands located within mucosal epithelia. Composed primarily of water, glycoproteins (mucins), electrolytes, and antimicrobial peptides, mucus forms a physical barrier that traps and immobilizes pathogens upon contact.

### Trapping of Pathogens

The mucus acts as a sticky matrix that entangles pathogens, preventing their movement and adherence to underlying epithelial cells. The viscoelastic properties of the mucus facilitate the formation of a protective barrier, reducing the likelihood of pathogen invasion and tissue damage.

### Clearance Mechanisms

Mucociliary clearance is a critical mechanism for removing trapped pathogens from mucosal surfaces. Ciliated epithelial cells lining the respiratory tract and portions of the gastrointestinal tract propel mucus and entrapped pathogens toward the oral or anal openings, where they are expelled from the body through coughing, sneezing, or swallowing.

## Antimicrobial Peptides: Broad-Spectrum Defense Against Pathogens

### Production and Secretion

Mucosal epithelial cells produce and secrete a diverse array of antimicrobial peptides, including defensins, cathelicidins, and lysozyme. These peptides are constitutively expressed or induced in response to microbial colonization or infection, providing rapid and localized defense against invading pathogens [8].

### Mechanisms of Action

Defensins and cathelicidins exert antimicrobial activity through various mechanisms, including disruption of microbial cell membranes, inhibition of cell wall synthesis, and modulation of immune responses. By targeting essential components of bacterial, viral, and fungal pathogens, antimicrobial peptides exhibit broad-spectrum activity and contribute to the maintenance of mucosal homeostasis.

## *Regulation of Immune Responses*

In addition to their direct antimicrobial effects, antimicrobial peptides modulate immune responses and contribute to the orchestration of host defense mechanisms.

Defensins and cathelicidins can recruit immune cells, such as neutrophils and macrophages, to sites of infection, enhancing pathogen clearance and resolution of inflammation.

## Cellular Effectors

### *Macrophages*

Macrophages are phagocytic cells that patrol tissues, scavenging for pathogens and cellular debris. In poultry, macrophages are distributed throughout various organs, including the spleen, liver, lungs, and intestines. Upon encountering pathogens, macrophages engulf and digest them through phagocytosis, effectively clearing the infection. Phagocytosis and the intracellular destruction of microbes by enzymes is one of the body's most basic defense mechanisms. Metchnikoff identified two main types of cells responsible for engulfing and digesting microorganisms: macrophages and microphages. Macrophages originate from bone marrow and develop from monocytes or similar cells. Monocytes in the blood are immature macrophages, constantly being released from the bone marrow. Certain bone marrow-derived cells, resembling monocytes, can differentiate into specialized cells such as Kupffer cells in the liver, osteoclasts in bones, and Langerhans cells in the skin. Macrophages are equipped with receptors for C3b, an activated component of the complement system. This system can be activated by bacterial cell wall components, such as the outer membrane proteins (OMPs) of Salmonella and coliform bacteria, as well as certain tumor cells. After a pathogen is engulfed, it is broken down by the fusion of phagocytic vacuoles with lysosomes. Occasionally, undigested material is released outside the cell, but it often persists and can lead to chronic inflammation, as seen with Mycobacterium infections. These immune responses are marked by the release of proinflammatory cytokines and increased production of nitric oxide (Fig. **4**) [9].

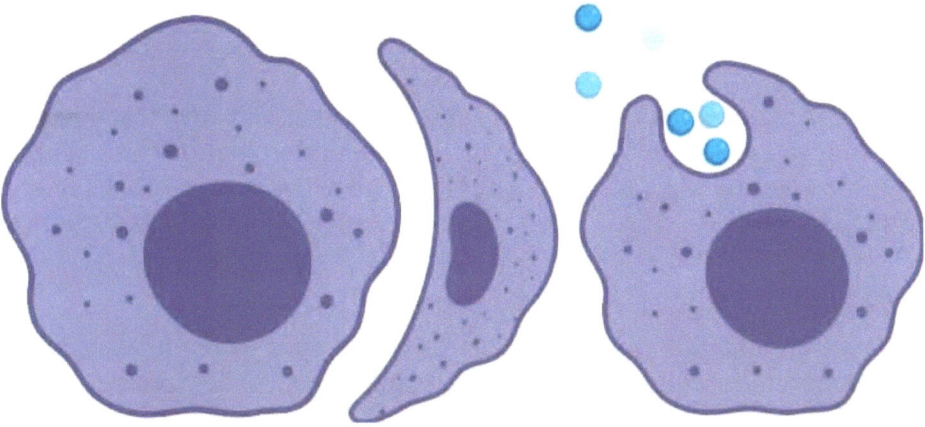

**Fig. (4).** Structure of microphages.

## *Heterophils*

Heterophils, the avian counterparts of mammalian neutrophils, represent a critical component of the innate immune system in poultry. This section provides a comprehensive exploration of heterophils, highlighting their structural and functional characteristics, their role in combating microbial threats, and their contribution to acute inflammatory reactions (Fig. **5**) [10, 11].

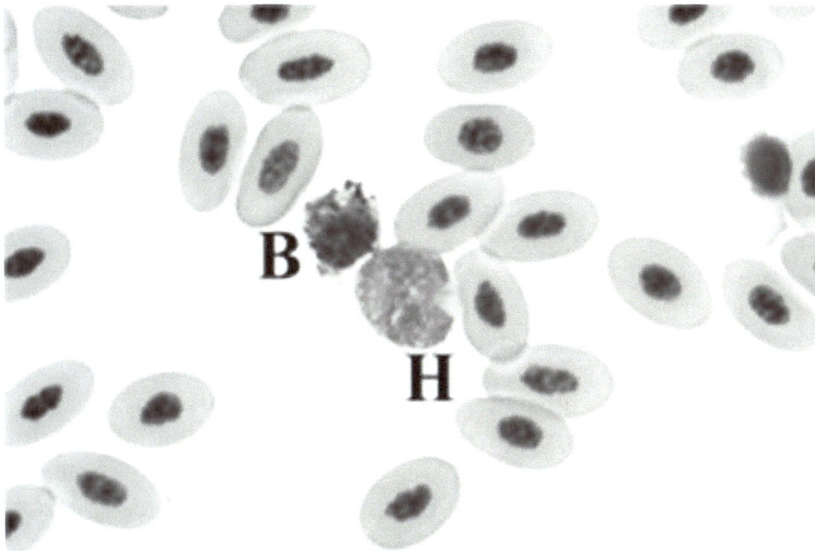

**Fig. (5).** Structure of Heterophil (H).

## Structural and Functional Characteristics of Heterophils

### Granulocytic Leukocytes

Heterophils are granulocytic leukocytes characterized by the presence of cytoplasmic granules containing enzymes and antimicrobial proteins. These cells derive from the myeloid lineage in the bone marrow and are released into the bloodstream as mature effector cells ready to combat microbial invaders.

### Abundance in Blood and Tissues

Heterophils are abundant in the circulation and tissues of poultry, constituting a significant proportion of the total leukocyte population. Their presence in tissues ensures rapid response to local infections and injuries, facilitating the initiation of immune defense mechanisms.

### Comparison to Mammalian Neutrophils

Heterophils, though functionally similar to mammalian neutrophils, have distinct characteristics. They contain enzymes such as acid phosphatase and β-glucuronidase but lack peroxidase and alkaline phosphatase, which are commonly found in mammalian neutrophils.

## Functional Role in Immune Defense

### Phagocytic Activity

Heterophils play a crucial role in phagocytosis, the process by which they engulf and internalize microbial pathogens, foreign particles, and cellular debris. Upon encountering pathogens, heterophils extend pseudopodia to engulf the invaders, forming phagosomes that subsequently fuse with lysosomes to form phagolysosomes, where pathogens are destroyed by antimicrobial proteins and reactive oxygen species [12].

### Antimicrobial Activity

Heterophils produce and release various antimicrobial proteins and peptides, including lysozyme, lactoferrin, and defensins, which exhibit potent antimicrobial activity against bacteria, fungi, and viruses. These antimicrobial molecules disrupt microbial cell walls, inhibit protein synthesis, and induce microbial lysis, contributing to the elimination of pathogens.

## Regulation of Inflammatory Responses

Heterophils play a pivotal role in the initiation and regulation of inflammatory responses, particularly acute inflammatory reactions. Upon activation by microbial stimuli or inflammatory mediators, heterophils release pro-inflammatory cytokines, chemokines, and lipid mediators, recruiting other immune cells to the site of infection and promoting the resolution of inflammation.

## *Contribution to Acute Inflammatory Reactions*

### Dominance in Acute Inflammation

Heterophils are the primary phagocytic cells involved in acute inflammatory responses in poultry. Their quick recruitment to areas of infection or tissue damage, along with their strong antimicrobial and pro-inflammatory abilities, enables them to launch an effective immune defense against microbial invaders.

### Enzymatic and Microbicidal Activity

The presence of acid phosphatase and β-glucuronidase enzymes in heterophils contributes to their microbicidal activity and the breakdown of microbial components.

While lacking peroxidase and alkaline phosphatase, heterophils rely on alternative mechanisms, such as the generation of reactive oxygen species, to combat pathogens and contribute to tissue sterilization [13].

## *Natural Killer (NK) Cells*

Natural Killer (NK) cells, an essential component of the innate immune system, play a pivotal role in detecting and eliminating virus-infected or transformed cells. This section delves into the structural and functional characteristics of NK cells in poultry, highlighting their unique mechanisms of action, their involvement in antiviral immunity, and their potential contribution to disease resistance, particularly in the context of Marek's disease (Fig. **6**) [14].

## *Structural and Functional Characteristics of Avian NK Cells*

### Innate Lymphoid Cells

NK cells belong to the family of innate lymphoid cells (ILCs), which lack antigen-specific receptors and respond rapidly to infection or cellular stress. In poultry, NK cells represent a distinct population of lymphocytes with cytotoxic activity against target cells, particularly those infected with viruses or undergoing malignant transformation.

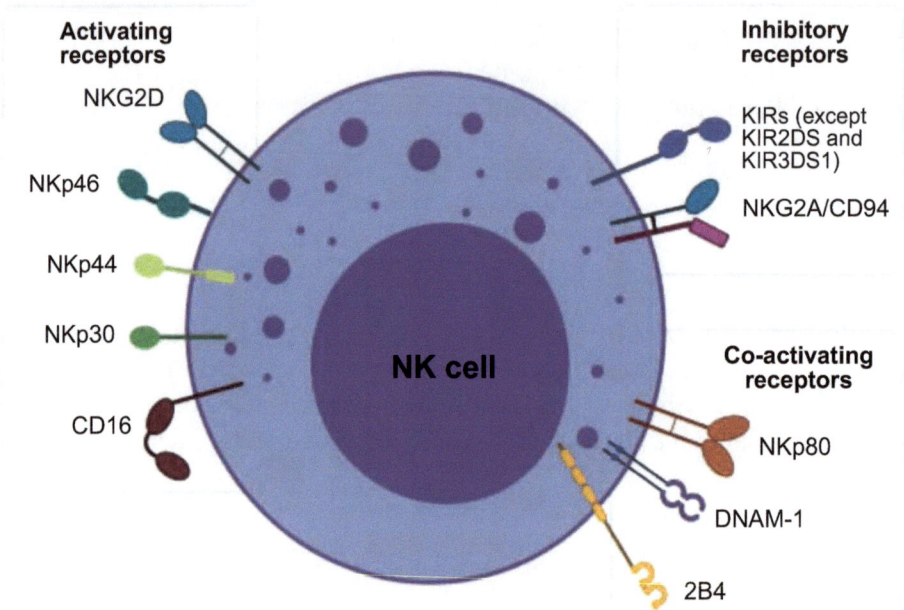

**Fig. (6).** Structure of Natural Killer cell.

## *Glycoprotein Recognition*

NK cells possess the ability to recognize carbohydrate determinants on the surface of target cells, enabling them to distinguish between healthy and aberrant cells based on their glycoprotein profiles. Cells displaying incompatible or incomplete glycoproteins are targeted for elimination by NK cells, thereby contributing to immune surveillance and host defense mechanisms.

## *Developmental Stage and Tissue Localization*

Avian NK cells are described as a population of cells found in the chicken embryonic spleen at a developmental stage preceding the migration of T cells to the periphery.

This unique localization suggests that NK cells may play a crucial role in early immune surveillance and defense during embryonic development, providing innate protection against pathogens before the adaptive immune system matures.

## Role in Antiviral Immunity

### Cytotoxic Activity

NK-like cells in poultry exhibit potent cytotoxic activity against virus-infected cells, releasing cytolytic granules containing perforin and granzymes upon recognition of target cells. Perforin forms pores in the target cell membrane, facilitating the entry of granzymes into the cytoplasm, where they induce apoptosis and cell death [15].

### Rapid Clearance of Infected Cells

NK cells play a crucial role in early antiviral immunity, contributing to the rapid clearance of infected cells before the adaptive immune response is fully activated.

By eliminating virus-infected cells at the early stages of infection, NK cells help limit viral replication and dissemination, thereby reducing the severity and duration of viral infections.

## Contribution to Immune Memory

While traditionally considered part of the innate immune system, recent evidence suggests that NK cells may also contribute to the establishment of immune memory and the generation of adaptive immune responses. NK cells interact with dendritic cells and other antigen-presenting cells, influencing the activation and differentiation of T cells and shaping the adaptive immune response to viral pathogens.

## Implications for Marek's Disease Resistance

### Marek's Disease

Marek's disease, caused by Marek's disease virus (MDV), is a highly contagious viral disease affecting poultry, particularly chickens. The disease is characterized by lymphoproliferative tumors, neurological symptoms, and immunosuppression, leading to significant economic losses in the poultry industry.

### Role of NK Cells in Disease Resistance

NK cells likely play a role in both natural and vaccine-induced resistance to Marek's disease, contributing to the early detection and elimination of MDV-infected cells. By targeting virus-infected cells and limiting viral spread, NK cells may help prevent the establishment of Marek's disease and reduce the severity of clinical symptoms in infected birds.

## Potential Therapeutic Targets

Insight into the mechanism of NK cells in Marek's disease resistance opens avenues for the development of novel therapeutic strategies targeting NK cell activation and function. Immunomodulatory interventions aimed at enhancing NK cell activity may complement existing vaccination strategies and improve disease control in poultry flocks [16].

## Pattern Recognition Receptors (PRRs)

## Toll-like Receptors (TLRs)

Toll-like receptors (TLRs) stand at the forefront of the innate immune response, serving as sentinel molecules that detect specific molecular patterns associated with pathogens. In the context of parasitic infections in poultry, TLRs play a crucial role in recognizing pathogen-associated molecular patterns (PAMPs) derived from various parasitic organisms. This comprehensive review explores the structural and functional characteristics of TLRs, their expression and activation in poultry, and their significance in initiating the innate immune response against parasitic infections. Toll-like receptors (TLRs) are a family of transmembrane receptors that play a fundamental role in host defense against microbial pathogens. These receptors are primarily expressed on immune cells, including macrophages, dendritic cells, and B lymphocytes, but may also be found on non-immune cells. TLRs recognize conserved molecular patterns associated with microbial pathogens, such as lipopolysaccharides (LPS), lipoproteins, and nucleic acids, through their extracellular domains [17].

## Structure and Ligand Recognition

TLRs are characterized by an extracellular leucine-rich repeat (LRR) domain responsible for ligand recognition, a transmembrane domain, and an intracellular Toll/IL-1 receptor (TIR) domain involved in signaling. Each TLR exhibits specificity for distinct PAMPs derived from bacteria, viruses, fungi, and parasites, allowing for the detection of a wide range of microbial invaders (Fig. **7**).

## Expression and Activation of TLRs in Poultry

**TLR Expression Profile**: In poultry, TLRs are expressed on various immune cells, including macrophages, dendritic cells, and heterophils, as well as epithelial cells lining mucosal surfaces.

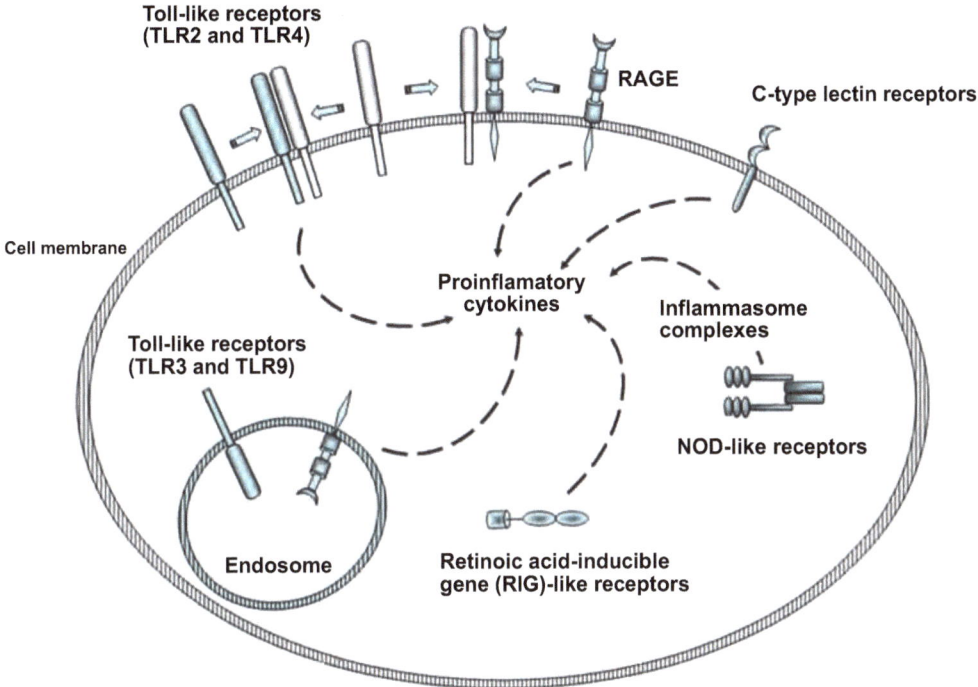

**Fig. (7).** Structure of Toll-like Receptors (TLRs).

The expression profile of TLRs may vary depending on the tissue type, developmental stage, and immunological context, reflecting the diverse roles of these receptors in host defense mechanisms.

**Recognition of Parasite-Derived PAMPs**: Parasitic organisms release a variety of molecular patterns, including lipids, glycoproteins, and nucleic acids, which serve as ligands for TLR recognition.TLRs in poultry are capable of detecting PAMPs derived from parasitic organisms such as protozoa, helminths, and ectoparasites, triggering intracellular signaling cascades and initiating the innate immune response.

**Activation and Signaling Pathways**: The binding of PAMPs to the extracellular domain of TLRs induces conformational changes that lead to the recruitment of adaptor proteins, such as MyD88 and TRIF, to the intracellular TIR domain. This initiates downstream signaling cascades, including the activation of transcription factors NF-κB and IRF, resulting in the production of pro-inflammatory cytokines, chemokines, and antimicrobial peptides [11].

## Role of TLRs in Parasitic Infections in Poultry

**Protozoan Infections**: Protozoan parasites such as *Eimeria* spp. and *Cryptosporidium* spp. release PAMPs that can be recognized by TLRs, triggering immune responses against these pathogens.

Activation of TLR signaling pathways in response to protozoan infections leads to the production of pro-inflammatory cytokines and chemokines, recruitment of immune cells, and elimination of intracellular parasites.

**Helminthic Infections**: Helminth parasites release excretory-secretory products containing PAMPs that are recognized by TLRs, eliciting immune responses against these pathogens. TLR activation in response to helminthic infections promotes the production of Th2 cytokines, such as IL-4, IL-5, and IL-13, which mediate eosinophil recruitment, mucus production, and antibody responses against helminth parasites.

**Ectoparasitic Infestations**: Ectoparasites such as *Dermanyssus gallinae* and *Cnemidocoptes mutans* release salivary proteins and exoskeletal components that may serve as ligands for TLR recognition. TLR activation in response to ectoparasitic infestations triggers cutaneous immune responses, including the production of antimicrobial peptides, recruitment of immune cells, and induction of inflammation at the site of infestation [9].

## Implications for Disease Resistance and Control

**Genetic Variation in TLRs**: Genetic polymorphisms in TLR genes may influence the susceptibility or resistance of poultry to parasitic infections, affecting the magnitude and efficacy of TLR-mediated immune responses. Elucidation of the genetic basis of TLR variation in poultry populations may inform breeding strategies aimed at enhancing disease resistance and resilience to parasitic infections.

**Immunomodulatory Interventions**: Targeting TLR signaling pathways through immunomodulatory interventions, such as TLR agonists or antagonists, may hold promise for enhancing host defense mechanisms against parasitic infections in poultry. By modulating TLR activity, it may be possible to enhance immune responses, reduce pathogen burden, and improve disease resistance in poultry flocks [8].

**Vaccine Development:** Exploiting TLR agonists as adjuvants in vaccine formulations may enhance the efficacy of vaccines against parasitic infections in poultry. TLR agonists can boost vaccine-induced immune responses, promote antigen presentation, and enhance the generation of protective immunity, leading to improved vaccine efficacy and disease control.

## *Nucleotide-binding Oligomerization Domain (NOD)-like Receptors (NLRs)*

Nucleotide-binding oligomerization domain (NOD)-like receptors (NLRs) are a family of cytoplasmic pattern recognition receptors (PRRs) that play a pivotal role in innate immunity. These receptors are characterized by the presence of a central nucleotide-binding domain (NBD or NACHT), a C-terminal leucine-rich repeat (LRR) domain, and an N-terminal effector domain, which may include a caspase activation and recruitment domain (CARD) or a pyrin domain (PYD) (Fig. **8**) [5, 6].

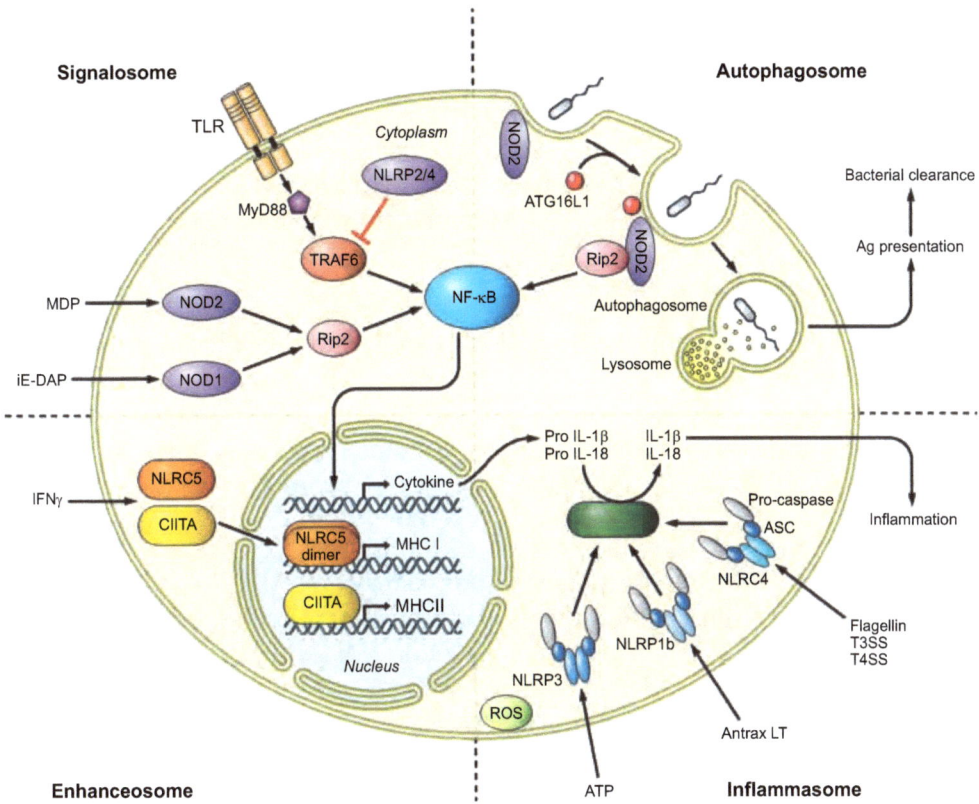

**Fig. (8).** Structure of Nucleotide-binding Oligomerization Domain (NOD)-like receptors.

**Sensing Intracellular PAMPs and Danger Signals:** NLRs function as sensors of intracellular pathogen-associated molecular patterns (PAMPs) or danger signals released during cellular stress or injury. Upon activation by PAMPs or danger signals, NLRs undergo conformational changes and oligomerize to form signaling platforms, leading to the activation of pro-inflammatory pathways and the induction of immune responses [10].

## Structural and Functional Characteristics of NLRs

**Domain Structure**: The domain structure of NLRs consists of a central NACHT domain responsible for nucleotide binding and oligomerization, a C-terminal LRR domain involved in ligand recognition, and an N-terminal effector domain, which determines downstream signaling events. Depending on the presence of specific effector domains, NLRs are classified into different subfamilies, including NLRCs (NLRs containing a CARD domain), NLRPs (NLRs containing a PYD domain), and NLRBs (NLRs lacking a CARD or PYD domain).

**Oligomerization and Signaling**: Activation of NLRs leads to their oligomerization and the formation of multiprotein complexes, termed inflammasomes or signaling platforms. Oligomerized NLRs recruit and activate downstream signaling molecules, such as caspases or kinases, leading to the processing and secretion of pro-inflammatory cytokines, including interleukin-1$\beta$ (IL-1$\beta$) and interleukin-18 (IL-18), and the induction of antimicrobial responses.

## Role of NLRs in Poultry Immunity

**Detection of Intracellular Pathogens**: In poultry, NLRs play a critical role in detecting intracellular pathogens, including viruses and intracellular bacteria, by sensing their nucleic acids, cell wall components, or virulence factors. Activation of NLRs by intracellular PAMPs triggers immune responses aimed at restricting pathogen replication and dissemination, as well as promoting pathogen clearance [11].

**Initiation of Immune Responses**: Upon activation, NLRs initiate immune responses by activating pro-inflammatory signaling pathways, such as the NF-$\kappa$B and MAPK pathways, leading to the production of cytokines, chemokines, and antimicrobial peptides. NLR-mediated immune responses contribute to the recruitment and activation of immune cells, such as macrophages, dendritic cells, and lymphocytes, to the site of infection, where they coordinate the elimination of pathogens.

**Regulation of Inflammatory Responses:** NLRs play a crucial role in regulating inflammatory responses to prevent excessive inflammation and tissue damage. Negative regulators of NLR signaling, such as NLR-associated protein 1 (NLRP1), suppress inflammasome activation and cytokine production, maintaining immune homeostasis and preventing immunopathology.

## *Implications for Disease Resistance and Control*

**Genetic Variation in NLRs**: Genetic polymorphisms in NLR genes may influence the susceptibility or resistance of poultry to infectious diseases, including viral and bacterial infections. Modulating NLR signaling pathways through immunomodulatory interventions or therapeutic agents may hold promise for enhancing host defense mechanisms against intracellular pathogens in poultry. Targeting specific NLRs or downstream effectors may help fine-tune immune responses and improve disease control strategies in poultry production systems [12].

**Vaccine Development**: Exploiting NLRs as adjuvants or vaccine targets may enhance the efficacy of vaccines against intracellular pathogens in poultry. NLR agonists or vaccine formulations designed to activate NLR-mediated immune responses could boost vaccine-induced immunity and improve protection against infectious diseases.

## ADAPTIVE IMMUNITY

Poultry possess both cellular and humoral components of adaptive immunity.

T lymphocytes (T cells) coordinate cell-mediated immune responses, while B lymphocytes (B cells) produce antibodies to neutralize extracellular pathogens.

Immunoglobulin classes in poultry include IgM, IgY (equivalent to mammalian IgG), IgA, and IgE, each with distinct roles in immune defense. Regulatory T cells (Tregs) and cytokine feedback mechanisms maintain immune homeostasis and prevent excessive inflammation [6, 8].

### Lymphoid tissues

Lymphoid tissues originate from either epithelial sources, such as the thymus and bursa of Fabricius, or mesenchymal sources, like the spleen and bone marrow, and are colonized by hematopoietic cells *via* the bloodstream. The primary lymphoid organs—the thymus and bursa of Fabricius—are populated by hematopoietic stem cells that differentiate into immune cells. These mature immune cells re-enter the bloodstream and migrate to peripheral lymphoid organs, including the spleen, cecal tonsils, Peyer's patches, Meckel's diverticulum, the Harderian gland, and various lymphoid tissues in the gut, bronchi, skin, nasal passages, and reproductive organs. In peripheral tissues, T cells and B cells localize within specific areas known as T- and B-dependent zones, respectively (Fig. **9**) [1 - 3].

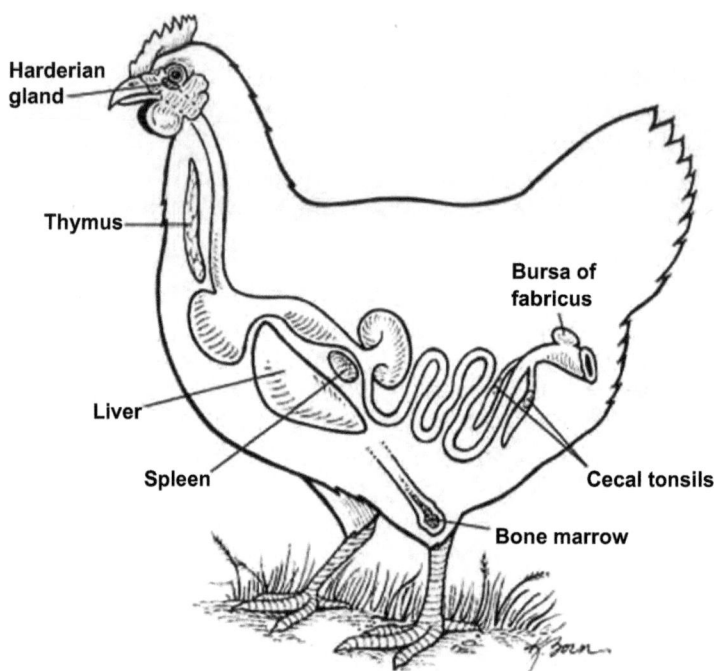

**Fig. (9).** Structure of lymphoid tissue in bird.

## *Primary Lymphoid Organs*

1. **Thymus**: The thymus emerges on the 5th day of embryonic development and continues to grow post-hatching until around 3-4 months of age, after which it gradually shrinks as sexual maturity nears. Its activity is most pronounced during the early stages of life. The thymus is essential for the maturation and differentiation of stem cells into thymus-dependent lymphocytes, or T-cells, which are critical for cell-mediated immunity.

2. **Bursa of Fabricius (Cloacal Bursa):** The bursa of Fabricius is a lymphoepithelial, hollow, round, or oval sac-like structure that extends from the hindgut. It is located in the caudal body cavity and connects to the dorsal region of the cloaca *via* a short duct. Its mucosal surface features 11-13 longitudinal folds. The bursa is responsible for the maturation and differentiation of stem cells into bursal-dependent lymphocytes, or B-cells, which are essential for antibody-mediated immunity.

## *Secondary Lymphoid Organs*

The matured B and T-cells are migrated to these sites from the primary or maturation lymphoid organs in a process known as immune migration or immune peripheralization. They include:

## Gut-Associated Lymphoid Tissue (GALT)

GALT is a critical component of secondary lymphoid organs, encompassing all lymphoid structures and cell aggregations found in the digestive tract. In conjunction with secretory IgA, GALT plays a vital role in local mucosal immunity within the digestive system, which is among the most significant immune mechanisms. GALT includes [13]:

**Submucosal Lymphoid Cell Aggregations:** These extensive clusters of lymphoid cells are located within the digestive tract. The esophageal tonsil, a newly identified component of mucosal-associated lymphoid tissue (MALT), is found at the entrance of the proventriculus. It comprises 6 to 8 individual units encased in a thin fibrous capsule, functioning as 'tonsillar crypts.' The stratified squamous epithelium is infiltrated by lymphoid cells, including T cells, plasma cells, macrophages, and dendritic cells, but not B cells, forming a lymphoepithelium (LE). In the subepithelial lymphoid tissue, T- and B-dependent regions are organized into interfollicular areas and germinal centers, respectively [11].

**Gastric tubular glands**: These branched tubular glands, located in the submucosa of the proventriculus, open into the mucosal surface. They contain numerous secretory tubules lined with cuboidal cells, each leading to a duct that connects to the main collecting duct, which opens onto the luminal surface.

**Meckel's diverticulum**: This is a pouch located at the junction between the intestine and the umbilical cord.

**Lymphoid or annular rings**: Found at the end of the jejunum and the beginning of the ileum, these structures are well-developed in waterfowl.

**Caecal tonsils**: Representing the largest aggregation of GALT, caecal tonsils are situated at the ileocecal junction. They are not present at hatching but develop shortly thereafter. By 10 days of age, they are easily identifiable, and their size continues to increase until approximately 12 weeks [10]. Caecal tonsils contain an equal proportion of T-lymphocytes (50%) and B-lymphocytes (50%), along with numerous immature and mature plasma cells. As the organism matures, the number of B-lymphocytes and plasma cells increases, contributing to antibody production and cell-mediated immune responses.

**Peyer's patches**: Located in the intestinal mucosa [11], these structures are similar in function to caecal tonsils. They exhibit significant B-dependent lymphocyte infiltration beneath the epithelium. Peyer's patches in chickens share various characteristics with those in mammals.

**Lymphoid aggregates**: Present in the urodeum and proctodeum of the cloaca, these aggregates are also part of the GALT [9].

## *Head-Associated Lymphoid Tissue (HALT)*

HALT is a crucial component of secondary lymphoid organs, encompassing all lymphoid structures and extensive lymphoid cell aggregations found in the head region. HALT includes:

**Harderian/Harder's/Paraocular Gland:** The Harderian gland (HG) is an immune-endocrine organ situated in the orbit behind the eye. It appears and develops post-hatching and contains numerous plasma cells that primarily produce and secrete IgA and other immunoglobulins. This gland serves as the major secondary lymphoid organ within HALT, with B-cells making up 80% of the lymphoid cell population and T-cells comprising the remaining 20%.

**Conjunctival-Associated Lymphoid Tissue (CALT):** This extensive aggregation of lymphoid cells is located beneath the mucosa of the conjunctiva. While it is not prominent in specific pathogen-free (SPF) birds, CALT is particularly well developed in poultry, especially in turkeys.

**Paranasal Glands, Lacrimal Duct, and Lateral Nasal Ducts:** These structures also contribute to the overall lymphoid tissue present in the head region.

## *Bronchial-Associated Lymphoid Tissues (BALT)*

BALT plays a crucial role in initiating respiratory humoral immune responses in chickens and turkeys. It is one of the most significant components of secondary, peripheral, or seeding lymphoid organs, representing all lymphoid structures present in the respiratory tract. In conjunction with secretory IgA, BALT is responsible for establishing respiratory local or mucosal immunity, a vital immune mechanism. BALT includes:

**Sub-mucosal Lymphoid Cell Aggregation**: These aggregates are located throughout the respiratory tracts.

**Bronchial Epithelium:** The bronchial epithelium primarily consists of nonciliated squamous cells that transition to more columnar and ciliated cells as the animal ages.

**Lymphoid Nodules**: These nodules are found in the lungs, specifically associated with the primary bronchi.

## Skin-Associated Lymphoid Tissues (SALT)

Lymphocytes are distributed throughout various tissues, including the intestinal epithelium, lamina propria, skin, liver, gonads, and pancreas. SALT encompasses all lymphoid structures and large aggregates of lymphoid cells situated beneath the skin [8].

## Spleen

The spleen, the largest secondary lymphoid organ, is composed of white and red pulp, which together make up about 80% of its tissue. The white pulp surrounds the blood vessels within the spleen and includes distinct morphological regions. Periarteriolar lymphoid sheaths (PALS) envelop the central arteries, while peri-ellipsoid lymphoid sheaths (PELS), comparable to the marginal zone in mammals, encircle the penicillary capillaries. Germinal centers are situated at arterial bifurcations, near the origins of the PALS [9].

## Mural Lymphoid Nodules

Mural lymphoid nodules are organized clusters of lymphoid tissue that can be circular, elongated, or oval in shape. They are non-capsulated and contain diffuse lymphoid tissue, typically featuring three or four germinal centers located either within or in close proximity to lymphatic vessels, particularly those found in the limbs and neck.

## Pineal Gland

The pineal gland is situated between the cerebral hemispheres and the cerebellum. Avian pineal glands can maintain rhythmic activity for several days under *in vitro* conditions. Various physical factors, such as light, temperature, and magnetic fields, along with biochemical inputs like vasoactive intestinal polypeptide (VIP), norepinephrine, and pituitary adenylate cyclase-activating polypeptide (PACAP), influence the release of melatonin. This functionality *in vitro* makes the explanted avian pineal gland an excellent model for studying the circadian biological clock [10].

## Bone Marrow

Bone marrow is fundamentally a primitive lymphoid organ; however, following immune migration, it also functions as a secondary immune organ. As a secondary lymphoid organ, it houses B-lymphocytes, mononuclear cells, and T-lymphocytes.

## *Bursa of Fabricius*

Serving as both a primary and secondary lymphoid organ, the bursa of Fabricius is essential for the diversification and maturation of avian B cells, which respond to alimentary and environmental antigens found within its lumen. As a secondary lymphoid organ, it comprises B-lymphocytes, mononuclear cells, and T-lymphocytes. Notably, birds lack traditional lymph nodes, with the exception of primitive lymph nodes observed in aquatic birds, such as cervicothoracic nodes located at the thoracic inlets. These structures are relatively simple, and lymph flows swiftly through them, likely due to the presence of a main or central sinus that may function as an intranodal lymphatic vessel [11]

### *Regulatory T cells (Tregs)*

Regulatory T cells (Tregs) are a specialized subset of CD4+ T cells recognized for their immunosuppressive functions and capacity to maintain immune tolerance. Tregs play a vital role in modulating excessive immune responses, preventing autoimmune diseases, and ensuring immune homeostasis.

## *Suppressive Mechanisms of Tregs*

Tregs exert their suppressive effects through multiple mechanisms, including the secretion of anti-inflammatory cytokines such as interleukin-10 (IL-10) and transforming growth factor-beta (TGF-$\beta$). Additionally, Tregs can directly inhibit the proliferation and effector functions of other immune cells, including T cells, B cells, dendritic cells, and macrophages, through cell-to-cell interactions and the expression of inhibitory receptors such as CTLA-4 and PD-1.

## MODULATION OF IMMUNE RESPONSES IN PARASITIC DISEASES OF POULTRY

Parasitic diseases of poultry, including coccidiosis, helminthiasis, and ectoparasitic infestations, trigger complex immune responses characterized by the activation of both innate and adaptive immunity. While an appropriate immune response is necessary for pathogen clearance, excessive inflammation, and tissue damage must be prevented to maintain host health and welfare.

### Role of Tregs in Parasitic Infections

Tregs play a crucial role in modulating immune responses to parasitic infections in poultry, balancing pathogen clearance with tissue protection and repair.

By suppressing excessive inflammation and immunopathology, Tregs help prevent tissue damage caused by the host immune response, promoting host survival and recovery from parasitic diseases.

## Cytokine Feedback Mechanisms in Immune Regulation

Cytokines are small signaling molecules secreted by immune cells that orchestrate immune responses and regulate inflammation. Pro-inflammatory cytokines, such as interleukin-1 (IL-1), interleukin-6 (IL-6), and tumor necrosis factor-alpha (TNF-α), promote inflammation and immune activation, while anti-inflammatory cytokines, such as IL-10 and TGF-β, suppress inflammation and promote immune tolerance [6].

### *Role of Cytokine Feedback Loops*

Cytokine feedback mechanisms play a crucial role in maintaining immune homeostasis and preventing excessive inflammation. Anti-inflammatory cytokines, such as IL-10 and TGF-β, act as negative regulators of inflammation by suppressing the production and activity of pro-inflammatory cytokines, thus limiting the magnitude and duration of immune responses.

## Interplay between Tregs and Cytokine Feedback Mechanisms

### *Treg-mediated Cytokine Regulation*

Tregs play a central role in orchestrating cytokine feedback mechanisms by secreting anti-inflammatory cytokines such as IL-10 and TGF-β. These cytokines act locally to suppress the production of pro-inflammatory cytokines by effector immune cells, limiting tissue inflammation and damage during parasitic infections.

### *Regulation of Treg Function by Cytokines*

Cytokines produced during parasitic infections can modulate Treg function and stability, influencing the balance between immune activation and suppression. Pro-inflammatory cytokines may impair Treg function or induce the differentiation of pro-inflammatory T cell subsets, whereas anti-inflammatory cytokines enhance Treg suppressive activity and promote immune tolerance.

## Implications for Parasitic Disease Control in Poultry

### *Therapeutic Targeting of Tregs and Cytokine Pathways*

Modulating Treg function or cytokine signaling pathways may offer potential therapeutic strategies for controlling parasitic diseases in poultry. Targeting Tregs or cytokine feedback mechanisms could help mitigate excessive inflammation and tissue damage while preserving host immune responses against parasitic pathogens [10].

### *Vaccine Development and Immune Regulation*

Incorporating Treg-inducing antigens or cytokine adjuvants into vaccines may promote immune tolerance and enhance vaccine efficacy against parasitic diseases in poultry.

Harnessing the immunomodulatory properties of Tregs and cytokines could lead to the development of novel vaccine formulations that induce protective immunity while minimizing immunopathology.

## Immunomodulatory Mechanisms

Immunomodulatory mechanisms play a crucial role in regulating immune responses in poultry, ensuring an appropriate and balanced reaction to pathogens while preventing excessive inflammation or immunopathology. Immuno-modulatory molecules encompass a broad range of substances that regulate the activity and function of immune cells in poultry. These molecules can be endogenous or exogenous and may exert their effects through various mechanisms, including direct cell-to-cell interactions, cytokine signaling, and modulation of immune cell activation or differentiation [9].

### *Types of Immunomodulatory Molecules*

**Cytokines:** Interleukins (ILs), interferons (IFNs), and tumor necrosis factors (TNFs) are among the key cytokines involved in modulating immune responses in poultry.

**Chemokines:** Chemokines regulate immune cell trafficking and recruitment to sites of infection or inflammation.

**Antimicrobial peptides**: These molecules possess both antimicrobial and immunomodulatory properties, contributing to host defense and immune regulation.

## *Functions of Immunomodulatory Molecules*

### *Regulation of Immune Cell Function*

Immunomodulatory molecules modulate the function and activity of immune cells, including T cells, B cells, macrophages, dendritic cells, and natural killer (NK) cells.

They can enhance or suppress immune cell activation, proliferation, differentiation, and effector functions, depending on the context of the immune response.

### *Communication Between Immune Cells*

Immunomodulatory molecules facilitate communication and crosstalk between different immune cell subsets, coordinating the overall immune response to pathogens.

They regulate the secretion of cytokines, chemokines, and other signaling molecules, orchestrating the recruitment and activation of immune cells at sites of infection or inflammation [13].

## *Key Immunomodulatory Cytokines in Poultry*

### *Interleukins (ILs)*

Interleukins are a diverse group of cytokines involved in immune cell communication and regulation. IL-2 promotes T cell proliferation and differentiation, while IL-10 suppresses pro-inflammatory cytokine production and promotes immune tolerance.

### *Interferons (IFNs)*

Interferons are essential for antiviral defense and immune regulation. Type I IFNs (IFN-α and IFN-β) induce an antiviral state in infected cells, while type II IFN (IFN-γ) enhances macrophage activation and Th1 immune responses.

### *Tumor Necrosis Factors (TNFs)*

Tumor necrosis factors are multifunctional cytokines with diverse roles in inflammation and immunity. TNF-α promotes inflammation and activates immune cells, while TNF-β regulates lymphocyte proliferation and differentiation.

## Regulatory Mechanisms in Immune Homeostasis

### Balanced Immune Response

Regulatory mechanisms ensure a balanced immune response in poultry, preventing excessive inflammation or immunopathology. Negative feedback loops, such as the production of anti-inflammatory cytokines or the induction of regulatory T cells (Tregs), help dampen immune responses and maintain homeostasis [11].

### Prevention of Autoimmunity and Immunopathology

Immunomodulatory molecules and regulatory mechanisms play a crucial role in preventing autoimmunity and immunopathology in poultry. They suppress aberrant immune responses against self-antigens and limit tissue damage caused by excessive inflammation or immune-mediated pathology.

### Implications for Poultry Health and Disease Resistance

### Disease Resistance and Immune Competence

The proper functioning of immunomodulatory mechanisms is essential for disease resistance and immune competence in poultry. The dysregulation of immune responses or deficiencies in immunomodulatory pathways can predispose poultry to infectious diseases and impair overall health and productivity.

### Immunopathology in Poultry Diseases

### Infectious Diseases

Infectious agents such as viruses, bacteria, fungi, and parasites can trigger immunopathological responses in poultry. Examples include avian influenza, infectious bronchitis, Marek's disease, coccidiosis, and histomonosis. Immunopathology in infectious poultry diseases often involves excessive inflammation, tissue necrosis, and organ dysfunction, contributing to morbidity and mortality in affected birds.

### Non-infectious Diseases

Non-infectious factors such as toxins, pollutants, nutritional deficiencies, and metabolic disorders can also induce immunopathological changes in poultry. Examples include mycotoxicosis, heavy metal toxicity, vitamin deficiencies, and metabolic syndromes. Immunopathological responses to non-infectious factors may manifest as inflammatory lesions, organ damage, or systemic dysfunction, impairing bird health and performance.

## *Parasitic Diseases*

Parasitic infections, including ectoparasites (*e.g.*, mites, lice) and endoparasites (*e.g.*, protozoa, helminths), elicit immunopathological responses in poultry. Examples include poultry red mite infestation, coccidiosis, and helminthiasis. Immunopathology in parasitic diseases of poultry often involves a combination of tissue damage caused by the parasites themselves and inflammatory reactions mounted by the host immune system, leading to lesions, hemorrhage, and impaired organ function.

## Diagnostic Significance of Immunopathology

### *Histopathological Evaluation*

Histopathological examination of tissues allows for the detection and characterization of immunopathological changes, including inflammation, necrosis, granuloma formation, and fibrosis. Histopathological findings provide valuable diagnostic information, aiding in the identification of specific diseases, assessment of disease severity, and evaluation of treatment efficacy in poultry.

### *Immunological Biomarkers*

Measurement of immunological biomarkers, such as cytokines, acute-phase proteins, and immunoglobulins, can provide insights into the immunopathological processes occurring in diseased poultry. Alterations in the levels of specific biomarkers may indicate immune activation, inflammation, or immunosuppression, guiding diagnostic and therapeutic decisions in poultry health management [10].

## Management and Control of Immunopathological Diseases

Immunopathological diseases pose significant challenges to poultry health and productivity, necessitating effective management and control strategies to minimize their impact on bird welfare and production outcomes.

## Prevention Strategies

### *Biosecurity Protocols*

Implementation of biosecurity protocols is fundamental for preventing the introduction and spread of infectious agents associated with immunopathological diseases. Biosecurity measures may include restricted access to poultry facilities, visitor control, disinfection procedures, and proper waste management practices to minimize the risk of pathogen transmission.

## Vaccination Programs

Vaccination plays a crucial role in preventing immunopathological diseases by stimulating protective immunity against specific pathogens. Vaccination programs should be tailored to the epidemiological context and disease prevalence in poultry populations, incorporating appropriate vaccine formulations, administration routes, and schedules to maximize vaccine efficacy.

## Environmental Management Practices

Environmental factors, such as housing conditions, ventilation systems, and litter management, can influence the susceptibility of poultry to immunopathological diseases. Optimal environmental management practices, including adequate ventilation, temperature control, and litter quality maintenance, help minimize stressors and enhance the resilience of birds against infectious and non-infectious challenges [11].

## Treatment Modalities

### Antimicrobial Therapy

Antimicrobial therapy is often utilized in the treatment of immunopathological diseases associated with bacterial infections. The selection of appropriate antimicrobial agents, based on susceptibility testing and pharmacokinetic considerations, is essential for achieving therapeutic efficacy and minimizing the development of antimicrobial resistance.

### Anti-inflammatory Agents

Anti-inflammatory drugs, such as nonsteroidal anti-inflammatory drugs (NSAIDs) and corticosteroids, may be employed to mitigate inflammation and tissue damage associated with immunopathological responses. Careful consideration of dosage, duration of treatment, and potential side effects is necessary to optimize the therapeutic benefits of anti-inflammatory agents while minimizing adverse effects.

### Supportive Care

Supportive care measures, including fluid therapy, nutritional support, and stress reduction strategies, are essential for maintaining the health and well-being of poultry during disease outbreaks. Adequate provision of nutrients, vitamins, and electrolytes helps support immune function and facilitate recovery from immunopathological diseases.

## Nutritional Interventions

Nutritional interventions aimed at optimizing immune function and minimizing the impact of immunopathological diseases may include dietary supplementation with immune-modulating compounds, such as vitamins, minerals, and probiotics. Balanced nutrition, tailored to the specific requirements of poultry species and production stages, contributes to overall health and resilience against infectious and non-infectious challenges.

## Integrated Approaches

### Multifaceted Management Strategies

Integrated approaches that combine preventive measures, treatment modalities, and holistic management practices are essential for effectively managing and controlling immunopathological diseases in poultry.

### One Health Perspective

Adopting a One Health approach that considers the interconnectedness of human, animal, and environmental health is crucial for addressing complex immunopathological diseases and their broader implications. Collaboration among veterinary professionals, poultry producers, public health authorities, and environmental stakeholders facilitates the implementation of integrated disease control strategies and promotes sustainable poultry production systems [12].

## Research Perspectives and Future Directions

Research in the field of immunopathology in poultry diseases is essential for understanding the complex interactions between pathogens and the host immune system. This section delves into future directions and research perspectives aimed at advancing our knowledge of poultry immunopathology and developing innovative strategies for disease control and prevention.

### Mechanistic Studies

Further research is needed to elucidate the underlying mechanisms of immunopathology in poultry diseases. This includes investigating the roles of specific immune cells, cytokines, chemokines, and signaling pathways involved in the host response to infectious agents and the development of pathological conditions [9].

## Role of Immune Cells

Investigating the function and regulation of immune cells, such as macrophages, dendritic cells, T cells, B cells, and innate lymphoid cells, in the context of poultry immunopathology will provide insights into disease pathogenesis and immune dysregulation.

## Cytokine Dynamics

Studying the expression patterns, kinetics, and functional significance of cytokines, chemokines, and other immunomodulatory molecules in poultry diseases will enhance our understanding of host immune responses and their impact on disease outcomes.

## Signaling Pathways

Exploring intracellular signaling pathways, including Toll-like receptor (TLR), NOD-like receptor (NLR), and inflammasome signaling, will uncover the molecular mechanisms underlying immune activation, inflammation, and tissue damage in poultry immunopathology.

## Advances in Molecular and Cellular Techniques

Leveraging cutting-edge molecular and cellular techniques, such as transcriptomics, proteomics, metabolomics, flow cytometry, and single-cell analysis, will facilitate the in-depth characterization of host-pathogen interactions and immune dysregulation in poultry diseases.

## Omics Approaches

Applying omics approaches to profile global changes in gene expression, protein abundance, and metabolite levels in response to infectious agents and immunomodulatory interventions will identify novel biomarkers and therapeutic targets for poultry immunopathology.

## Vaccine Development

## Targeting Immunopathological Diseases

The development of vaccines targeting specific immunopathological diseases in poultry represents a promising approach to disease control and prevention. By stimulating protective immunity against key pathogens and modulating host immune responses, vaccines can reduce disease incidence, severity, and transmission within poultry populations [12].

## *Innovative Vaccine Formulations*

Novel vaccine formulations incorporating immunomodulatory adjuvants, delivery systems, or antigens have the potential to enhance vaccine efficacy, reduce immunopathology, and improve immune responses in poultry populations.

## *Adjuvant Development*

Research focused on the identification and characterization of novel adjuvants capable of enhancing vaccine-induced immune responses while minimizing adverse reactions will advance the field of poultry vaccinology [13].

## CONCLUDING REMARKS

The immunopathological dynamics of parasitic infections in poultry represent a multifaceted relationship between the immune responses of the host and the evasion tactics employed by parasites, significantly influencing the health, productivity, and welfare of these birds. Infections caused by organisms such as *Eimeria spp., Ascaridia galli*, and *Histomonas meleagridis* elicit a spectrum of immune reactions, ranging from innate mechanisms that include physical barriers and phagocytic activity to adaptive responses characterized by the engagement of T cells, B cells, and the generation of specific antibodies. While these immune mechanisms are crucial for controlling pathogens, they can also result in tissue damage and inflammation, manifesting in clinical symptoms like diarrhea, weight loss, and anemia, which ultimately diminish productivity and elevate mortality rates.

Gaining a comprehensive understanding of the immunopathological processes associated with parasitic infections in poultry is vital for the formulation of more effective management strategies. Current research indicates that the equilibrium between pro-inflammatory and regulatory immune responses plays a pivotal role in influencing the outcomes of these infections. An overactive immune response may cause significant tissue damage, whereas an insufficient response could fail to eliminate the parasite, leading to chronic infections. The identification of specific immune markers that correlate with either resistance or susceptibility to infections could provide valuable insights for selective breeding initiatives aimed at improving genetic resistance against parasitic threats. Furthermore, recent advancements in immunomodulatory approaches, including vaccines and dietary supplements, present promising opportunities to alleviate the impacts of parasitic infections. Vaccines designed to target critical antigens involved in the interactions between host and parasite have shown potential in mitigating the severity of infections; however, challenges related to efficacy, cost, and delivery methods persist. Additionally, the incorporation of innovative nutritional strategies, such as the use of phytochemicals, probiotics, and prebiotics, has shown promise in bolstering immune function and enhancing resilience against parasitic challenges.

# REFERENCES

[1]   Abdelhamid MK, Hess C, Bilic I, *et al.* A comprehensive study of colisepticaemia progression in layer chickens applying novel tools elucidates pathogenesis and transmission of *Escherichia coli* into eggs. Sci Rep 2024; 14(1): 8111.
[http://dx.doi.org/10.1038/s41598-024-58706-3] [PMID: 38582950]

[2]   Abo-Samaha MI, Sharaf MM, El Nahas AF, Odemuyiwa SO. Innate immune response to double-stranded RNA in American heritage chicken breeds. Poult Sci 2024; 103(2): 103318.
[http://dx.doi.org/10.1016/j.psj.2023.103318] [PMID: 38064884]

[3]   Tiwari A, Swamy M, Mishra P. Avian immunity and immunopathology of avian diseases. J Entomol Zool Stud 2020; 8(5): 484-92.

[4]   Barathiraja S, Mathivathani C, Gangadhara P A V, Sujatha V, Saminathan M, Seshuram P. Natural Killer (NK) Cells: An innate defense shield against respiratory viral infections. J Immunol Immunopathol. 2024;24(1):9-18.

[5]   Chauhan RS, Malik YS, Saminathan M, Tripathi BN. Basic concepts in immunology. Essentials of veterinary immunology and immunopathology. Singapore: Springer Nature Singapore 2024; pp. 1-30.

[6]   Dunislawska A, Pietrzak E, Bełdowska A, Siwek M. Health in poultry- immunity and microbiome with regard to a concept of one health. Phys Sci Rev 2024; 9(1): 477-95.
[http://dx.doi.org/10.1515/psr-2021-0124]

[7]   Fellah JS, Jaffredo T, Nagy N, Dunon D. Development of the avian immune system. In: Schat KA, Kaspers B, Kaiser P, Eds., Avian immunology. Academic Press 2014; pp. 45-63.
[http://dx.doi.org/10.1016/B978-0-12-396965-1.00003-0]

[8]   Gao Y, Sun P, Hu D, *et al.* Advancements in understanding chicken coccidiosis: from *Eimeria* biology to innovative control strategies. One Health Advances 2024; 2(1): 6.
[http://dx.doi.org/10.1186/s44280-024-00039-x]

[9]   Guo X, Rosa AJM, Chen DG, Wang X. Molecular mechanisms of primary and secondary mucosal immunity using avian infectious bronchitis virus as a model system. Vet Immunol Immunopathol 2008; 121(3-4): 332-43.
[http://dx.doi.org/10.1016/j.vetimm.2007.09.016] [PMID: 17983666]

[10]  Kumar V, Stewart JH IV. cGLRs join their cousins of pattern recognition receptor family to regulate immune homeostasis. Int J Mol Sci 2024; 25(3): 1828.
[http://dx.doi.org/10.3390/ijms25031828] [PMID: 38339107]

[11]  Maxwell M, Söderlund R, Härtle S, Wattrang E. Single-cell RNA-seq mapping of chicken peripheral blood leukocytes. BMC Genomics 2024; 25(1): 124.
[http://dx.doi.org/10.1186/s12864-024-10044-4] [PMID: 38287279]

[12]  Rolland A, Douard V, Lapaque N. Role of pattern recognition receptors and microbiota-derived ligands in obesity. Front Microbiomes 2024; 3: 1324476.
[http://dx.doi.org/10.3389/frmbi.2024.1324476]

[13]  Song Y, Mehl F, Zeichner SL. Vaccine strategies to elicit mucosal immunity. Vaccines (Basel) 2024; 12(2): 191.
[http://dx.doi.org/10.3390/vaccines12020191] [PMID: 38400174]

[14]  Tharmalingam J, Liu D. Host immune responses to *Taenia* infection. In: Tang YW, Hindiyeh MY, Liu D, Sails A, Spearman P, Zhang JR, Eds, Molecular Medical Microbiology. Academic Press 2024; pp. 3191-203.

[http://dx.doi.org/10.1016/B978-0-12-818619-0.00004-6]

[15]    Umar S, Munir MT, Ahsan U, *et al.* RETRACTED ARTICLE: Immunosuppressive interactions of viral diseases in poultry. Worlds Poult Sci J 2017; 73(1): 121-35.
[http://dx.doi.org/10.1017/S0043933916000829]

[16]    Wang J, Zhang J, Wang Q, *et al.* A heterophil/lymphocyte-selected population reveals the phosphatase PTPRJ is associated with immune defense in chickens. Commun Biol 2023; 6(1): 196.
[http://dx.doi.org/10.1038/s42003-023-04559-x] [PMID: 36807561]

[17]    Yoshimura Y, Nii T, Isobe N. Innate immune training in chickens for improved defense against pathogens: A review. J Poult Sci 2024; 61(0): 2024008.
[http://dx.doi.org/10.2141/jpsa.2024008] [PMID: 38481975]

**CHAPTER 6**

# Diagnostic Methods of Parasitic Diseases of Poultry

**Saroj Kumar[1], Pradeep Kumar[2,\*], R.L. Rakesh[3], Alok Kumar Singh[4], Vivek Agarwal[5], Krishnendu Kundu[1]** and **Renu Singh[6]**

[1] *Department of Veterinary Parasitology, Faculty of Veterinary and Animal Sciences, Institute of Agricultural Sciences, Banaras Hindu University, Varanasi 221005, Uttar Pradesh, India*

[2] *Department of Veterinary Parasitology, Uttar Pradesh Pandit Deen Dayal Upadhyaya Pashu Chikitsa Vigyan Vishwavidyalaya Evam Go-Anusandhan Sansthan, Mathura 281001, Uttar Pradesh, India*

[3] *Department of Veterinary Parasitology, Veterinary College, Hassan 573202, KVAFSU, Bidar, India*

[4] *Department of Veterinary Parasitology, College of Veterinary Science & Animal Husbandry, Kuthuliya, Rewa 486001, Madhya Pradesh, India*

[5] *Department of Veterinary Parasitology, College of Veterinary Sciences & A.H, Nanaji Deshmukh Veterinary Science University, Mhow, Indore 453446, Madhya Pradesh, India*

[6] *Department of Veterinary Pathology, Uttar Pradesh Pandit Deen Dayal Upadhyaya Pashu Chikitsa Vigyan Vishwavidyalaya Evam Go-Anusandhan Sansthan, Mathura 281001, Uttar Pradesh, India*

**Abstract:** The use of diagnostic methods for the diagnosis of parasitic diseases in poultry has been almost constant over the past few decades. Since the introduction of PCR, few major advances have been adopted in clinical diagnostic tests. Many diagnostic tests that form the backbone of the "modern" microbiology laboratories rely on very old and labour-intensive technologies such as microscopy for the diagnosis of parasites including helminths, protozoans, arthropods, and haemoprotozoans. Urgent needs include more rapid tests without compromising the sensitivity, value-added tests, and point-of-care tests for both high- and low-resource settings. In recent years, research has been focused on alternative methods to improve the diagnosis of parasitic diseases. These include molecular technique-based approaches, immunoassays and proteomics using mass spectrometry platforms technology. This chapter discusses the progress of several approaches in parasite diagnosis and some of their silent characteristics.

**Keywords:** ELISA, Microscopic examination, McMaster chamber, PCR, Poultry parasites.

---

\* **Corresponding author Pradeep Kumar:** Department of Veterinary Parasitology, Uttar Pradesh Pandit Deen Dayal Upadhyaya Pashu Chikitsa Vigyan Vishwavidyalaya Evam Go-Anusandhan Sansthan, Mathura 281001, Uttar Pradesh, India; E-mail: drpkdiwakar@gmail.com

**Tanmoy Rana (Ed.)**
**All rights reserved-© 2025 Bentham Science Publishers**

# INTRODUCTION

The poultry industry is one of the leading and fast-growing sectors that support protein nutrition globally. The consumption of chicken is becoming more popular across the world due to consumer perceptions of its health benefits, low price, ease of preparation, and lack of religious constraints [1 - 4]. Approximately, 90 million tons of broiler meat is produced annually from 21 billion broiler chicks worldwide, accounting for 89% of total meat production in the world. It has been predicted that the world's meat consumption will rise exponentially from 330 to 455 million tons annually by 2050 due to increased consumer demand for meat products and the accelerated growth of the world's human population (present 7.6 billion population predicted to reach 9.8 billion by 2050). Meanwhile, 40% of the increased demand will be covered by broiler chicken meat [5 - 7]. In addition to the production costs in the present and strategic future of the poultry industry, the health of birds is a vital factor that influences the growth and global competition of the poultry industry. Accordingly, infectious diseases brought on by a variety of pathogens, including bacteria, viruses, parasites, and fungus, either by themselves or in conjunction with other microorganisms, can have a detrimental impact on the productivity and well-being of the poultry sector, leading to a rise in mortality [6, 8]. Parasitic diseases are one of the proven factors that cause the most detrimental effects in poultry, causing high mortality, impaired growth, reduced feed efficacy, and anemia compared to other bacterial or viral diseases [9, 10]. Parasitic infections result in huge economic losses in terms of mechanical injuries, the effects of toxic compounds, nutritional deficiencies, and immunosuppression of the host [11]. The better housing management and hygiene and the prevalence of parasitic infection in poultry seem to have decreased significantly in indoor production systems as compared to deep litter/ free-range and backyard farming systems. However, parasitic infections are still a major concern in both commercial deep litter and free-range systems. These traditional systems of poultry rearing around the world are infected with several parasites, which contribute significantly to reduced productivity. The commonly reported parasites in poultry are *Eimeria spp., Ascaridia galli, Heterakis gallinarum, Raillietina spp, Echidnophaga gallinacea, Dermanyssus gallinae, Histomonas meleagridis, Plasmodium sp., Leucocytozoon* sp. and *Haemoproteus* sp. *etc.* An early and accurate diagnosis of the causative agents is a crucial step for the prevention and control of any diseases. This chapter discusses the different approaches to parasite diagnosis with its salient features (Table **1**).

All the parasites of poultry are divided into three major groups with subgroups. These groups include Endoparasites, Ectoparasites, and Haemoparasites. A list of the most common pathogenic and economically important parasites that affect poultry is tabulated in the given Table **1, 2 & 3** [12]. For a comprehensive list of poultry parasites please refer to the book Helminths, arthropods and Protozoa of Domesticated Animals by E.J.L. Soulsby [13] or other books as mentioned under the reference section (Tables **2** and **3**).

Table 1. Some important endoparasites of poultry.

| Parasite | Hosts | Site of Predilections |
|---|---|---|
| **Trematodes:** | | |
| *Prosthogonimus* spp. | Fowls, ducks, geese | Bursa fabricius, oviduct, cloaca, rectum |
| *Echinostoma revolutum* | Duck, geese | Caeca, rectum |
| **Cestodes:** | - | - |
| *Davainea proglottina* | Fowls, pigeons | Small intestine |
| *Raillietina* spp. | Chicken, guinea fowl, turkey, pigeons | Small intestine |
| *Cotugnia* spp. | Fowls, duck | Small intestine |
| *Choanotaenia infundibulum* | Fowls, turkeys | Small intestine |
| *Amoebotaenia sphenoides* | Fowls | Small intestine |
| *Hymenolepis carioca* | Fowls | Small intestine |
| **Nematodes:** | - | - |
| *Heterakis gallinarum* | Chickens, guinea fowl, turkey, duck, goose, pea fowl | Caeca |
| *Ascaridia galli* | Chickens, guinea fowl, turkey, goose | Small intestine |
| *Subulura brumpti* | Chickens, turkey, guineafowl | Caeca |
| *Oxyspirura mansoni* | Chickens, turkey, guineafowls, pea fowls | Nictitating membrane of eye, lacrimal duct |
| *Syngamus trachea* | Chickens, turkeys, guineafowls, pea fowls, geese, quails | Trachea, lungs |
| *Dispharynx spiralis* | Chickens, turkeys, pigeons, guinea fowl, pheasant | Wall of proventriculus and esophagus |
| *Hartertia gallinarum* | Fowl, wild bustards | Small intestine |
| *Ornithostrongylus quardriradiatus* | Pigeon | Crop, proventriculus, and small intestine |
| *Gongylonema ingluvicola* | Chickens, turkey, quails, pheasant | Crop |
| *Cheilospirura (Acuaria) hamulosa* | Chickens, turkey, guinea fowl, pheasant, grouse, quails | Gizzard |
| *Tetrameres americana* | Chickens, turkey, duck, geese, guinea fowl, pigeon, grouse, quails | Proventriculus |
| *Capillaria* spp. | Chicken, turkey, guinea fowl, geese, quail, pigeon | Intestine |

(Table 1) cont.....

| Parasite | Hosts | Site of Predilections |
|---|---|---|
| **Protozoa:** | - | - |
| *Eimeria* spp. | Chicken, duck, turkey | Intestine |
| *Histomonas meleagridis* | Turkey, chicken | Liver, caeca |

**Table 2. Some important ectoparasites of poultry.**

| Parasite | Hosts | Site of Predilections |
|---|---|---|
| **Lice:** *Goniocotes gallinae* (Fluff louse), *Lipeurus caponis* (Wing louse), *Cuclotogaster (Liperus) heterographus* (Head louse), *Menopon gallinae* (Shaft louse), *Menacanthus stramineus* (Body louse) *and Columbicola columbae* | Chickens, pigeon, turkey and other birds | Wings, head, body |
| **Flea:** *Echidnophaga gallinacea* (Stick tight flea) | Chicken and other birds | Head |
| **Ticks:** *Argas persicus*(Fowl tick) | Chicken, turkey, pigeon, duck | Skin |
| **Mites:** *Dermanyssus gallinae* (Red mite), *Ornithonyssus bursa* (Tropical fowl mite), *O. sylviarum* (Northern fowl mite) | Chicken, turkey, duck and wild birds | Skin |
| **Mites:** *Cnemidocoptes mutans* (Scaly leg mite) | Chicken, turkey | Under the skin of legs, comb and wattles |

**Table 3. Some important haemoparasites of poultry.**

| Parasite | Hosts | Site of Predilections |
|---|---|---|
| *Leucocytozoon spp.* | Chickens, duck, turkey, geese | Leucocytes, erythrocytes |
| *Haemoproteus spp.* | Duck, geese, chicken | Erythrocytes |
| *Plasmodium spp.* | Chicken, turkey | Erythrocytes |
| *Aegyptianella spp.* | Chickens, turkey, duck, geese | Erythrocytes |
| *Trypanosoma gallinarum* | Chicken | Blood |

# DIAGNOSTIC METHODS FOR PARASITIC DISEASES IN POULTRY

The diagnosis of poultry parasitic infections is a very laborious and time-consuming task but can be done with the aid of basic diagnostic techniques and tools. This chapter discusses the present diagnostic techniques that most laboratories can use for the identification and quantification of parasitic infections through clinical and post-mortem examinations, as well as the examination of fecal samples, blood smears, and skin scraping. So far, very limited immunological and molecular biological techniques have been reported for the diagnosis of poultry parasitic diseases [12 - 15]. Diagnostic techniques have been developed to diagnose protozoan parasitic infections in poultry, especially with

*Eimeria spp.* and *Histomonas spp.* Molecular PCR-based tests are frequently used in research and are helpful in the confirmation of parasite species at the time of diagnosis. Various techniques such as Enzyme-linked immunosorbent assay (ELISA), Western blot, and other molecular tests are commonly used in research [16, 17].

## Clinical Examination of Poultry Birds

Clinical examination of individual birds might be of limited value. However, it is often beneficial to examine some random birds while investigating a disease condition in a poultry flock. Certain information regarding the flock and previous history of disease should be noted before the examination begins. These include the size of the flock, management practices, vaccinations, feeding practices, other poultry in the flock, symptoms before death, clinical signs, number of dead birds, time of death, *etc* [14, 15].

## MICROSCOPIC FECAL EXAMINATION FOR THE PARASITIC EGGS/OOCYSTS/CYSTS

This includes several methods or techniques for the identification or detection of parasitic stages (eggs/cysts/ oocysts) in feces. It is a quick and simple method for diagnosing a variety of parasitic infections and these methods also give information about the level of infections in both individual and flock populations. The eggs/oocysts of every gastrointestinal parasitic infection must find a mechanism to become available for a new susceptible host. The GI parasitic eggs/oocysts of poultry pass out through the feces. Freshly deposited feces contain eggs which may be un-embryonated or embryonated cysts, oocysts *e.g.*, *Ascaris* sp., *Heterakis* sp., *Tetrameres* sp., *Syngamus* sp., *Acuaria hamulosa* and *Gongylonema ingluvicola, Histomonas* sp. and *Eimeria* spp. Poultry feces do not contain hatched larvae. Therefore, the Baermann technique is not applied for the separation of parasitic larvae as it is not part of a complete fresh fecal examination of poultry feces [18].

The microscopic fecal examination includes several methods that are discussed below:

**1. Qualitative fecal examination:** By this method, we can know about the presence/absence of any parasitic stages (parasitic stages (eggs/cysts/ oocysts) in the fecal samples.
**2. Quantitative fecal examination:** By this method, we can get an idea about the level of infection/ worm burden in the host. This means the intensity of the infection can be detected by this method.

## Collection of Fecal Samples

The fecal sample collected for diagnosis of different infections (Fig. **1**):

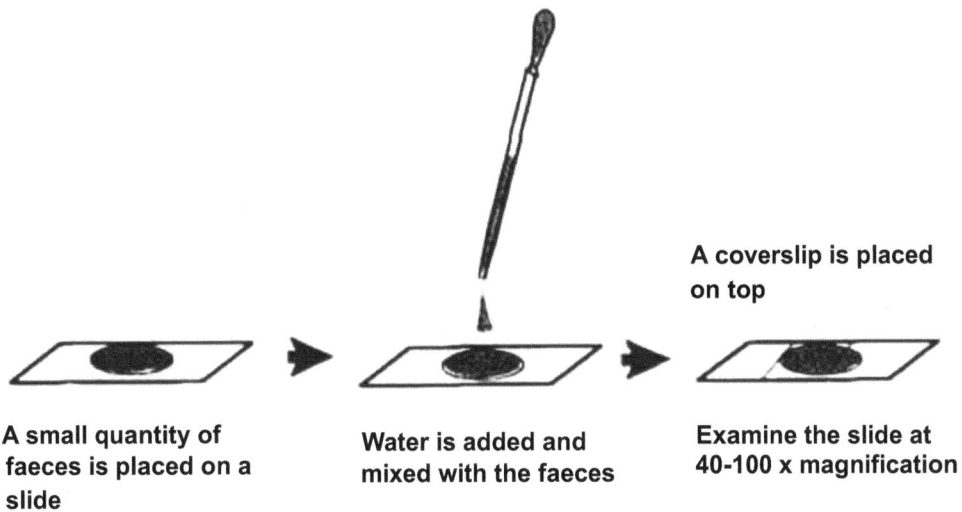

**Fig. (1).** Direct smear examination (Adopted from Permin and Hansen [12]).

## Interpretation of Direct Microscopic Examination

No egg in the whole sample Negative (-)

Few eggs in the whole sample Moderate infection (+)

Few eggs in each microscopic field Medium infection (+ +)

Many eggs in each microscopic field Heavy infection (+ + +)

### *Concentration Method*

The concentration method is used to separate the parasitic stages from the bulk of the materials in the fecal sample. The concentration of the parasitic eggs/oocyst from fecal samples is done either by sedimentation or flotation techniques. The flotation technique is the most widely used method for concentrating the parasite eggs. The specific gravity of the majority of the nematode eggs, cestode eggs, and coccidian oocysts are lower than that of the other residues in the feces, the eggs may be separated from other fecal particles by mixing the feces with a flotation fluid in which the eggs float while other fecal particles settle down. Trematode eggs are typically heavier and larger. Thus, unable to float in commonly used flotation solutions. Therefore, these trematode eggs are concentrated by sedimentation techniques, however, they are not fully effective and have variability in their sensitivity [12, 13].

## Concentration by Sedimentation Technique

Sedimentation techniques are performed to settle down the parasitic eggs/ oocysts present in the fecal samples by gravitational force or by centrifugation. As mentioned above, the eggs of trematodes do not float in commonly used flotation solutions due to their high specific gravity but can be concentrated by the sedimentation technique. Revolving around poultry, this technique applies to the recovery of *Prosthogonimus* spp. and *Echinostoma revolutum* trematode eggs. This technique is reliable for all types of eggs but essential for heavy trematode eggs. However, it is a time-consuming technique, it is not suitable for lightweight eggs and protozoan infections, and it is not efficient and variable in their sensitivity [12, 18].

## *Procedure*

- Transfer approx. 3-5 g of feces to a plastic container or falcon tube.
- Add approx. 50-100 ml of tap water into a container/ tube and mix thoroughly with a spatula or glass rod until all of the fecal material is broken down.
- Mix the fecal material and tap water by stirring or vortexing the tube.
- Immediately after stirring, pour the fecal suspension through a tea strainer into a conic sedimentation beaker, and fill up the beaker with tap water.
- Alternatively, pour the fecal suspension through a strainer into the different plastic containers, then transfer about 10 ml of the filtered suspension into a test tube that is placed in a test tube rack and either allowed to sediment the fecal particles/parasitic eggs for 10 minutes or centrifuge the tubes at 1500-2000 rpm for 2 min.
- Gently remove the supernatant in one steady movement (conic sedimentation beakers) or with the help of a pipette (test tube sedimentation). This process should be treated very carefully to avoid resuspending the sediment. The supernatant mustbe discarded.
- Repeat this procedure at least 2-3 times to remove debris as much as possible.
- Transfer a few drops of the sediment onto to microscopic slide by using a pipette, put the coverslip over it, and examine the sample under the microscope at 40-100X magnification.
- Repeat the last step until all the sediments have been examined. If nematode eggs are present in the fecal sample, some of the nematode eggs may be detected in the sediment, but the recovery rate is extremely low and sedimentation cannot replace the floatation technique where nematodes are concerned.

- For improvement of egg examination, add 1-2 drops of Methylene Blue or Malachite Green. The fecal particles will stain deeply blue/green by both dyes, while the trematode eggs remain unstained. This contrast staining allows the brownish eggs to be detected more easily (Fig. **2**).

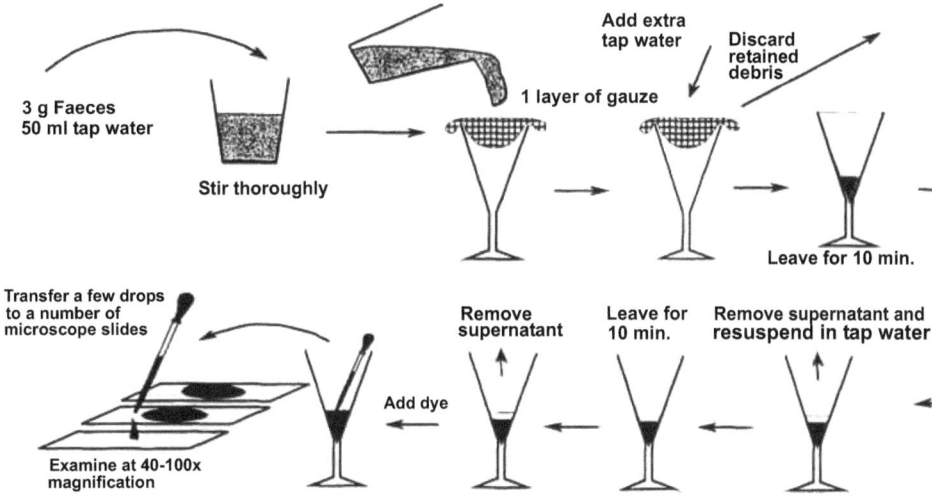

**Fig. (2).** Sedimentation technique (Adopted from Permin and Hansen [12]).

## *Concentration by Flotation Technique*

This is a qualitative fecal examination technique used for the detection of most of the nematode, cestode eggs, and coccidian oocysts present in the feces that float in commonly used flotation solutions. Unfortunately, the helminth eggs differ in their specific gravity. The majority of nematode and cestode eggs will float in saturated salt (NaCl) while certain nematode and cestode species' eggs will float only in fluids with higher specific gravities, like saturated $MgSO_4$ or saturated NaCl + glucose (sugar). Since very little is known about this fact about poultry helminths, it is recommended to standardize and consistently use only one of the flotation fluids with high specific gravity, such as a saturated salt and sugar solution. This flotation technique is the best and the simplest test for the detection of infection with light eggs and protozoan oocysts/ cysts, parasitic stages are concentrated and unmixed with debris to be easily detectable. However, it is not a suitable technique for heavy trematode eggs and it requires a flotation solution [12 - 14, 18, 19].

## *Procedure*

- Transfer approx. 3-5 g of feces to a plastic container or falcon tube.
- Add approx. 50-100 ml flotation solution into a container/ tube and mix thoroughly with a spatula or glass rod until all the fecal material is broken down.
- Mix the fecal material by stirring or vortexing the tube and immediately after vortexing pour the fecal suspension through a tea strainer into another beaker or tube.
- Pour the filtrate suspension into the test tube up to its brim, so that it has a convex meniscus at the top and carefully place the clean cover slip on the brim of the tube.
- Allow floating and accumulated parasitic eggs/ oocysts near the meniscus of the flotation solution for at least 10-20 minutes.
- **Alternatively:** Pour the filtered suspension into a test tube, but not up to the rim, tighten it with by cap carefully. Place the tube in a centrifuge machine and centrifuge the tubes at 1500-2000 rpm for 5 minutes.
- After the process of centrifugation, pick up the tube gently and keep it in a vertical position in the tube rack for 2-3 minutes.
- Pick the coverslip gently and put it over a clean glass slide for examination or take 0.5 ml of fluid from the top of the solution and put 2-3 drops of it on the clean glass slide and examine the slide sample under microscope at 40-100X magnification (Fig. **3**).

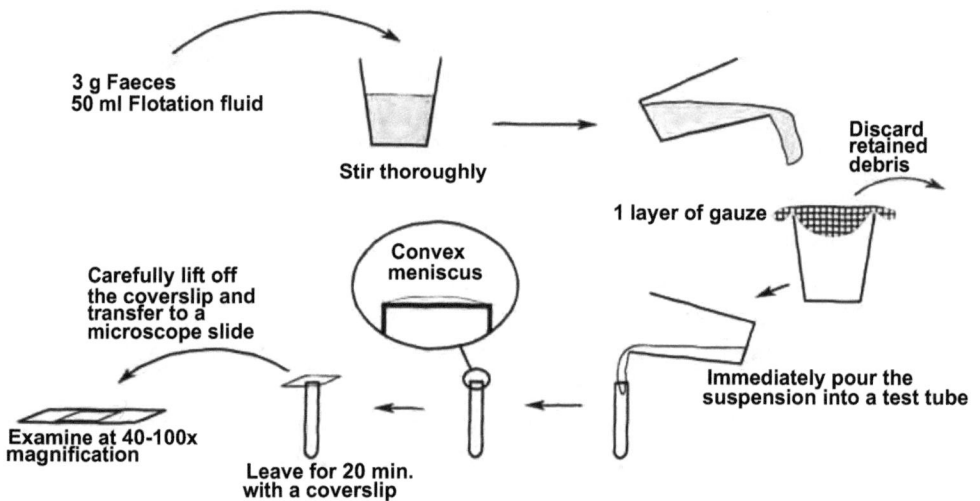

**Fig. (3).** Flotation technique (Adopted from Permin and Hansen [12]).

## Quantitative Fecal Examinations

Quantitative fecal examinations give the actual degree/ level of parasitic infection in animals [12 - 14]. It can be estimated by the use of a special counting chamber that is called the McMaster counting chamber. The qualitative flotation techniques used for the detection of nematodes, cestode eggs, and protozoan cysts/oocysts, have been developed to become quantitative when the parasitic eggs/oocysts, present in positive samples, are allowed to float in the specialized McMaster counting chambers. The McMaster counting chamber is made up of two glass plates that are separated by two or three narrow 1.5 mm thick strips of glass plates placed transversely. This creates 2 or 3 spaces between the two slides that have 1.5 mm depth. An area of 1 sq. cm is ruled over each chamber space on the upper slide. Therefore, the area underneath will have a capacity of 0.15 ml (1.5 mm x 1 sq. cm). The McMaster technique procedures can be executed with several modifications and the basic McMaster technique will be as follows:

### *Procedure*

- Weigh 4.0 g of feces and transfer it into a plastic tube or container.
- Add 56 ml of flotation solution into it. The amount of flotation solution should be changed according to the weight of the feces (14 ml flotation solution to 1.0 g feces). This ratio ensures that 1.0 g of feces is equivalent to 15 ml of the resulting fecal suspension.
- Mix the feces and flotation solution by vortexing or stirring the tube.
- Immediately after stirring or vortexing, pour the fecal suspension through a tea strainer into another tube/ container, and discard the retained fecal debris.
- Take the filtrate suspension in a Pasteur pipette immediately after mixing the filtrate.
- Fill both chambers of the McMaster slide with the help of the Pasteur pipette. The chmabers should be charged carefully to avoid air bubbles forming in them.
- Keep the filled McMaster chamber on the table for 3-5 minutes so that the eggs or oocysts might float to the upper surface of the McMaster chamber. Then, count the total number of eggs or oocysts present under each chamber.
- To determine the number of eggs per gram (EPG) of feces, multiply the number of eggs or oocysts in one chamber of the McMaster counting chamber by **100**. if both chambers of the McMaster counting chamber are counted then multiply by **50**. Example: If 22 eggs are counted on the first side of the chamber, and 28 eggs are counted on the second side, then

Eggs per gram (EPG) = (22+28) x 50 =2500

- The McMaster counting chamber should be washed under running tap water after each counting. It should be shaken to remove most of the water trapped inside the chamber, and then dried with a cotton cloth outside and a strip of filter paper inside the chamber (Fig. **4**).

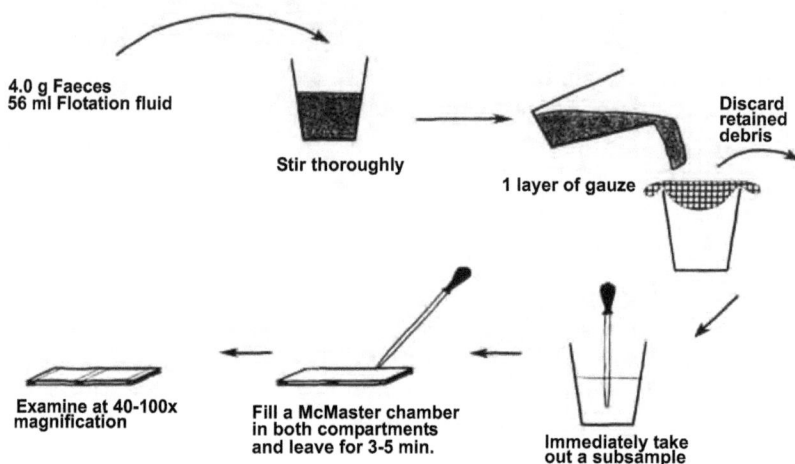

**Fig. (4).** McMaster counting chamber technique (Adopted from Permin and Hansen [12]).

## IDENTIFICATION OF PARASITIC EGGS/OOCYSTS/CYSTS

The identification of parasites, eggs, protozoan oocysts, and cysts found in poultry may have a characteristic appearance that is necessary for the unambiguous identifications to diagnose the parasitic stages. In Fig. (**5**), some of the most prevalent parasitic stages are shown. As coccidian parasitic infections are quite common in poultry and several species of the genus *Eimeria* have been reported [20] as shown in Fig. (**6**). Furthermore, for a more thorough description of parasites and their eggs/ oocysts please refer to the book Helminths, arthropods and protozoa of domesticated animals by E.J.L. Soulsby [13], FAO, Animal Health Manual, 1998 or other books as mentioned under reference section.

## DIAGNOSIS OF HAEMOPARASITES

For many years, microscopy has been a reliable tool in fieldwork and is the standard method for diagnosing blood parasites. The common blood parasites such as *Plasmodium* species, *Haemoproteus* species. *Leucocytozoon* species, *Babesia* species, and *Aegyptianella* species are affecting poultry. The basis for diagnosing these infections is the direct microscopy detection of schizonts or gametocytes and initial bodies (*Aegyptianella* spp.) in erythrocytes or leucocytes in thin blood smears. The stained blood smears from the infected bird may reveal large gametocytes that are pigmented in mature RBCs (*Haemoproteus* sp., *Leucocytozoon* spp), piroplasmic bodies inside RBC (*Babesia* sp.) or as one or more round or irregularly shaped, signet-ring (0.3-4 μm) bodies in RBC's

(*Aegyptinella* spp.). Large gametocytes of *Leucocytozoon* spp. grossly distort the infected host cells (particularly immature erythrocytes), making it difficult to identify parasitized cells. In contrast to this, the mature gametocytes of *Haemoproteus* spp. typically occupy more than 50% of the erythrocyte's cytoplasm, partially encircling the host cell nucleus in a characteristic "halter shape" and causing minimal displacement of the nucleus [13]. The conventional diagnosis of blood parasites by using microscopy is a readily available and cost-effective diagnostic tool, it is also essential to confirm the diagnosis using the bird's RBC profile, such as by determining the packed cell volume (PCV) for blood parasites like *Haemoproteus* sp., Plasmodium spp., *Leucocytozoon* spp., and *Babesia* sp. that cause severe anemia.

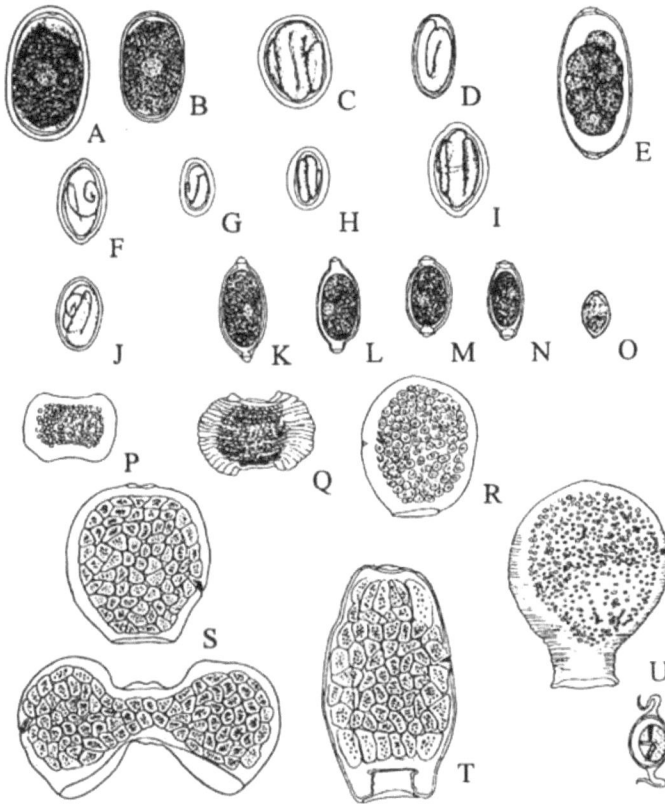

**Fig. (5).** Important helminth eggs and segments of cestodes. (**A**) *Ascaridia galli,* (**B**) *Heterakis gallinarum,* (**C**) *Allopada suctoria,* (**D**)*Strongyloides avium,* (**E**) *Syngamus trachea,* (**F**) *Tetrameres americana,* (**G**) *Acuaria* spp., (**H**) *Acuaria hamulosa,* (**I**) *Gongylonema ingluvicola,* (**J**) *Oxyspirura mansoni,* (**K**) *Capillaria annulata,* (**L**) *Capillaria anatis,* (**M**) *Capillaria obsignata,* (**N**) *Capillaria contorta,* (**O**) *Prosthogonimus* spp., (**P-U**) Segments of cestodes, **P.***Amoebotaenia cuneata,* (**Q**) *Hymenolepis carioca,* (**R**) *Raillietina cesticillus,* (**S**) *Raillietina echinobothrida,* (**T**) *Raillietina echinobothrida,* (**U**) Segment of *Choanotaenia infundibulum* and a single egg. (Adopted from Soulsby [13]).

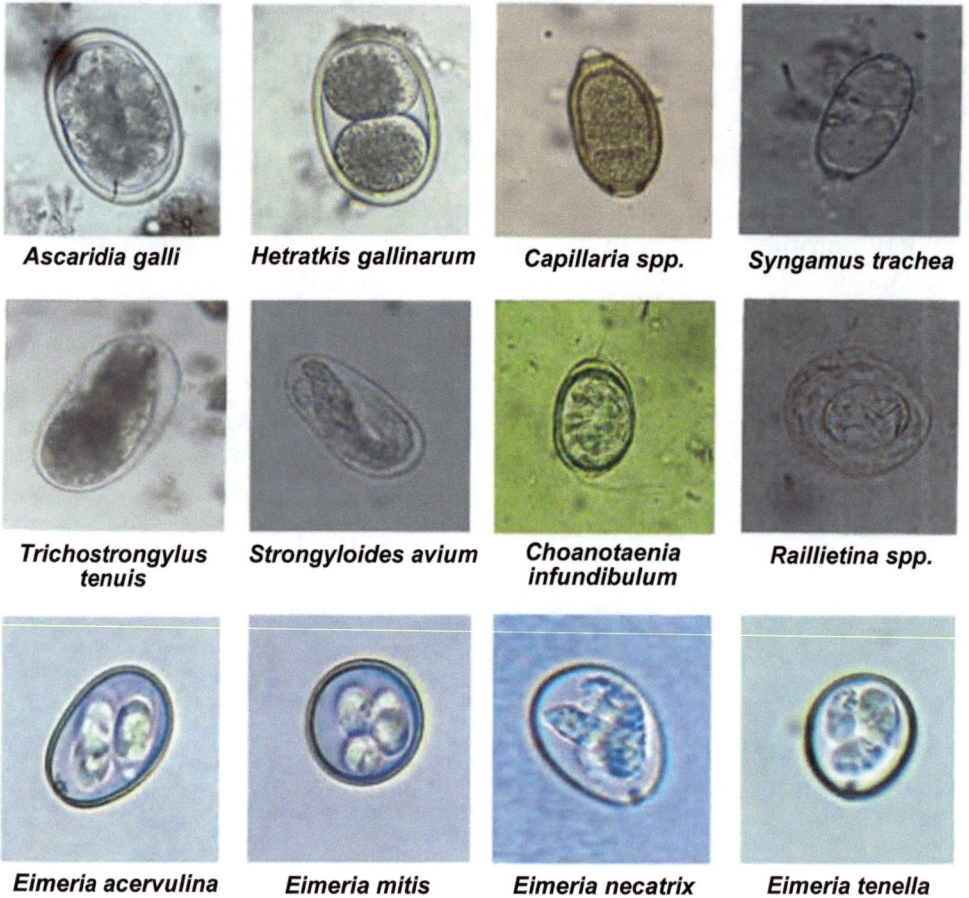

**Fig. (6).** Eggs/Oocysts of gastrointestinal parasites identified in poultry dropping samples (Adopted from Kumar *et al.* [20]).

## Blood Smear Examination

The most common medium for recovery of various stages of haemoprotozoan parasites of animals and birds is blood. To search for blood parasites, the blood should be collected from affected animals/birds and a smear for microscopic examination.

## Blood Smear Preparation

### *Procedure*

- The animal's details and the date of sampling are written in the frosted area of the glass slide with the help of a diamond pencil.
- The two glass slides are cleaned by being rinsed in 95% alcohol and and are wiped with clean cotton/ paper.
- The glass slide (Examination slide, A) is placed horizontally and a small quantity of blood is dropped at one end of the slide.
- The edge of the other slide (Spreader slide, B) is placed over the blood drop which allows the blood to spread over the entire margin. The angle between the spreader slide and examination slide should at an angle of 30°-45°.
- The spreader slide (B) is moved forward along the examination slide (A) with steady and quick movement dragging the blood behind it to spread the drop evenly on the first slide.
- After that, examination slide (A) is dried by either waving it in the air or putting it upright in a box.
- After drying, the blood film is fixed by pouring the absolute methyl alcohol/ methanol onto the slide or dipping the slide in 100% methyl alcohol/ methanol for 1-2 minutes.
- The slide is held upright in order for the alcohol to naturally evaporate.

## Blood Smear Staining by Giemsa's Stain

### *Procedure*

- A 1:10 dilution of stock Giemsa stain is prepared with a Phosphate Buffer Solution (or distilled water) pH6.76 for avian blood.
- The dilution has to be standardized for each batch of stock prepared.
- The diluted stain is poured on the blood smear (one slide contains a maximum of 2.5 ml of solution).
- The slides are left for 30-45 minutes for the best staining result.
- After that, the stain solution and the slides are washed quickly with running tap water or buffered distilled water.
- The slide is kept in an upright position to drain out the remaining water and allow it to air dry.
- After drying, the slide is to be examined with a light microscope under an oil immersion objective (100X).
- If the staining does not work well enough, the slides can be stained again (Figs. 7 and **8**).

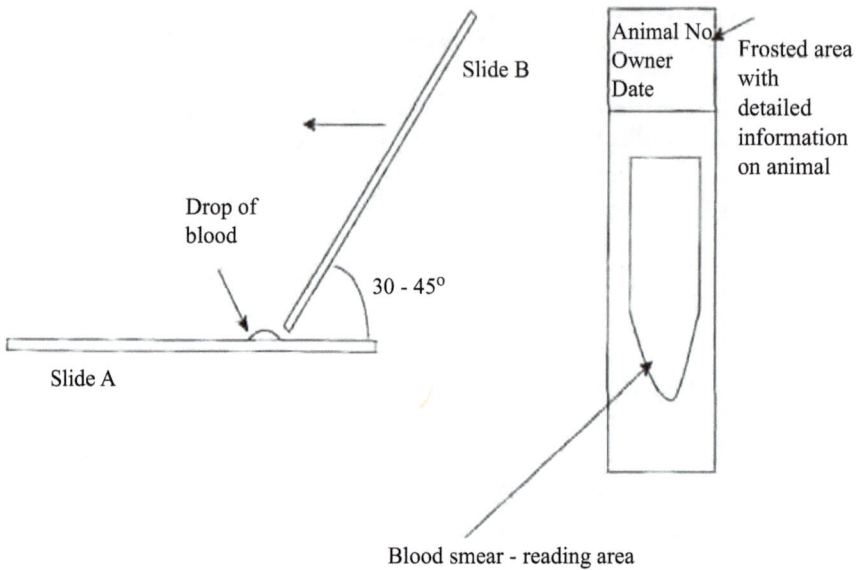

Fig. (7). Preparation of a blood smear (Adopted from Permin and Hansen [12]).

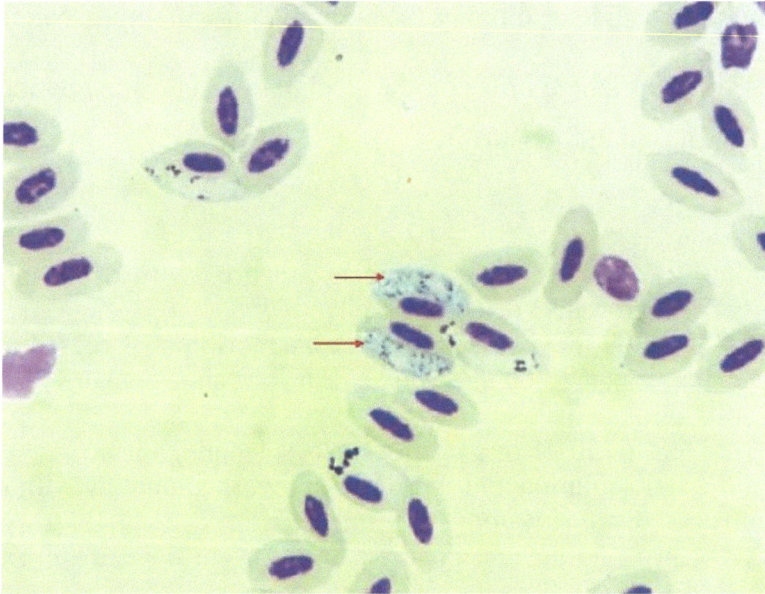

Fig. (8). Gametocytes (red arrow) of *Haemoproteus* spp. inside the erythrocytes of pigeons.

**Note:** Poultry erythrocytes have a nucleus thus it could be challenging for the inexperienced researcher to produce thin blood smears. Therefore, it is recommended to practice before making a blood smear for examination.

## DIAGNOSIS OF ECTOPARASITES

The ticks, mites, fleas, and lice are examples of ectoparasites, which are identified by distinguishing between body divisions, the head, thorax, and legs [21]. The conventional method for detecting parasitic mites from animal and poultry birds relies on the skin-scrapping method, which includes superficial or deep skin scrapping from the margin of affected areas. For deep skin scrapping, a dulled rounded scalpel blade (# 10) and the area to be scraped are coated with mineral oil, and the scraped skin materials are to be examined directly or after 10% KOH digestion [21, 22].

### Direct Microscopic Examination of Sample for Ectoparasites

The infected feathers and fur are collected from the vent or beneath the wings and are placed in a screw-capped glass or plastic bottle. The presence of ectoparasites (lice, fleas, or their nits) is directly examined under the stereo zoom microscopes. A few ectoparasites can be picked up with a needle, transferred in saline or Berlese's fluid, and identified in the laboratory by examining under a light microscope. It is convenient to mount the specimens for direct examination using the Berlese's fluid. Some species of lice were recovered from poultry are shown in Fig. (**9**) [23].

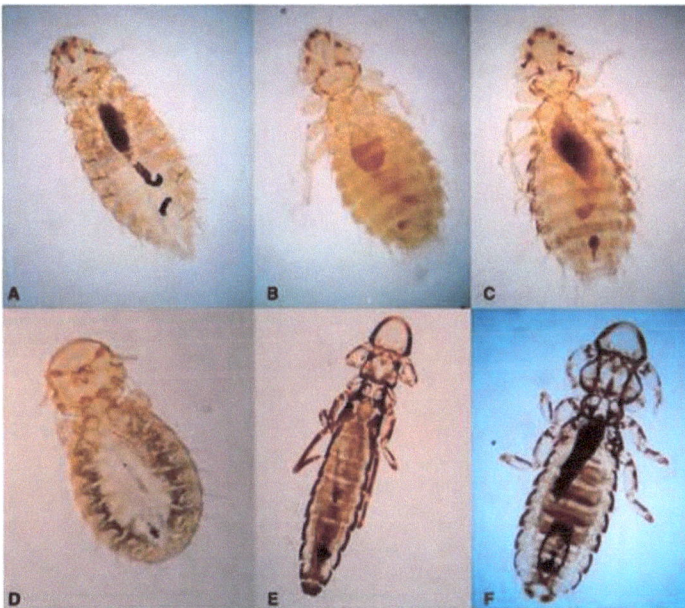

**Fig. (9).** Lice found in the poultry: (**A**)*Menopon gallinae*, (**B**)*Menacanthus cornutus*, (**C**) *Menacanthus stramineus*, (**D**)*Goniocotes gallinae*, (**E**)*Lipeurus caponis*, and (**F**)*Cuclotogaster heterographus* (Adopted from Murillo and Mullens [23]).

## Skin Scraping for Mites

Skin scrapings from the affected area of poultry are examined for the presence of mites. The samples must be collected from a moist part near the edge/ periphery of the lesion avoiding the inclusion of a large amount of dry crust or small feathers and examined directly or after 10% KOH treatment under the light microscope.

### *Procedure*

- Scraped skin is collected from the edge of the affected areas.
- Feathers should be removed from the chosen areas.
- The skin should be moistened with liquid paraffin before scraping to ensure that all scraping materials stick to the scalpel.
- The skin surface is scraped until a small amount of blood oozes out from the surface.
- After transferring the scraping material on the slide, a few drops of 10% KOH are added and the specimen should be left to clear for 5-10 minutes.
- A glass coverslip is placed on and examined under the microscope at 40-100X magnification (Fig. **9**).

## POST-MORTEM EXAMINATION OF POULTRY

- During PM examination, first of all, the general body condition of birds and the skin, feathers, plumage, legs, wings, *etc.* is examined for the presence of ectoparasites. Then, the body of the bird is disected and examinations are carried out for the presence of parasites (larynx and trachea for *Syngamus trachea* proventriculus, gizzard for *Gongylonema ingluvicola*, *Amidostomum anseris* and *Tetrameres* spp. and intestinal parts such as duodenum, middle part of intestine, rectum and cloaca for the trematode, cestodes, nematodes, and coccidian oocysts/cysts). The embedded parasites in the intestinal mucosa layer are collected in a petri dish after washing the mucosa is carefully stored in 70% ethyl alcohol for the final identification of parasites.
- For identification, a representative sample of collected helminths is examined under a light microscope with 40-100X magnification after clearing with lactophenol/ lactic acid.

## DIAGNOSIS OF COCCIDIOSIS IN POULTRY

The best methods for the diagnosis of coccidiosis infection in poultry are microscopic examination of dropping from affected birds and necropsy of dead/ euthanized infected birds. The serosal surface of the entire digestive tract should be examined first, followed by the mucosal surface. The microscope should be required to view the endogenous developmental forms on questionable lesions. Microscopic examination of the intestinal scraping reveals the presence of a few oocysts, which suggests the existence of an infection but does not diagnose the clinical coccidiosis. When further confirmation is needed, PCR molecular diagnosis is frequently used. In a practical situation, the presence of severe gross lesions only supports the diagnosis of coccidiosis. The clinical diagnosis of coccidiosis should be based on finding the lesions during necropsy of representative birds of the flock and further confirmed by the presence of microscopic stages of coccidia [14, 15, 24].

## Microscopic Examination of Mucosal scrapping/Faecal Sample

The developmental stages of *Eimeria* spp. include schizonts, gametocytes, and oocysts can be seen during microscopic examination of smears made from mucosal scraping from the suspected lesions. A small amount of mucosal scraping was put on the glass slide, diluted with saline or distilled water, and examined under a microscope after putting the coverslip. During the examination, oocysts or macrogametes are most easily visible, but in many cases, maturing schizont may be visible. Diagnostic characteristics of coccidiosis that are of significant value include the different sizes of schizonts/ rounded oocysts of *Eimeria* spp. Due to the considerable overlapping of size and shape of oocysts among the different *Eimeria* species, oocysts size, and shape are not useful diagnostic features. However, the combination of the oocyst's size, shape, location in the gut, and the appearance of lesions gives enough confidence in the diagnosis of coccidiosis.

The *Eimerian* oocysts excreted feces of infected chicken can be detected by qualitative fecal examination method, which is the most convenient and least expensive method for the diagnosis of coccidiosis in chickens [25]. The most common qualitative fecal examination techniques for diagnosing coccidiosis in chickens include microscopic examination of a fecal smear prepared from emulsified feces or the use of the floatation technique to determine the concentration/number of floated oocysts [26, 27].

The number of oocysts counts per gram of feces (OPG count), sporulation rate, and oocyst dimensions are determined by performing a quantitative fecal examination [14, 26 - 30]. The OPG counts can be performed by either the McMaster chamber method or the Hemocytometer chamber method (Fig. **10**).

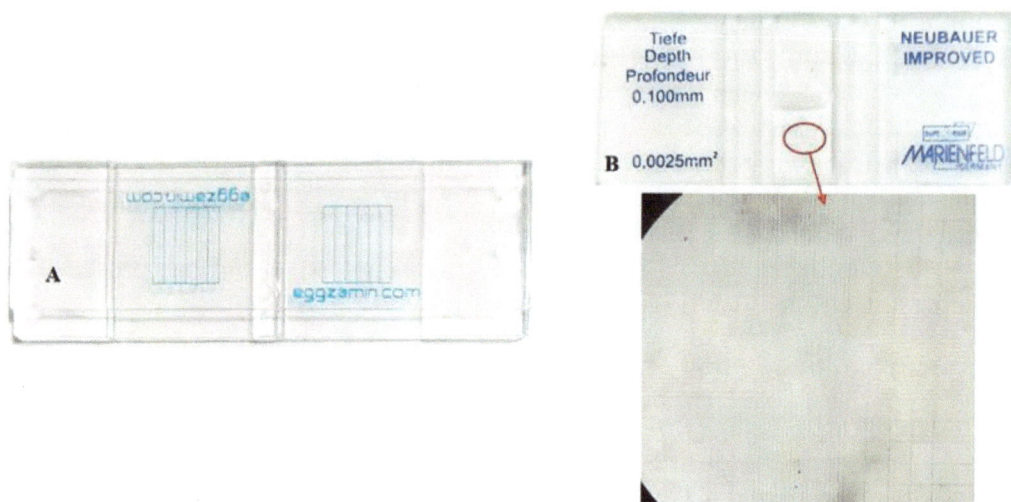

**Fig. (10). (A)** McMaster counting chamber, **(B)** Neubauer type hemocytometer chamber.

## Lesion Scoring Method

The severity of lesions developed in coccidiosis is roughly proportional to the quantity of sporulated oocysts ingested by birds. Other parameters such as reduced body weight, higher feed conversion ratio, and death are correlated with the severity of the lesions. Johnson and Reid [31] have developed a postmortem examination scoring system to determine the severity of poultry coccidiosis based on the macroscopically visible lesions in the gut caused by *Eimeria* spp. The scoring system ranges from 0 to +4 (*i.e.*, 0= No lesion, +1 = mild lesions, +2 = moderate lesions, +3 = severe lesions, and +4 = extremely severe lesions) (Table **4**; Fig. **11**). The lesion score is determined by the size or extent of the gross lesion, and the species of *Eimeria* can be identified by examining the predilection site of lesions (because species are highly host and site-specific; Table **5**). The lesion scoring method requires a high level of specialized expertise and it is very labor-intensive, subjective, and time-consuming [32]. Johnson and Reid's method is more suitable and accurate in diagnosing chicken coccidiosis under controlled experimental infections rather than the actual farming conditions in fields, where the challenge dose of oocysts and species of *Eimeria* are known. However, it has been used by many veterinarians and parasitologists to evaluate the severity of natural infection of *Eimeria* spp. in field conditions [15, 28] (Tables **4** and **5**).

## Histopathology Methods

Histopathology is a good method for routine examination of intestinal tissues infected with coccidia. The tissue sections stained with Haematoxylin and Eosin (H&E) or other common histological stains can show the developmental stages of coccidia and based on these microscopic lesions, the scoring method was developed for coccidiosis infections [24, 34]. Specific phases of developmental stages can be identified by specialized techniques. For example, polysaccharide associated with the refractile body and the wall-forming bodies in the macrogamete gives a brilliant red color when stained with Schiff reagent. Monoclonal antibodies coupled with fluorescent markers such as fluorescein can be very helpful in advanced research and it makes it very easy to identify the specific developmental stages of parasites (Fig. **12**).

**Table 4. Johnson and Reid method; scoring system for lesions caused by** *Eimeria tenella***.**

| Lesion Score | Description |
|---|---|
| 0 | No lesion or absence of gross lesions. |
| +1 | Normal caecal content is visible, absence of thickening of the caecal wall with few scattered petechiae. |
| +2 | Moderate thickening of caecal walls with numerous lesions and noticeable blood in the caecal content. |
| +3 | Thickened caecal walls, there is a lot of blood and caecal cores, absence of normal caecal contents, and unopened caecal serosa show petechia on the entire surface. |
| +4 | Marked thickening of caecal walls, enlarged caeca with a lot of blood, and fecal debris mixed with the caecal core, the distal end of caeca gets shrunken and ruptured. Dead birds were also given a score of +4. |

(Adopted from Johnson and Reid [31])

**Table 5. Characteristics of lesions caused by** *Eimeria* **species infections and its predilection sites.**

| *Eimeria* species | Predilection site | Characteristics of lesions |
|---|---|---|
| Eimeria acervuline | Upper part of the intestine. | Whitish spots are present on the serosal surface of the intestine, hemorrhagic streaks and whitish lesions on the intestinal surface, and mucoid enteritis. |
| Eimeria brunetti | Lower part of the intestine. | Thin-walled distended intestine, mucoid necrotic discharge. |
| Eimeria maxima | The middle part of the intestine | Distended intestine with hemorrhagic spots and mucoid discharge. |
| Eimeria necatrix | The middle part of the intestine | Severe hemorrhage with mucoid discharge, whitish and red spots on the surface of the intestine. |
| Eimeria tenella | Caeca | Severe hemorrhage with white to red spots on the surface of the intestine. |
| Eimeria praecox | Duodenum | No evident lesion is present but the duodenal surface has a slightly hemorrhagic appearance with a little mucoid discharge. |

(Adopted from Abebe and Gugsa [33])

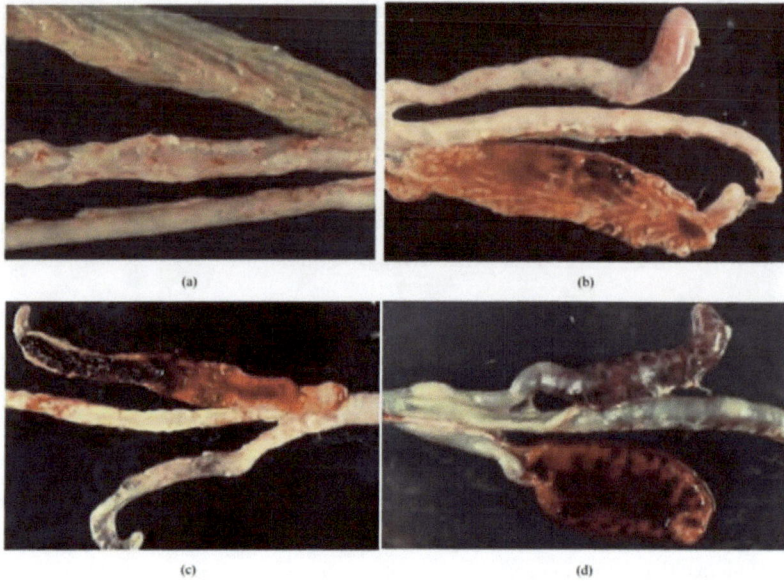

**Fig. (11).**   Scoring of lesions caused by *Eimeria tenella*, **(a)** +1; **(b)** +2; **(c)** +3 and **(d)** +4. (Adopted from Conway and McKenzie [14]).

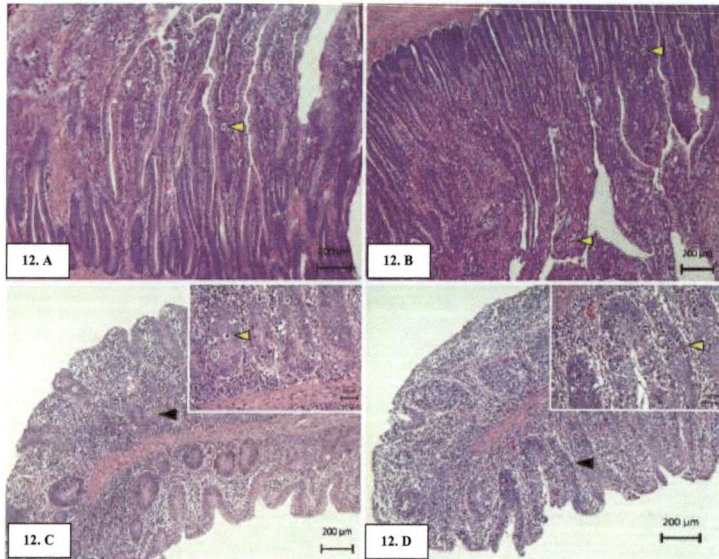

**Fig. (12). (A-D)** Histopathological characterization of *Eimeria* spp. infection in chickens: **(A)** Duodenum: Score 2 lesion with a moderate number of immature oocysts in less than ten villi (yellow arrowhead). **(B)** Jejunum: Score 2 lesion with a moderate number of immature oocysts in less than ten villi (yellow arrowhead). **(C)** Cecum: Score 1 lesion with a discrete number of parasites (black arrowhead) in less than ten crypts. The immature oocysts (yellow arrowhead) are highlighted. **(D)** Cecum: Score 3 lesions with a large number of parasites (black arrowhead) in more than ten crypts. The immature oocysts (yellow arrowhead) are highlighted. (Adopted from Balestrin *et al*. [24]).

## IMMUNOLOGICAL AND MOLECULAR DIAGNOSIS OF PARASITIC DISEASES

To prevent and control parasitic diseases, next-generation laboratory diagnostic methods are essential when compared to the aforementioned traditional methods for identification of the exact species of *Eimeria* responsible for the coccidiosis infection. Furthermore, using laboratory-developed diagnostic methods that are species-specific and have a higher rate of sensitivity and accuracy might help to overcome the limitations of traditional methods [6, 28].

The poultry parasites are diagnosed immunologically by using the enzyme-linked immunosorbent assay (ELISA). Currently, polyclonal antibody-based ELISA has been shown to have high sensitivity (93%) and specificity (100%) in the diagnosis of ascariasis infection in poultry [35]. This is a simple and reliable biochemical assay for diagnosing coccidiosis, which detects epitope-specific antibodies (IgG and IgM) of *Eimeria* species present in the serum [17, 36]. Furthermore, Onaga *et al.* [37] reported that ELISA can be used to ascertain the exposure rate of vaccinated birds as well as the degree of exposure of *Eimeria* spp. to the flock. Nevertheless, the cross-reactivity of antibodies across the multiple *Eimeria* spp. sporozoites and merozoites in chicken serum may cause biases in the results of ELISA [38]. The serological diagnosis for common blood parasites *Plasmodium* sp. and *Haemoproteus* sp. can be achieved by antigen-based ELISA. Merozoite surface protein-1 (or MSP-1) has been used to diagnose *Plasmodium relictum* infection in birds [39].

Molecular diagnostic tools like Polymerase chain reaction (PCR) are highly specific and accurate in diagnosing the parasites of animals. The molecular diagnosis has the advantage of being able to detect even low populations of particular species, even when affected birds do not show clinical signs or obvious gross lesions. Depending on the requirements, there are different PCR formats for the diagnosis of parasites such as nested PCR, allele-specific PCR, multiplex PCR, RT PCR, LAMP, *etc.* The differential diagnosis of certain poultry parasites, such as the differential diagnosis of *Ascardiia galli* and *Herakis gallinarum* eggs can be done by the use of dd PCR or droplet digital PCR targeting the ITS-2 gene has exhibited some feasibility [40]. Furthermore, the use of a Triplex PCR assay for the differential diagnosis of three species of *Raillietina* species has proven to be a reliable diagnostic tool for intestinal cestodiasis in poultry [41].

The diagnosis of the most important parasites of poultry *i.e.*, *Eimeria* spp. can be made by using PCR based technique. The DNA sequence of each *Eimeria* species is unique and is used to design the specific oligonucleotide primers for PCR selective amplification. Molecular-based techniques targeting multiple genes such as ribosomal RNA internal transcribed spacer regions 1 or 2 (ITS-1, ITS-2) [6, 30, 42 - 45] or sequence characterized amplified region (SCAR), which are found using a technique called Random amplified polymorphic DNA (RAPD) [16, 30, 46 - 48], are used for detection and differentiation of *Eimeria* species. The multiplex PCR techniques have been described that can be performed by adding all primers of each *Eimeria* species either in a single tube or two tubes [30, 42, 47, 49]. Most recent technology includes real-time PCR (quantitative) [50 - 53] and loop-mediated isothermal amplification (LAMP) [54, 55] as alternatives to gel electrophoresis. Currently, the molecular PCR assay is available for the diagnosis of commonly prevalent haemo-parasites of poultry such as *Plasmodium* sp., *Haemoproteus* sp., and *Leucocytozoon* spp. Sometimes these assays become non-specific in the diagnosis of parasites due to the presence of multiple species under the same genus, thus the modified forms of PCR such as multiplex PCR can help detect single and mixed infections from three genera *Plasmodium, Haemoproteus*, and *Leucocytozoon*sp [56].

The DNA or nucleic acid extraction process is one of the most crucial steps for the molecular PCR assay, whether the source of parasites is intestinal tissue, blood, fecal dropping, or litter samples. The DNA from the parasitic materials can be extracted by conventional methods following the protocols of Sambrook *et al.* [57] or commercially available DNA extraction kits [30]. The extracted DNA or nucleic acid can be stored at -20°C until used for PCR.

The correct and prompt diagnosis of parasitic diseases is needed for the prevention and control of parasitic infections in animals. In recent years, the research has been focused on the development of an alternative method to improve the diagnosis of parasitic disease. These could include advanced molecular techniques, immunoassays, and proteomics approaches to develop more reliability with high specificity and sensitivity and easy to perform on doorsteps.

**List of Some Chemicals and Reagents used During the Diagnosis of Samples**

**Flotation solutions:**

This section describes how to prepare different flotation solutions. Depending on the availability of reagents, either of them can be used for the flotation method.

## A. Saturated salt solution: (Specific gravity: 1.20)

Sodium chloride: 400 g

Water: 1000 ml

## B. Saturated sugar solution: (Specific gravity: 1.12 – 1.20)

White sugar: Q.S.

Water: 1000 ml

Add the sugar until it is saturated as indicated by the presence of sugar particles at the bottom of the container after 15 minutes of stirring. Stir well before use.

## C. Salt/Sugar solution: (Specific gravity: 1.28)

Sodium chloride: 400 g

Water: 1000 ml

White sugar: 500 g

First of all, dissolve the all salt in the water, thereafter add the sugar to the solution and constantly stir the solution to dissolve the sugar.

**2. Berlese's fluid:** Used for preservation and identification of ectoparasites.

Gum acacia: 30 g

Choral hydrate: 200 g

Glycerin: 20 g

Distilled water: 50 g

After soaking the Gum acacia in water for 12 hours, the glycerin is added. First of all, the Gum acacia is soaked in water for 12 hours, thereafter glycerin is added and the mixture (not boiled) is heated and stirred until all the gum is dissolved. After this, the chloral hydrate is added and dissolved in this mixture. When the bubbles start to appear, the fluid must be put aside and kept warm until they disappear. After that, the medium is stored for future use.

## 3. Preparation of Giemsa's Stain: (Stock solution)

Stain powder: 1 g

Glycerol: 66 ml

Methanol (acetone free): 66 ml

**Working Giemsa Stain:** It is a 10% solution of prepared stock Giemsa stain.

Distilled water or Tap water buffered to pH 6.76 (avian blood): 900 ml

Giemsa stock stain: 100 ml

## CONCLUDING REMARKS

The use of suitable diagnostic methods is the urgent need of the healthcare community for prompt and accurate diagnosis of parasitic diseases, which is very necessary to make a strategy for the prevention and control of parasitic infections in animals. For a long time, the diagnosis of parasitic diseases in poultry has been almost constant with very limited advances such as the introduction of PCR and a rapid Immunochromatographic Test (ICT) have been adopted in clinical diagnostic tests. The microscopical/microbiological-based diagnostic tests are very old, labor-intensive, and time-consuming, and require the expertise of the subject for the diagnosis of parasites including helminths, protozoans, arthropods, and haemoprotozoans. So, in the current scenario, research has been focused on advanced molecular technique approaches, immunoassays, and proteomics to achieve more reliability with high specificity and sensitivity for diagnostic tests.

## REFERENCES

[1]     Attia YA, Al-Harthi MA, Korish MA, Shiboob MM. Fatty acid and cholesterol profiles, hypocholesterolemic, atherogenic, and thrombogenic indices of broiler meat in the retail market. Lipids Health Dis 2017; 16(1): 40.
        [http://dx.doi.org/10.1186/s12944-017-0423-8] [PMID: 28209162]

[2]     Petracci M, Soglia F, Madruga M, Carvalho L, Ida E, Estévez M. Wooden-breast, white striping, and spaghetti meat: causes, consequences and consumer perception of emerging broiler meat abnormalities. Compr Rev Food Sci Food Saf 2019; 18(2): 565-83.
        [http://dx.doi.org/10.1111/1541-4337.12431] [PMID: 33336940]

[3]     Pouta E, Heikkilä J, Forsman-Hugg S, Isoniemi M, Mäkelä J. Consumer choice of broiler meat: The effects of country of origin and production methods. Food Qual Prefer 2010; 21(5): 539-46.
        [http://dx.doi.org/10.1016/j.foodqual.2010.02.004]

[4]     Wideman N, O'Bryan CA, Crandall PG. Factors affecting poultry meat colour and consumer preferences - A review. Worlds Poult Sci J 2016; 72(2): 353-66.
        [http://dx.doi.org/10.1017/S0043933916000015]

[5]     Blake DP, Tomley FM. Securing poultry production from the ever-present *Eimeria* challenge. Trends Parasitol 2014; 30(1): 12-9.
        [http://dx.doi.org/10.1016/j.pt.2013.10.003] [PMID: 24238797]

[6]     Fatoba AJ, Adeleke MA. Diagnosis and control of chicken coccidiosis: a recent update. J Parasit Dis 2018; 42(4): 483-93.
        [http://dx.doi.org/10.1007/s12639-018-1048-1] [PMID: 30538344]

[7]     Izar-Tenorio J, Jaramillo P, Griffin WM, Small M. Impacts of projected climate change scenarios on heating and cooling demand for industrial broiler chicken farming in the Eastern U.S. J Clean Prod 2020; 255: 120306-14.
[http://dx.doi.org/10.1016/j.jclepro.2020.120306]

[8]     Hafez HM, Attia YA. Challenges to the poultry industry: current perspectives and strategic future after the COVID-19 outbreak. Front Vet Sci 2020; 7: 516.
[http://dx.doi.org/10.3389/fvets.2020.00516] [PMID: 33005639]

[9]     Ruff MD. Important parasites in poultry production systems. Vet Parasitol 1999; 84(3-4): 337-47.
[http://dx.doi.org/10.1016/S0304-4017(99)00076-X] [PMID: 10456422]

[10]    Kaufman PE, Koehler PG, Butler JF. External parasites of poultry. Published by Entomology and Nematology Department, Florida Cooperative Extension Service, Institute of Food and Agricultural Sciences, University of Florida 2006; pp. 1-13.

[11]    Garcia LS, Arrowood M, Kokoskin E, *et al.* Practical guidance for clinical microbiology laboratories: laboratory diagnosis of parasites from the gastrointestinal tract. Clin Microbiol Rev 2017; 31(1): 1-81.
[PMID: 29142079]

[12]    Permin A, Hansen JW. Epidemiology, diagnosis and control of poultry parasites. Rome: FAO Manual, Food and Agriculture Organization of the United Nations 1998; pp. 1-154.

[13]    Soulsby EJL. Helminths, Athropods and Protozoa of Domesticated Animals. 7th ed., London, UK: Baillière Tindall 1982.

[14]    Conway DP, McKenzie ME. Poultry Coccidiosis: Diagnostic and Testing Procedures. 3rd ed., State Avenue, Iowa, USA: Blackwell Publishing 2007.
[http://dx.doi.org/10.1002/9780470344620]

[15]    Cervantes HM. Revisiting intestinal lesion scoring techniques for coccidiosis. Proceedings of the 150th Annual Meeting of the American Veterinary Medical Association.

[16]    Cantacessi C, Riddell S, Morris GM, *et al.* Genetic characterization of three unique operational taxonomic units of *Eimeria* from chickens in Australia based on nuclear spacer ribosomal DNA. Vet Parasitol 2008; 152(3-4): 226-34.
[http://dx.doi.org/10.1016/j.vetpar.2007.12.028] [PMID: 18243560]

[17]    Constantinoiu CC, Molloy JB, Jorgensen WK, Coleman GT. Development and validation of an ELISA for detecting antibodies to *Eimeria tenella* in chickens. Vet Parasitol 2007; 150(4): 306-13.
[http://dx.doi.org/10.1016/j.vetpar.2007.09.019] [PMID: 17976915]

[18]    Calnek BW, Barnes HJ, Beard CW, Reid WM, Yoder HW Jr. Diseases of Poultry. 9th edition. Iowa State University Press/AMES. 1991; p. 929.

[19]    Chabaud AG. Keys to the genera of the supeifamilies Cosmocercoidea, Seuratoidea, Heterakoidea and Subuluroidea No. 6. In: Anderson , Ed. Keys to the Nematode parasites of Vertebrates. CAB International 1978.

[20]    Kumar S, Garg R, Ram H, Maurya PS, Banerjee PS. Gastrointestinal parasitic infections in chickens of upper gangetic plains of India with special reference to poultry coccidiosis. J Parasit Dis 2015; 39(1): 22-6.
[http://dx.doi.org/10.1007/s12639-013-0273-x] [PMID: 25698854]

[21]    Zajac AM, Conboy GA. Veterinary Clinical Parasitology. 8th ed., John Wiley & Sons 2012.

[22]    Bowman DD. Georgis' Parasitology for Veterinarian. 9th Editon, Saunders, Newyork, Saunders Elsevier. 2009; pp. 1-465.

[23]    Murillo AC, Mullens BA. Diversity and prevalence of ectoparasites on backyard chicken flocks in California. J Med Entomol 2016; 53(3): 707-11.
[http://dx.doi.org/10.1093/jme/tjv243] [PMID: 26753948]

[24]    Balestrin PWG, Balestrin E, Santiani F, *et al.* Comparison of macroscopy, histopathology and PCR for diagnosing *Eimeria* spp. in broiler chickens. *Pesq Vet Bras.* Pesq Vet Bras 2022; 42: e06968.

[25]    Mwale M, Masika PJ. Point prevalence study of gastro-intestinal parasites in village chickens of Centane district, South Africa. Afr J Agric Res 2011; 6(9): 2033-8.

[26]    Johnson WT. Coccidiosis of the chicken with special reference to species. Station Bulletin 1938; 358: 1-33.

[27]    Abo Alqomsan HM. Prevalence of caecal coccidiosis among broilers in Gaza strip. Dissertation, Gaza 2010; 1-78.

[28]    Singla LD. And Gupta SK. Advances in diagnosis of coccidiosis in poultry. In: Gupta RP, Garg SR, Nehra V, Lather D, Eds. Veterinary diagnostics Current trends. Delhi: Satish Serial Publishing House 2012; pp. 615-28.

[29]    Vadlejch J, Petrtýl M, Zaichenko I, *et al.* Which McMaster egg counting technique is the most reliable? Parasitol Res 2011; 109(5): 1387-94.
[http://dx.doi.org/10.1007/s00436-011-2385-5] [PMID: 21526406]

[30]    Kumar S, Garg R, Moftah A, *et al.* An optimised protocol for molecular identification of *Eimeria* from chickens. Vet Parasitol 2014; 199(1-2): 24-31.
[http://dx.doi.org/10.1016/j.vetpar.2013.09.026] [PMID: 24138724]

[31]    Johnson J, Reid WM. Anticoccidial drugs: Lesion scoring techniques in battery and floor-pen experiments with chickens. Exp Parasitol 1970; 28(1): 30-6.
[http://dx.doi.org/10.1016/0014-4894(70)90063-9] [PMID: 5459870]

[32]    Shirley MW, Smith AL, Tomley FM. The biology of avian *Eimeria* with an emphasis on their control by vaccination. Adv Parasitol 2005; 60: 285-330.
[http://dx.doi.org/10.1016/S0065-308X(05)60005-X] [PMID: 16230106]

[33]    Abebe E, Gugsa G. A review on poultry coccidiosis. Abyss J Sci Technol 2018; 3(1): 1-12.

[34]    Goodwin MA, Bounous DI, Brown J, Dekich MA. Clinical application of a light microscopic scoring method to make decisions regarding the pharmacotherapy of an *Eimeria maxima* abatement programme. Avian Pathol 1999; 28(3): 305-8.
[http://dx.doi.org/10.1080/03079459994803] [PMID: 26915387]

[35]    Oladosu OJ, Hennies M, Gauly M, Daş G. A copro-antigen ELISA for the detection of ascarid infections in chickens. Vet Parasitol 2022; 311: 109795.
[http://dx.doi.org/10.1016/j.vetpar.2022.109795] [PMID: 36108471]

[36]    Smith NC, Bucklar H, Muggli E, Hoop RK, Gottstein B, Eckert J. Use of IgG- and IgM-specific ELISAs for the assessment of exposure status of chickens to *Eimeria* species. Vet Parasitol 1993; 51(1-2): 13-25.
[http://dx.doi.org/10.1016/0304-4017(93)90191-O] [PMID: 8128576]

[37]    Onaga H, Saeki H, Hoshi S, Ueda S. An enzyme-linked immunosorbent assay for serodiagnosis of coccidiosis in chickens: use of a single serum dilution. Avian Dis 1986; 30(4): 658-61.
[http://dx.doi.org/10.2307/1590564] [PMID: 3814003]

[38]    Uchida T, Hasbullah , Nakamura T, Nakai Y, Ogimoto K. Cross reactivity of serum antibodies from chickens immunized with three Eimerian species. J Vet Med Sci 1994; 56(5): 1021-3.
[http://dx.doi.org/10.1292/jvms.56.1021] [PMID: 7865576]

[39]    Zhang X, Meadows SNA, Martin T, *et al. Plasmodium relictum* MSP-1 capture antigen-based ELISA for detection of avian malaria antibodies in African penguins (*Spheniscus demersus*). Int J Parasitol Parasites Wildl 2022; 19: 89-95.
[http://dx.doi.org/10.1016/j.ijppaw.2022.08.009] [PMID: 36090665]

[40]    Tarbiat B, Enweji N, Baltrusis P, *et al.* A novel duplex ddPCR assay for detection and differential diagnosis of *Ascaridia galli* and *Heterakis gallinarum* eggs from chickens feces. Vet Parasitol 2021;

296: 109499.
[http://dx.doi.org/10.1016/j.vetpar.2021.109499] [PMID: 34144378]

[41]   Panich W, Nak-on S, Chontananarth T. High-performance triplex PCR detection of three tapeworm species belonging to the genus *Raillietina* in infected poultry. Acta Trop 2022; 232: 106516.
[http://dx.doi.org/10.1016/j.actatropica.2022.106516] [PMID: 35580638]

[42]   Lew AE, Anderson GR, Minchin CM, Jeston PJ, Jorgensen WK. Inter- and intra-strain variation and PCR detection of the internal transcribed spacer 1 (ITS-1) sequences of Australian isolates of *Eimeria* species from chickens. Vet Parasitol 2003; 112(1-2): 33-50.
[http://dx.doi.org/10.1016/S0304-4017(02)00393-X] [PMID: 12581583]

[43]   Jenkins MC, Miska K, Klopp S. Improved polymerase chain reaction technique for determining the species composition of *Eimeria* in poultry litter. Avian Dis 2006; 50(4): 632-5.
[http://dx.doi.org/10.1637/7615-042106R.1] [PMID: 17274306]

[44]   Haug A, Thebo P, Mattsson JG. A simplified protocol for molecular identification of *Eimeria* species in field samples. Vet Parasitol 2007; 146(1-2): 35-45.
[http://dx.doi.org/10.1016/j.vetpar.2006.12.015] [PMID: 17386979]

[45]   Hamidinejat H, Shapouri MS, Mayahi M, Borujeni MP. Characterization of *Eimeria* species in commercial broilers by PCR based on ITS1 regions of rDNA. Iran J Parasitol 2010; 5(4): 48-54.
[PMID: 22347266]

[46]   Fernandez S, Costa AC, Katsuyama ÂM, Madeira AMBN, Gruber A. A survey of the inter- and intraspecific RAPD markers of *Eimeria* spp. of the domestic fowl and the development of reliable diagnostic tools. Parasitol Res 2003; 89(6): 437-45.
[http://dx.doi.org/10.1007/s00436-002-0785-2] [PMID: 12658454]

[47]   Fernandez S, Pagotto AH, Furtado MM, Katsuyama AM, Madeira AM, Gruber A. A multiplex PCR assay for the simultaneous discrimination and detection of the seven *Eimeria* species that infect domestic fowl. Parasitol 2003; 12: 317-25.
[http://dx.doi.org/10.1017/S0031182003003883] [PMID: 14636018]

[48]   Fernandez S, Katsuyama AM, Kashiwabara AY, Madeira AM, Durham AM, Gruber A. Characterization of SCAR markers of *Eimeria* spp. of domestic fowl and construction of a public relational database (The *Eimeria* SCARdb). FEMS Microbiol Lett 2004; 238(1): 183-8.
[PMID: 15336420]

[49]   Ogedengbe JD, Hunter DB, Barta JR. Molecular identification of *Eimeria* species infecting market-age meat chickens in commercial flocks in Ontario. Vet Parasitol 2011; 178(3-4): 350-4.
[http://dx.doi.org/10.1016/j.vetpar.2011.01.009] [PMID: 21295915]

[50]   Kawahara F, Taira K, Nagai S, Onaga H, Onuma M, Nunoya T. Detection of five avian *Eimeria* species by species-specific real-time polymerase chain reaction assay. Avian Dis 2008; 52(4): 652-6.
[http://dx.doi.org/10.1637/8351-050908-Reg.1] [PMID: 19166058]

[51]   Blake DP, Qin Z, Cai J, Smith AL. Development and validation of real-time polymerase chain reaction assays specific to four species of *Eimeria*. Avian Pathol 2008; 37(1): 89-94.
[http://dx.doi.org/10.1080/03079450701802248] [PMID: 18202955]

[52]   Morgan JAT, Morris GM, Wlodek BM, *et al.* Real-time polymerase chain reaction (PCR) assays for the specific detection and quantification of seven *Eimeria* species that cause coccidiosis in chickens. Mol Cell Probes 2009; 23(2): 83-9.
[http://dx.doi.org/10.1016/j.mcp.2008.12.005] [PMID: 19141318]

[53]   Kundu K, Kumar S, Banerjee PS, Garg R. Quantification of *Eimeria necatrix, E. acervulina* and *E. maxima* genomes in commercial chicken farms by quantitative real time PCR. J Parasit Dis 2020; 44(2): 374-80.
[http://dx.doi.org/10.1007/s12639-019-01188-2] [PMID: 32419744]

[54]   Allen PC, Fetterer RH. Recent advances in biology and immunobiology of *Eimeria* species and in

diagnosis and control of infection with these coccidian parasites of poultry. Clin Microbiol Rev. 2002 Jan;15(1):58-65.
[http://dx.doi.org/10.1128/CMR.15.1.58-65.2002]

[55]    Barkway CP, Pocock RL, Vrba V, Blake DP. Loop-mediated isothermal amplification (LAMP) assays for the species-specific detection of *Eimeria* that infect chickens. J Vis Exp 2015; 96(96): e52552.
[http://dx.doi.org/10.3791/52552] [PMID: 25741643]

[56]    Ciloglu A, Ellis VA, Bernotienė R, Valkiūnas G, Bensch S. A new one-step multiplex PCR assay for simultaneous detection and identification of avian haemosporidian parasites. Parasitol Res 2019; 118(1): 191-201.
[http://dx.doi.org/10.1007/s00436-018-6153-7] [PMID: 30536121]

[57]    Sambrook J, Russell DW, Irwin N, Janseen KA. Molecular cloning-A laboratory manual. 3rd ed. New York: Cold Sping Harbor Laboratory Press 2001; pp. 6.1-6.62.

# CHAPTER 7

# Anthelminthic Drug Resistance and One Health Approach

**Manoj Kumar Singh**[1] and **Jinu Manoj**[2,*]

[1] *Department of Livestock Production and Management, College of Veterinary and Animal Sciences, Sardar Vallabhbhai Patel University of Agriculture and Technology, Meerut 250110, Uttar Pradesh, India*

[2] *Department of Veterinary Public Health & Epidemiology, College Central Laboratory, Lala Lajpat Rai University of Veterinary and Animal Sciences, Hisar 125004, Haryana, India*

**Abstract:** Anthelminthic resistance (AR) is a significant global concern in both human and veterinary medicine. Understanding the types of AR resistance is crucial for designing effective parasite control strategies to preserve the efficacy of available anthelmintics as well as to minimize the risk of resistance development. The development of anthelminthic resistance is an interdisciplinary process influenced by factors such as host, parasite, anthelminthic type, management practices, and environmental conditions. Diagnosis of AR is possible by both *in vivo* and *in vitro* methods and early detection of resistance allows for timely intervention strategies. The research and surveillance programs are important for its prevention and management. The promotion of good hygiene practices, education, and awareness can reduce the spread of AR. AR issue requires coordinated efforts at local, national, and international levels. Implementation of policies and regulations to control the use of anthelminthic drugs in both human and veterinary medicine is necessary by adopting the one health approach.

**Keywords:** Anthelminthic resistance, Livestock, One health, Stewardship.

## INTRODUCTION

Anthelmintics are crucial in managing parasitic infections in livestock. Liver flukes, lungworms and gastrointestinal nematodes are the helminths that parasitize livestock. These infections are among the most significant worldwide production-limiting illnesses and they have the potential to cause serious illness and decrease productivity in every category of animals [1].

---

* **Corresponding author Jinu Manoj:** Department of Veterinary Public Health & Epidemiology, College Central Laboratory, Lala Lajpat Rai University of Veterinary and Animal Sciences, Hisar 125004, Haryana, India; E-mail: drjinumanoj@gmail.com

Anthelminthic drug resistance refers to the phenomenon where parasites, particularly helminths, develop reduced susceptibility or complete resistance to anthelminthic drugs used to treat or control them. The development of anthelmintic drug resistance is a significant concern in both human and veterinary medicine, as it can lead to treatment failure, decreased productivity, increased disease transmission, and economic losses in agriculture. Anthelminthic resistance (AR) has been reported in various animal species including livestock (cattle, sheep, goats, and pigs), horses, pets (dogs and cats) and wildlife. This resistance can occur in various types of parasites, including roundworms, lungworms and liver flukes and poses a significant challenge in the control and management of parasitic infections in animals. The most common parasites associated with anthelminthic resistance in veterinary medicine include *Haemonchus contortus* (barber's pole worm), *Trichostrongylus* spp., *Cooperia* spp. and *Ostertagia* spp.

## COMMON ANTHELMINTHICS

Three kinds of anthelminthics are most widely used among livestock.

**Benzimidazoles (BZs):** This class includes drugs like albendazole and fenbendazole. They act by disrupting the parasite's ability to maintain cellular integrity, leading to paralysis and death. Resistance to BZs has become widespread due to their long history of use and the development of resistance mechanisms by parasites [2].

**Macrocyclic lactones (MLs):** MLs such as ivermectin and doramectin exert their anthelminthic effects by interfering with nerve transmission in parasites, ultimately causing paralysis and death. While resistance to MLs was initially less common, it has been increasingly reported, particularly in gastrointestinal nematodes.

**Cholinergic agonists**: Levamisole acts by stimulating nicotinic acetylcholine receptors in the parasite, leading to paralysis and expulsion. Resistance to levamisole has also been documented, although it tends to be less prevalent compared to BZs and MLs.

## GLOBAL PREVALENCE

The development of anthelmintic resistance is a global phenomenon affecting various helminths across multiple animal species and affecting both developed and developing countries. The key points for the widespread nature of AR are diverse helminth species, multiple anthelminthic classes, diverse environments and management practices, wide animal range as host, and easy global distribution.

It has been reported in various regions and across different livestock production systems. The prevalence of anthelminthic resistance varies depending on factors such as the type of parasite, geographical location, drug usage patterns, and farming practices. Some regions, such as parts of Europe, Australia, and the Americas, have reported significant levels of anthelminthic resistance in livestock, particularly in sheep and cattle. Anthelminthic resistance is indeed a concern in Asia, particularly in countries where there's extensive use of anthelminthic drugs in agriculture and animal husbandry. While specific data on the prevalence of anthelminthic resistance in Asia may vary by country and region, there have been reports of resistance emerging in various livestock species, including cattle, sheep, and goats [3].

## TYPES OF RESISTANCE

Cross-resistance, side resistance and multiple resistance are three different types of anthelminthic resistance. These types of anthelminthic resistance underscore the complex interactions between parasites and anthelminthics, as well as the adaptability of parasites to develop resistance mechanisms. Understanding these types of resistance is crucial for designing effective parasite control strategies that minimize the risk of resistance development and preserve the efficacy of available anthelmintics.

**Cross Resistance:** In cross-resistance, a parasite strain develops tolerance to therapeutic doses of anthelmintics that are chemically unrelated or have different mechanisms of action. This means that resistance to one type of anthelminthic confers resistance to others, even if they belong to different classes. For example, a parasite strain resistant to benzimidazoles may also exhibit resistance to macrocyclic lactones or cholinergic agonists. Cross-resistance highlights the ability of parasites to develop broad resistance mechanisms that affect multiple drug classes.

**Side Resistance**: Side resistance occurs when resistance to one anthelminthic is conferred by the selection pressure exerted by another anthelminthic having an analogous mode of functioning. In other words, exposure to one anthelminthic results in the emergence of resistance to another anthelminthic with a comparable mode of action. An example of side resistance is seen among benzimidazole anthelmintics, where strains resistant to one benzimidazole may also show resistance to another benzimidazole due to shared mechanisms of action.

**Multiple Resistance**: Multiple resistance refers to the development of resistance to two or more anthelmintics, either belonging to the same class or different classes, due to independent selection pressures or side resistance mechanisms. This type of resistance represents a significant challenge in parasite control because it reduces the effectiveness of multiple drug classes, limiting treatment options. For instance, a parasite strain may exhibit resistance to both benzimidazoles and macrocyclic lactones, rendering these anthelmintics ineffective against the infection.

## FACTORS FOR ANTHELMINTHIC RESISTANCE

The development of anthelminthic resistance is an interdisciplinary process influenced by various factors. The interplay between host, parasite, anthelminthic type, management practices, and environmental conditions creates a multifaceted landscape where resistance can emerge and spread [4].

**Host Factors**: The genetic makeup and immune status of the host animal can affect its susceptibility to parasitic infections and the effectiveness of anthelminthic treatments. In some cases, repeated exposure to anthelminthic drugs may disrupt the balance between host immunity and parasite survival, leading to the emergence of resistance. Animals with genetic resistance to parasites may require fewer treatments, reducing the selection pressure for resistance. Hosts with weakened immune systems may be less able to clear infections increasing the risk of treatment failure and the selection of resistant parasites [5].

**Parasite Factors**: Some parasite populations may possess inherent genetic variations that can contribute to differences in susceptibility to anthelmintics and the development of resistance. Parasites may develop cross-resistance to multiple classes of anthelminthic drugs due to shared mechanisms of action or similar drug targets. These genetic factors can be passed down through generations, contributing to the spread of resistance within parasite populations. Mutations in genes associated with drug targets or drug metabolism can confer resistance. Factors such as high rates of reproduction, genetic diversity within parasite populations, and migration of parasites between hosts can influence the spread of resistance alleles within parasite populations [6].

**Environmental factors**: Climatic characteristics such as temperature, humidity, rainfall and soil type can affect the survival and transmission of parasite larvae on pasture. Certain environmental factors may facilitate the persistence and spread of resistant parasite strains, particularly in areas with high parasite burdens. Climatic conditions also influence the seasonal patterns of parasite infections, which may impact the timing and frequency of anthelminthic treatments.

**Indiscriminate use of Anthelminthics**: One of the primary drivers of anthelminthic resistance is the overuse and misuse of anthelminthic drugs in both human and veterinary medicine. The extensive use of these drugs can also contribute to the development of resistance in parasite populations. Different classes of anthelmintics exert their effects through distinct mechanisms, and the frequency and timing of their use can impact the development of resistance. Frequent or inappropriate administration of these drugs can exert selective pressure on parasite populations, favoring the survival and reproduction of resistant individuals.

**Inadequate Treatment Regimens**: Incorrect dosing of anthelminthic drugs, such as underdosing or overdosing, can contribute to the development of resistance. Underdosing may not eliminate all parasites, allowing resistant individuals to survive and propagate, while overdosing can increase the selection pressure for resistance [7].

**Lack of Rotation and Alternation**: Repeated use of the same class of anthelminthic drugs without rotation or alternation can lead to the selection of resistant parasites. Rotating between different classes of drugs with distinct mechanisms of action can help delay the development of resistance by reducing the frequency of exposure to any single drug.

**Animal Management Practices**: Management practices such as stocking density, grazing rotation and quarantine protocols can influence parasite exposure and transmission rates. Practices that reduce parasite burden and minimize stress on the host animals can help mitigate the risk of AR.

## DIAGNOSIS OF ANTHELMINTHIC RESISTANCE

Diagnosing anthelminthic resistance requires a combination of field and laboratory-based techniques to accurately assess drug efficacy and resistance status in parasite populations for effective monitoring.

### *In Vivo* Methods

Fecal Egg Count Reduction Test (FECRT): The FECRT is the standard *in vivo* method for assessing anthelminthic efficacy in livestock. It involves collecting fecal samples from a group of animals before and after treatment with an anthelminthic drug. Fecal samples are analyzed to determine the number of parasite eggs per gram (EPG) of feces. A significant reduction in EPG following treatment indicates that the drug was effective against the parasites present. If the reduction in EPG is less than expected (usually <95%), it suggests the presence of anthelmintic resistance. The time between treatment and the second egg count differs based on the anthelminthic drug group. A post-treatment egg count for benzimidazoles needs to be undertaken within 10-14 days of anthelminthic administration. If there is suspicion of levamisole resistance, fecal samples must be obtained no later than seven days post-treatment [8].

**Dose Confirmation Test:** In cases where resistance is suspected based on FECRT results, a dose confirmation test may be conducted to verify the resistance phenotype. This involves administering a higher dose of the suspected anthelminthic drug to a separate group of animals and then performing FECRT to assess efficacy. If the higher dose fails to achieve the expected reduction in EPG, it provides further evidence of anthelminthic resistance.

*In Vitro* **Methods**

**Egg Hatch Assay (EHA):** The EHA is a laboratory-based test (*in vitro*) used to assess the susceptibility of parasite eggs to anthelminthic drugs. Fecal samples are processed to isolate parasite eggs, which are then incubated in the presence of various concentrations of the anthelminthic drug in question. The percentage of eggs that successfully hatch in the presence of the drug is compared to control samples to determine drug efficacy and resistance status. This method has been developed to identify resistance to the Benzimidazoles class of anthelmintics. Imidazothiazoles, macrocyclic lactones and tetrahydropyrimidines are not ovicidal, hence the test is not appropriate for their usage.

**Larval Development Assay (LDA):** The LDA evaluates the susceptibility of parasite larvae to anthelminthic drugs. Larvae are collected from fecal samples and cultured *in vitro* in the presence of different drug concentrations. A solid or liquid nutritive medium can be used for incubation. The development and viability of larvae are assessed to determine drug efficacy and resistance status. Using this method, AR against the majority of anthelminthic categories is identified. The test's LD50 (larval 50% death) has been found to vary according to when the infection occurs, particularly when macrocyclic lactones are used.

**Larval Motility Test (LMT):** Larvae are cultured in the dark at 25°C for 24 hours at different medication doses. These are then allowed to remain in light for twenty minutes to stimulate the ones who are not paralyzed. Subsequently, the percentage of nonmotile larvae relative to all larvae available at each medication concentration is computed [9].

**Molecular Techniques:** Molecular methods, such as polymerase chain reaction (PCR) assays, can be used to detect genetic markers associated with anthelminthic resistance. These techniques can provide rapid and sensitive detection of resistance-associated mutations in parasite populations, helping to confirm resistance status. This method facilitates the genotyping of susceptible or resistant adult worms and larvae. Genotyping for mutations on the β-tubulin gene, which is associated with benzimidazole resistance is reported using a PCR-based approach.

## PREVENTION METHODS

Preventing anthelminthic resistance involves several strategies aimed at preserving the effectiveness of anthelminthic medications over time. Ongoing surveillance and monitoring of resistance levels are also essential for early detection and appropriate management strategies.

**Research and Surveillance:** It is essential to conduct regular surveillance and monitoring to detect and manage resistance effectively, thereby preserving the effectiveness of anthelminthic drugs for future use. Ongoing research is essential to understand the mechanisms of anthelmintic resistance and develop new strategies for its prevention and management. Surveillance programs are also important for monitoring resistance levels and trends in parasite populations. Early detection of resistance allows for timely intervention strategies.

**Management Strategies:** To combat anthelminthic resistance, veterinarians and livestock producers employ several management strategies such as the rational use of anthelminthic medications, proper dosage, and administration based on weight, using combination therapies, rotation of different classes of anthelminthic drugs and targeted treatment based on diagnostic testing, breeding for resistance or resilience to parasites in livestock populations, *etc*. Additionally, maintaining good pasture and grazing management practices, such as rotational grazing, quarantine of infected animals, and avoiding overstocking, can help reduce parasite burdens and slow the development of resistance.

Promotion of good hygiene practices, including proper sanitation and waste disposal, can reduce the spread of parasitic infections in communities. Providing education and awareness to farmers, veterinarians, and the general public on responsible anthelminthic use, the risks of anthelminthic resistance, and alternative parasite control methods can prevent the development of AR. Implementation of policies and regulations to control the use of anthelminthic drugs in both human and veterinary medicine, including restrictions on over-the-counter sales and prescription requirements are to be enforced [10].

## ONE HEALTH APPROACH

The concept of a One Health approach emphasizes the interconnectedness of human, animal and environmental health. When it comes to addressing anthelminthic resistance, adopting a One Health approach is crucial because factors contributing to resistance development involve not only veterinary and agricultural practices but also human health considerations. Anthelminthic resistance poses a significant threat to animal health and welfare as well as to the sustainability of livestock production systems. By understanding the underlying factors driving resistance development, efforts can be directed toward implementing effective strategies to mitigate its impact. Addressing this issue requires a multifaceted approach involving collaboration between veterinarians, researchers, livestock producers, and regulatory agencies to implement effective control measures and preserve the efficacy of anthelminthic drugs.

Due to the global nature of AR, this issue requires coordinated efforts at local, national, and international levels. Organizations such as the World Health Organization (WHO) and the Food and Agriculture Organization (FAO) recognize the importance of addressing anthelminthic resistance and advocate for integrated parasite management strategies. Strategies such as responsible anthelminthic use, integrated parasite management, surveillance and monitoring programs, and research into alternative control methods are essential for managing AR effectively and preserving the efficacy of anthelminthics for future generations. The One Health approaches that can be applied to tackle anthelminthic resistance are as follows:

**Interdisciplinary Collaboration**: Veterinarians, physicians, public health officials, researchers, farmers, and environmental scientists need to collaborate to develop comprehensive strategies to address anthelminthic resistance. By pooling their expertise, these stakeholders can develop more effective interventions.

**Surveillance and Monitoring**: Implementing surveillance programs to monitor the prevalence and spread of anthelminthic resistance in both human and animal populations is essential. This involves collecting data on resistance patterns, identifying hotspots, and tracking trends over time [8].

**Education and Awareness**: Educating healthcare providers, veterinarians, farmers, and the public about the importance of responsible anthelminthic use, proper dosing, and the risks associated with resistance can help promote behavior change and adherence to best practices.

**Stewardship**: Promoting judicious use of anthelminthic drugs through stewardship programs can help reduce the selection pressure for resistance. This includes using the right drug at the right dose for the right duration and avoiding unnecessary or prophylactic treatments.

**Alternative Control Strategies**: Encouraging the development and adoption of alternative control strategies, such as integrated parasite management, biological control methods and genetic selection for resistance-resistant livestock breeds can help reduce reliance on anthelminthic drugs.

**Regulatory Measures**: Implementing regulations and guidelines for the use of anthelminthic drugs in both veterinary and human medicine can help ensure responsible use and minimize the emergence of resistance. This may include restrictions on over-the-counter sales, prescription requirements, and monitoring of drug residues in food products.

**Research and Innovation**: Investing in research to better understand the mechanisms of anthelmintic resistance, develop new drug compounds, diagnostics, and vaccines, and improve treatment regimens is essential for staying ahead of evolving resistance patterns [7].

By adopting a One Health approach, stakeholders can work together to address the complex and interconnected challenges posed by anthelminthic resistance, ultimately safeguarding human, animal, and environmental health.

## CONCLUDING REMARKS

The development of anthelmintic resistance is a complex process influenced by various factors such as the parasite, the animal treated, the type of anthelminthic used, and its application resulting from the extensive use of anthelmintics to manage helminths in livestock. The development of AR is significantly influenced by anthelminthic misuse, which includes underdosing, treating all animals simultaneously on the same farm, administering the same anthelminthic continuously, using anthelminthic of inferior quality, and using anthelminthic frequently. The main mechanisms of anthelminthic resistance are increased drug metabolism, modification of drug receptor sites that decrease drug binding or the functional consequences of drug binding, upregulation of cellular efflux mechanisms, and decreased drug receptor abundance through the reduced expression within the parasite. There are no other effective ways to control parasitic helminths except the application of anthelmintics. Additionally, the development of new anthelmintics to manage AR is a slow and costly process. For these reasons, it is critical to use anthelmintics that are currently available in a way that minimizes the impact of AR such as appropriate administration of anthelmintics and decreased dependence on anthelmintics, therefore, regular surveillance and monitoring of AR development are very critical.

## REFERENCES

[1]    Brown TL, Airs PM, Porter S, Caplat P, Morgan ER. Understanding the role of wild ruminants in anthelmintic resistance in livestock. Biol Lett 2022; 18(5): 20220057.
[http://dx.doi.org/10.1098/rsbl.2022.0057] [PMID: 35506237]

[2]    Charlier J, Hoste H, Sotiraki S. COMBAR – Combatting anthelmintic resistance in ruminants. Parasite 2023; 30: E1.
[http://dx.doi.org/10.1051/parasite/2023006] [PMID: 36762940]

[3]     Fissiha W, Kinde MZ. Anthelmintic resistance and its mechanism: a review. Infect Drug Resist 2021; 14: 5403-10.
[http://dx.doi.org/10.2147/IDR.S332378] [PMID: 34938088]

[4]     Macedo LO, Silva SS, Alves LC, Carvalho GA, Ramos RAN. An overview of anthelmintic resistance in domestic ruminants in Brazil. Ruminants 2023; 3(3): 214-32.
[http://dx.doi.org/10.3390/ruminants3030020]

[5]     Ng'etich AI, Amoah ID, Bux F, Kumari S. Anthelmintic resistance in soil-transmitted helminths: One-Health considerations. Parasitol Res 2024; 123(1): 62.
[http://dx.doi.org/10.1007/s00436-023-08088-8] [PMID: 38114766]

[6]     OIE. World Organisation for Animal Health. Responsible and prudent use of anthelmintic chemicals to help control anthelmintic resistance in grazing livestock species. Paris: OIE 2021.

[7]     Picot S, Beugnet F, Leboucher G, Bienvenu AL. Drug resistant parasites and fungi from a one-health perspective: A global concern that needs transdisciplinary stewardship programs. One Health 2022; 14: 100368.
[http://dx.doi.org/10.1016/j.onehlt.2021.100368] [PMID: 34957316]

[8]     Sangster NC, Cowling A, Woodgate RG. Ten events that defined anthelmintic resistance research. Trends Parasitol 2018; 34(7): 553-63.
[http://dx.doi.org/10.1016/j.pt.2018.05.001] [PMID: 29803755]

[9]     Waller PJ. The development of anthelmintic resistance in ruminant livestock. Acta Trop 1994; 56(2-3): 233-43.
[http://dx.doi.org/10.1016/0001-706X(94)90065-5] [PMID: 8203305]

[10]    Zekarias T, Toka T. A review of anthelmintic resistance in domestic animals. Acta Parasitologica Globalis 2019; 10(3): 117.

# CHAPTER 8

# Vaccines and Vaccination of Parasitic Diseases

**Furqan Munir[1], Amna Shakoor[2], Muhammad Tahir Aleem[3,\*] and Shahbaz Ul Haq[3]**

[1] *Department of Parasitology, Faculty of Veterinary Science, University of Agriculture, Faisalabad 38040, Pakistan*

[2] *Department of Anatomy, Faculty of Veterinary Science, University of Agriculture, Faisalabad 38040, Pakistan*

[3] *Department of Pharmacology, Shantou University Medical College, Shantou 515041, China*

**Abstract:** The poultry industry is one of the largest sources of meat and eggs for human consumption throughout the globe. For this, vaccination is needed due to the complexity of parasites and their life cycles. In addition, viral outbreaks in farmed stock are a very common occurrence and also a major source of concern for the industry. Mortality as well as morbidity in the flock during an outbreak can cause economic losses with a subsequent detrimental impact on the global food chain. Mass vaccination program is one of the main strategies to control viral infection in poultry. It can reduce husbandry costs. The vaccination protocol is essential to counteract emerging and re-emerging viral infectious diseases in poultry. Potential antigens for recombinant vaccines have also been incorporated for the viral infection. The book chapter describes viral vaccines and vaccination regimens available for common poultry viral infections.

**Keywords:** Poultry diseases, Production, Vaccine, Vaccination.

## INTRODUCTION

The production of meat and eggs from poultry farming is a crucial source of protein, making it a fundamental component of the global food business. The sector does, however, confront a number of difficulties, one of which is the risk of parasitic infections [1]. In chicken production, parasites are a major problem since they can cause lower output, higher mortality rates, and large financial losses. Numerous parasites, including helminths, ectoparasites, and protozoa, are responsible for these illnesses; each poses distinct difficulties for prevention and management [2]. Numerous types of protozoan parasites have the potential to

---

\* **Corresponding author Muhammad Tahir Aleem:** Department of Pharmacology, Shantou University Medical College, Shantou 515041, China; E-mail: dr.tahir1990@gmail.com

**Tanmoy Rana (Ed.)**

spread disease, making them a serious threat to poultry farms. *Eimeria*, the protozoan parasite that causes coccidiosis, is one of the most prevalent infections that affect poultry. A serious illness called coccidiosis can cause severe intestinal damage or even death in certain situations. The chicken industry makes extensive use of coccidiosis vaccines that have been produced. Usually administered as live attenuated or subunit vaccines, these shots offer defense against certain *Eimeria* species [3]. *Histomonas meleagridis*, another significant protozoan parasite, is the causative agent of histomoniasis, also referred to as blackhead sickness. In poultry, particularly in turkeys, histomoniasis can be a fatal condition with significant fatality rates. It is possible to prevent chickens from the disease histomoniasis by administering vaccines against it. Usually, these vaccinations are whole-cell vaccines that are killed or attenuated from live viruses to protect against *H. meleagridis*. Another protozoan disease that can afflict poultry is cryptosporidiosis. It is caused by *Cryptosporidium* spp. and affected birds may have diarrhea and weight loss. Research is currently concentrating on identifying appropriate antigens for vaccine development, as the development of vaccines against cryptosporidiosis is still in its early phases (Fig. **1**) [4].

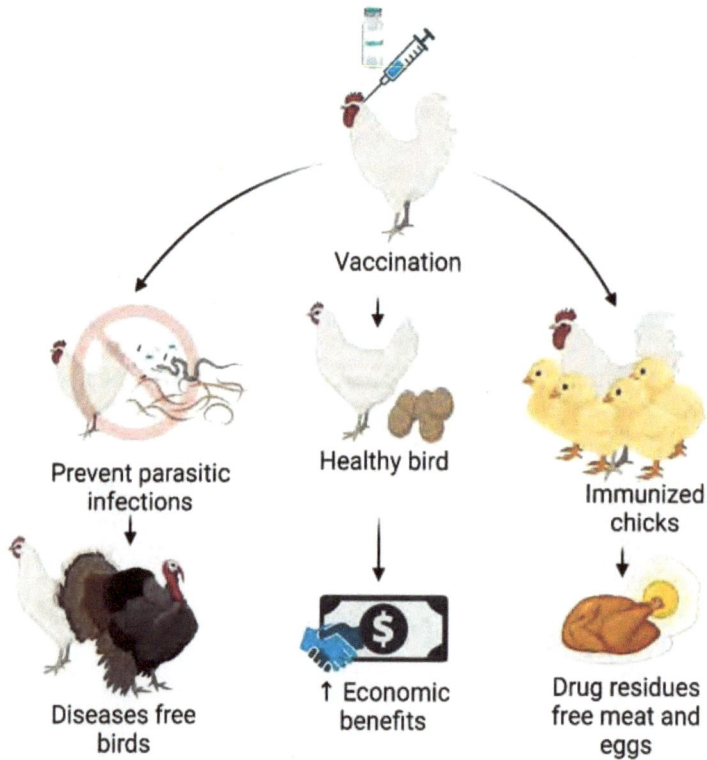

**Fig. (1).** Beneficial effects of vaccination in poultry.

Similarly, helminthic parasites, such as cestodes, nematodes, and trematodes, can severely increase the morbidity and mortality rate in chickens. In poultry, *Ascaridia galli* is the common helminth that causes ascaridiosis. Ascaridiosis vaccines have been developed and are used to protect poultry from the parasites. Usually, the recombinant antigens used in these vaccinations offer defense against *A. galli. Heterakis gallinarum* is the source of heteroakiasis, another significant helminthic infection in poultry. Heterakiasis vaccines have been developed and are used to protect birds from this parasite. Usually, the recombinant antigens used in these vaccines offer protection against *H. gallinarum* (Pleidrup *et al.*, [4]). Similarly, ectoparasites like fleas, lice, and mites are common in chickens and can lead to decreased egg production, skin irritation, and feather damage. *Dermanyssus gallinae*-caused mite infestations are a major problem in chicken husbandry. *D. gallinae* vaccines have been created and are used to keep poultry safe from this ectoparasite. Usually, recombinant antigens used in these vaccinations offer defense against *D. gallinae*. In chicken production, lice infestations brought on by *Menacanthus* and *Goniocotes* species are also a problem. In order to protect against these ectoparasites, recombinant antigens are demonstrating potential as a vaccine against lice infestations [5].

## TYPES OF POULTRY VACCINES

Vaccination is a vital part of managing flock health and preventing disease in poultry. Poultry are protected against a variety of bacterial, viral, and parasite infections using a variety of vaccines. These vaccinations are carefully chosen according to the particular needs of the poultry operation, the type of disease, and the age of the birds. Developing vaccination programs that effectively protect the health and welfare of chicken flocks requires an understanding of the various vaccine types and how they work [6]. In the poultry enterprise, live attenuated vaccines are a commonly used vaccine type. The disease-causing organism is present in these vaccinations in weaker forms that can replicate within the host but do not cause diseases. A robust immunological response is triggered by this vaccine, which results in the formation of lifelong immunity. Live attenuated vaccines can be administered to flocks of chickens in large quantities since they can be given orally. The Marek's disease vaccine, which offers protection against the highly contagious viral disease that can cause tumors and neurological abnormalities in chickens, is one of the most often used live attenuated vaccines in poultry [7]. Another significant vaccination utilized in poultry is inactivated vaccines, sometimes referred to as killed vaccines. The microorganisms in these vaccines have been rendered inactive or killed by radiation, heat, or chemicals. Since inactivated vaccines can not reproduce within the host, it usually takes more than one dosage to elicit a protective immune response. These vaccinations, which are used to prevent infections, including avian influenza and infectious bursal disease, are frequently given *via* injection [8].

More recently developed subunit vaccinations are playing a bigger role in the chicken business. Purified antigens or protein components obtained from the pathogen are present in these vaccinations. Because subunit vaccines do not include live or complete pathogens, there is a lower chance of side effects. To boost the immune response, they are frequently paired with adjuvants, however. Subunit vaccinations are used to prevent infections, including avian reovirus and chicken pox [9]. Vector vaccinations provide an additional cutting-edge method of immunizing chickens. These vaccinations transfer antigens from the target disease into the host by means of a safe virus or bacteria. As the carrier organism multiplies inside the host, the antigens trigger a potent immunological reaction. When it comes to targeting certain infections that are challenging to manage with conventional immunizations, vector vaccines are very helpful. For instance, the fowlpox virus vector vaccine is used to treat avian influenza, whereas the herpes virus of the turkey vector vaccine is used to treat Newcastle disease [10].

## MECHANISM OF VACCINES BEHIND THE GENERATION OF PROTECTIVE IMMUNITY

In veterinary medicine, one important discovery has been the development of vaccinations to prevent and control parasite infections in poultry. With the help of these vaccines, chickens' immune systems will be stimulated to identify and react to particular parasite antigens, protecting them from infection. These vaccines, which include DNA, subunit, inactivated, and live attenuated vaccines, have different modes of action based on their specific types. Live attenuated vaccines are produced from live parasites that have undergone attenuation or weakening in order to lessen their pathogenic potential. These vaccinations imitate natural illnesses in chickens, eliciting a strong and long-lasting immune response. Within the host, the live parasites multiply, inducing humoral and cell-mediated immunity. This kind of vaccination works especially well against parasites that break into host cells, like the *Eimeria* species that cause coccidiosis in chickens. A single dosage of live attenuated vaccines can confer lifetime immunity, but there is a chance that they could revert to a virulent form [11]. Using physical or chemical techniques, parasites are killed or rendered inactive in order to develop inactivated vaccines. Although these vaccinations are safe, in order to maximize the immune response, many doses and adjuvants are frequently needed. Vaccines that have been inactivated mainly generate humoral immunity, which includes the generation of antibodies. When compared to live vaccinations, inactivated vaccines often have a lower ability to induce cell-mediated immunity [12].

Subunit vaccines comprise certain proteins or antigens that are obtained from parasites. Although these vaccines are quite safe and well-purified, they might need adjuvants or different delivery methods to increase their immunogenicity. Subunit vaccinations mainly induce humoral immunity, which results in the production of anti-parasite antibodies. Subunit vaccinations can offer sustained immunity, although repeated doses may be necessary to sustain protection [13]. The direct injection of DNA-encoding parasite antigens into the host is the method used in DNA vaccinations. After that, the host cells translate and transcribe the DNA to create the parasite antigens, which trigger an immunological reaction. DNA vaccines are relatively simple and inexpensive to make, and they can induce both humoral and cell-mediated immunity. To improve their effectiveness, though, they might need to be administered *via* adjuvants or delivery methods. DNA vaccinations are a potential method of managing parasite infections in chickens, but further study is required to maximize their potency [14].

## Vaccines for Coccidiosis

In poultry, coccidiosis is a common and economically important disease that is brought on by *Eimeria*-genus protozoan parasites. The illness affects the hens' digestive systems, which results in decreased feed efficiency, stunted growth, and in extreme situations, death. Coccidiosis can only be controlled by vaccination, and the chicken industry uses a variety of vaccinations to manage and prevent the disease [15]. Among the most often used vaccinations for the prevention of coccidiosis in chickens are live attenuated vaccines. The live *Eimeria* parasites used in these vaccinations have been attenuated or weakened to lessen their toxicity while maintaining their capacity to elicit an immune response. Live attenuated vaccinations stimulate humoral immunity as well as cell-mediated immunity when given to chickens because they reproduce in the colon. These vaccinations offer robust and durable protection, which makes them an important instrument for programs aimed at controlling coccidiosis [16].

Certain proteins or antigens obtained from *Eimeria* parasites are included in subunit vaccinations against coccidiosis. After being refined, these antigens are given to chickens in an attempt to elicit an immunological response. Although adjuvants and numerous doses may be necessary to maximize the effectiveness of subunit vaccinations, they are safe and efficacious. For the best protection, these vaccines are frequently used in conjunction with live attenuated vaccines, which are especially helpful in targeting particular *Eimeria* species [17]. One kind of subunit vaccination made with recombinant DNA technology is the recombinant vaccine. The antigens in these vaccinations are created in labs with genetically modified organisms. Recombinant vaccines are frequently quite successful and can be modified to specifically target a certain type of *Eimeria*. Recombinant vaccines have a high degree of specificity and efficacy, as these vaccines present a viable strategy for controlling coccidiosis [16]. A more recent method of coccidiosis vaccination is vector vaccines. These vaccines transfer *Eimeria* antigens to the host's immune system using live viruses or bacteria as vectors. After the vector multiplies in the host, the immune system is triggered and the *Eimeria* antigens are expressed. Strong and enduring immunity can be produced *via* vector vaccinations, but in order to guarantee safety and effectiveness, the vector may need to be carefully chosen. These vaccinations present a fresh method for controlling coccidiosis, and they might be especially helpful in combating several *Eimeria* species at once [18].

Ionophore anticoccidials, although not vaccinations in the conventional sense, are frequently used to protect chickens against coccidiosis [19]. To regulate *Eimeria* populations in the colon, these substances—monensin and salinomycin, for example—are introduced to diet at low concentrations. Ionophores cause the parasite to die by upsetting its ion balance. They are a crucial part of programs to prevent coccidiosis and are frequently used in conjunction with vaccinations for the best possible management (Fig. **2**).

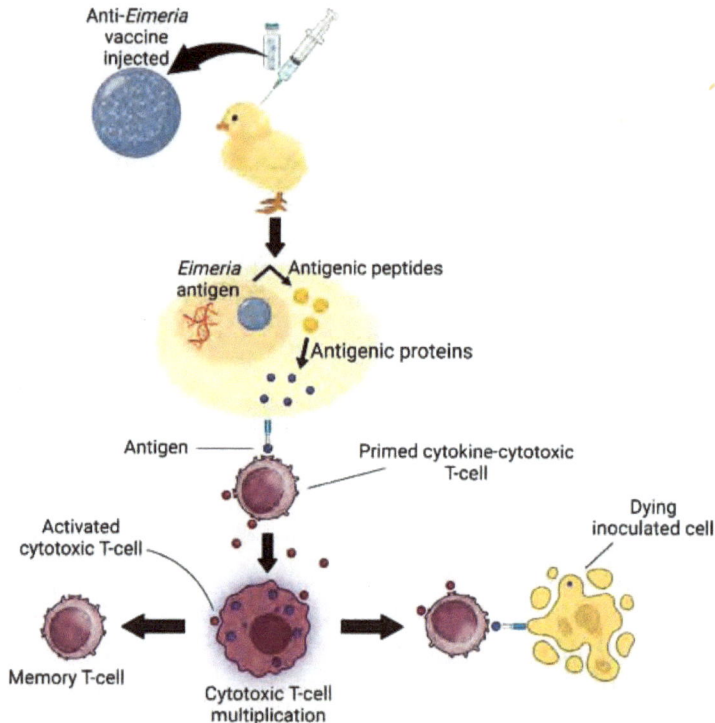

**Fig. (2).**  Mechanism of anti-*Eimeria* vaccine.

## Vaccine against *Histomonas meleagridis*

Blackhead disease, or histomoniasis, is a protozoan parasite that affects poultry. It is caused by *Histomonas meleagridis*. This illness poses a serious risk to the global chicken business, resulting in financial losses from mortality, lower egg yields, and lower-quality meat. Chemotherapeutic drugs, which are mostly dependent on current management measures, carry hazards of their own, including drug resistance and residues in poultry products. Thus, for the long-term management of histomoniasis in poultry, the creation of a secure and potent vaccine against *H. meleagridis* is essential [20]. The main species of domestic poultry affected by histomoniasis are turkeys, chickens, and other fowl. Lesions in the liver, ceca, and other organs are the disease's hallmark, and in extreme cases, it can be fatal. The intermediary host, the cecal worm *Heterakis gallinarum*, is the vehicle by which histomonads are spread. The histomonads cause tissue injury and inflammation when they invade the liver and ceca after being consumed by the bird [21].

Both innate immunity and adaptive immunity are involved in the complicated host immunological response to *H. meleagridis*. Pattern recognition receptors (PRRs) on innate immune cells identify hemomonads, which trigger the release of pro-inflammatory cytokines and the activation of phagocytic cells. The removal of the parasite is mostly dependent on adaptive immunity, especially cell-mediated immunity involving T cells. For maximum protection, innate and adaptive immune responses should be stimulated in the creation of an *H. meleagridis* vaccine [22]. Research on the immune response to histomonosis to date has mostly concentrated on various characteristics of the adaptive immune system. The interaction between innate and adaptive immune cells results from the activation of toll-like receptors, which has an impact on the clonal growth of B and T cells [23]. Controlling histomoniasis in chicken flocks depends on the development of a vaccination against the parasite *Histomonas meleagridis*. To tackle this parasite, a number of commercial vaccinations have been developed or are currently being developed. A live attenuated vaccine called Histostat, which contains a non-virulent strain of *H. meleagridis*, is one example. Orally given to day-old chicks, histostat stimulates a robust immune response that protects against histomoniasis. Another illustration is the vaccine Paracox, which has a mixture of coccidian parasite oocysts, including species of *Eimeria* known to offer partial cross-protection against *H. meleagridis* [24]. When given orally to chickens and turkeys, paracox has been demonstrated to lessen the severity of histomoniasis in animals that have received vaccinations. These commercial vaccines serve as an illustration of the continuous work being done to produce potent *H. meleagridis* vaccines and enhance the welfare and health of chickens across the globe.

## Vaccine against *Leucozytozoon caulleryi*

The protozoan parasite *Leucocytozoon caulleryi* is the source of leucocytozoonosis, a serious illness that primarily affects hens. The parasite spreads *via* the bites of Simulium-genus black flies, which act as the vector for the infection. Following transmission, the parasite goes through a convoluted life cycle in the avian host, resulting in a range of clinical symptoms as well as financial losses in the production of chickens [25]. Clinical indicators of *Leucocytozoon caulleryi* infection in chickens include fatigue, lethargy, decreased egg production, and pale wattles and comb. High fatality rates might arise from severe instances, particularly in juvenile birds. Anemia and other pathological alterations are caused by the parasite's merozoites, which are released from the liver and spleen when it matures into schizonts and infects red blood cells [26].

Multiple strategies are necessary for the control and prevention of leucocytozoonosis in poultry. Vector control, which includes using insecticides and environmental management techniques to eliminate fly breeding places, is essential to lowering exposure to infected black flies. It is also crucial to follow good management procedures, which include keeping chicken houses clean and hygienic, lowering stress levels, and boosting immunity through a healthy diet [27]. Leucocytozoonosis in chickens can be controlled and prevented in part *via* vaccination. Unfortunately, there are not any commercially accessible vaccinations that particularly target *L. caulleryi* as of yet. Effective vaccinations against this parasite are still being researched, including DNA, subunit, and live attenuated vaccines [28]. Due to the lack of effective treatment and prevention measures for this disease, an oil-adjuvanted recombinant vaccine (O-rR7) that targets the R7 protein of second-generation *L. caulleryi* schizonts was developed. By contrast, a single vaccine given at 45 days of age produced antibodies that were above 1600 ELISA units for 56 days after the shot, while a single immunization given at 130 days of age produced peak antibody titers that were over 1600 ELISA units for 35 days after the shot. Hens who received a booster immunization did not experience severe clinical disease from an experimental infection with *L. caulleryi* at 256 days when antibody titers had declined; however, hens that had a single vaccination did exhibit mild to severe disease [29].

## Vaccine against *Dermanyssus gallinae*

*Dermanyssus gallinae* is an ectoparasite that feeds on the blood of birds, especially chickens. It is often referred to as the poultry red mite. This mite poses a serious danger to the global chicken industry, resulting in financial losses from reduced egg production, stunted growth, and higher mortality rates in cases of severe infestations. Chemical acaricides have been the main means of controlling *D. gallinae*; however, worries about resistance, the impact on the environment, and residues in poultry products have driven the quest for alternate control methods. The development of vaccinations to prevent *D. gallinae* is one promising strategy [30]. The intricate biology and life cycle of *D. gallinae* present a number of obstacles to the development of a vaccine against it. Molecular biology and immunological method developments, however, have opened up new options for vaccine creation. Proteases, protease inhibitors, and structural proteins are among the several antigen possibilities that have been discovered. These substances are essential to the biology of the mite and its interactions with the host immune system. In experimental animals, these antigens have demonstrated the ability to trigger protective immune responses, which diminish mite infestation and related diseases [31].

The requirement for a formulation that can elicit a potent and sustained immune response is one of the most important factors in the development of a vaccine against *D. gallinae*. Oil-based formulations and particle delivery methods are examples of adjuvants that have been studied to increase the immunogenicity of antigens and extend their release, thus increasing vaccine efficacy. The timing, dosage, and mode of administration of the immunization all play a significant role in how well the vaccine works to control mite infestations [32]. When *D. gallinae* vaccines are tested in the field, a group of birds are usually vaccinated, and their production, health, and mite infestation levels are compared to those of an unvaccinated control group. The trials are carried out over a lengthy time to evaluate the vaccine's long-term safety and efficacy [33]. One such field trial that was effective was the one where vaccination against *D. gallinae* was used based on recombinant antigens. In this experiment, a control group of laying hens received no vaccination, and another group received the recombinant antigen vaccination. When compared to the control group, the vaccinated group's mite infestation levels were significantly lower. The inoculated hens also showed increased health and egg production, demonstrating the vaccine's efficacy in eradicating *D. gallinae* infestations [34]. An additional field trial examined the application of an adjuvant vaccination based on oil against *D. gallinae*. In this trial, a group of broiler chickens received the vaccine, while a control group was given a formulation that contained only adjuvants. The vaccination proved effective in reducing *D. gallinae* infestations in broiler production, as seen by the vaccinated group's enhanced weight growth and decreased mite infestation levels when compared to the control group [35].

## CHALLENGES WITH THE POULTRY PARASITIC VACCINES

It is difficult to develop vaccinations that are effective against parasites that affect poultry, such as *Dermanyssus gallinae*. The intricate biology and life cycle of these parasites present a significant obstacle. The complex ways in which parasites evade host immune responses make it challenging to choose appropriate targets for vaccines. Additionally, the absence of standardized challenge models and evaluation criteria impedes the development of vaccinations against poultry parasites. It can be difficult to reliably determine the efficiency of vaccines against parasites because they may not produce robust, readily detectable immune responses like bacterial or viral infections do [36]. Another noteworthy obstacle is the fluctuation in parasite numbers. The rapid evolution of parasites can result in the generation of resistant strains that can elude protection established by vaccinations. This means that in order to stay up with the evolving parasite landscape, vaccinations must be modified and surveillance must continue. Moreover, vaccinations against parasites in poultry may not be economically feasible. It may be more expensive and difficult to develop and produce vaccinations against parasites than against other infections, particularly in light of the comparatively low market value of individual poultry when compared to other livestock species [37]. There are also practical difficulties in vaccinating chickens. Typically, drinking water, spray, or injections are used to vaccinate poultry. Each method has its own set of difficulties with regard to vaccine durability, effective delivery, and stress on the animals. Furthermore, it can be difficult to guarantee vaccination safety and effectiveness in the field due to the significant variations in environmental factors and management techniques [38].

## FUTURE PERSPECTIVE

Advances in immunology, genetics, and vaccination technology promise a bright future for poultry anti-parasitic vaccines. The identification of novel vaccination targets and antigens using omics techniques, such as transcriptomics and proteomics, which can shed light on parasite biology and host-parasitic interactions, is a crucial component of future advances. By focusing on vital parasite proteins involved in invasion, feeding, or immune evasion, vaccination efficacy may be increased as a result of this information [35]. Additionally, a potential field of study is the application of adjuvants and delivery mechanisms to improve vaccine immunogenicity and stability. Strong immune responses can be induced by adjuvants, and vaccine absorption and release can be enhanced by innovative delivery methods such as nanoparticles or microparticles, which can result in extended immunity. These developments may lead to vaccinations that protect against chicken parasites for an extended period of time with fewer doses [31]. The creation of multi-stage or multi-species vaccinations that target various parasites or phases of a parasite's life cycle represents another potential path for the future. This strategy can simplify immunization regimens and cut expenses by providing greater protection and diminishing the need for repeated vaccinations. Furthermore, the generation of genetically attenuated parasites that can be utilized as live vaccines to provide safe and efficient protection against parasites may be made possible by the application of genetic manipulation techniques, such as gene editing [27].

## CONCLUDING REMARKS

The creation of strong anti-parasitic vaccinations for poultry is an important field of study with enormous potential rewards. Progress in this sector is still being driven by continual technological and scientific developments, despite the difficulties presented by the biology of parasites and the production and distribution of vaccines. The development of safe, effective, and affordable vaccines appears promising for the future. These vaccines would provide a long-term solution to the problem of poultry parasite management and enhance the general health and welfare of poultry. To fully realize the potential of chicken anti-parasitic vaccinations and overcome remaining obstacles, researchers, veterinarians, and the poultry industry must continue to collaborate.

## REFERENCES

[1]     Hauck R, Macklin KS. Vaccination against poultry parasites. Avian Dis 2023; 67(4): 441-9.
        [http://dx.doi.org/10.1637/aviandiseases-D-23-99989] [PMID: 38300662]

[2]     Fatoba AJ, Adeleke MA. Transgenic *Eimeria* parasite: A potential control strategy for chicken coccidiosis. Acta Trop 2020; 205: 105417.
        [http://dx.doi.org/10.1016/j.actatropica.2020.105417] [PMID: 32105666]

[3]     Thomas S, Abraham A, Rodríguez-Mallon A, Unajak S, Bannantine JP. Challenges in veterinary vaccine development. Methods Mol Biol 2022; 2411: 3-34.
        [http://dx.doi.org/10.1007/978-1-0716-1888-2_1] [PMID: 34816396]

[4]     Pleidrup J, Dalgaard TS, Norup LR, *et al. Ascaridia galli* infection influences the development of both humoral and cell-mediated immunity after Newcastle Disease vaccination in chickens. Vaccine 2014; 32(3): 383-92.
        [http://dx.doi.org/10.1016/j.vaccine.2013.11.034] [PMID: 24269617]

[5]     Win SY, Murata S, Fujisawa S, *et al.* Potential of ferritin 2 as an antigen for the development of a universal vaccine for avian mites, poultry red mites, tropical fowl mites, and northern fowl mites. Front Vet Sci 2023; 10: 1182930.2023;
        [http://dx.doi.org/10.3389/fvets.2023.1182930]

[6]     Poudel U, Dahal U, Upadhyaya N, Chaudhari S, Dhakal S. Livestock and poultry production in Nepal and current status of vaccine development. Vaccines (Basel) 2020; 8(2): 322.2020;
        [http://dx.doi.org/10.3390/vaccines8020322]

[7]     Bande F, Arshad SS, Hair Bejo M, Moeini H, Omar AR. Progress and challenges toward the development of vaccines against avian infectious bronchitis. J Immunol Res 2015; 2015: 1-12.
        [http://dx.doi.org/10.1155/2015/424860] [PMID: 25954763]

[8]     Oakeley RD. The limitations of a feed/water based heat-stable vaccine delivery system for Newcastle

disease-control strategies for backyard poultry flocks in sub-Saharan Africa. Prev Vet Med 2000; 47(4): 271-9.
[http://dx.doi.org/10.1016/S0167-5877(00)00169-0] [PMID: 11087958]

[9]     Hein R, Koopman R, García M, *et al.* Review of poultry recombinant vector vaccines. Avian Dis 2021; 65(3): 438-52.
[http://dx.doi.org/10.1637/0005-2086-65.3.438] [PMID: 34699141]

[10]    Bartlett BL, Pellicane AJ, Tyring SK. Vaccine immunology. Dermatol Ther 2009; 22(2): 104-9.
[http://dx.doi.org/10.1111/j.1529-8019.2009.01223.x] [PMID: 19335722]

[11]    Gaghan C, Adams D, Mohammed J, Crespo R, Livingston K, Kulkarni RR. Characterization of vaccine-induced immune responses against coccidiosis in broiler chickens. Vaccine 2022; 40(28): 3893-902.
[http://dx.doi.org/10.1016/j.vaccine.2022.05.043] [PMID: 35623907]

[12]    Porter KR, Raviprakash K. DNA vaccine delivery and improved immunogenicity. Curr Issues Mol Biol 2017; 22: 129-38.
[http://dx.doi.org/10.21775/cimb.022.129] [PMID: 27831541]

[13]    El-Shall NA, Abd El-Hack ME, Albaqami NM, *et al.* Phytochemical control of poultry coccidiosis: a review. Poult Sci 2022; 101(1): 101542.
[http://dx.doi.org/10.1016/j.psj.2021.101542] [PMID: 34871985]

[14]    Min W, Kim WH, Lillehoj EP, Lillehoj HS. Recent progress in host immunity to avian coccidiosis: IL-17 family cytokines as sentinels of the intestinal mucosa. Dev Comp Immunol 2013; 41(3): 418-28.
[http://dx.doi.org/10.1016/j.dci.2013.04.003] [PMID: 23583525]

[15]    Liu Q, Liu X, Zhao X, Zhu XQ, Suo X. Live attenuated anticoccidial vaccines for chickens. Trends Parasitol 2023; 39(12): 1087-99.
[http://dx.doi.org/10.1016/j.pt.2023.09.002] [PMID: 37770352]

[16]    Gumina E, Hall JW, Vecchi B, *et al.* Evaluation of a subunit vaccine candidate (Biotech Vac Cox) against *Eimeria* spp. in broiler chickens. Poult Sci 2021; 100(9): 101329.
[http://dx.doi.org/10.1016/j.psj.2021.101329] [PMID: 34333387]

[17]    Soutter F, Werling D, Nolan M, *et al.* A novel whole yeast-based subunit oral vaccine against *Eimeria tenella* in chickens. Front Immunol 2022; 13: 809711.
[http://dx.doi.org/10.3389/fimmu.2022.809711] [PMID: 35185896]

[18]    Clark S, Kimminau E. Critical review: Future control of blackhead disease (Histomoniasis) in poultry. Avian Dis 2017; 61(3): 281-8.
[http://dx.doi.org/10.1637/11593-012517-ReviewR] [PMID: 28957000]

[19]    Liebhart D, Hess M. Spotlight on Histomonosis (blackhead disease): a re-emerging disease in turkeys and chickens. Avian Pathol 2020; 49(1): 1-4.
[http://dx.doi.org/10.1080/03079457.2019.1654087] [PMID: 31393162]

[20]    Tykałowski B, Śmiałek M, Kowalczyk J, Dziewulska D, Stenzel T, Koncicki A. Phytoncides in the prevention and therapy of blackhead disease and their effect on the turkey immune system. J Vet Res (Pulawy) 2021; 65(1): 79-85.
[http://dx.doi.org/10.2478/jvetres-2021-0010] [PMID: 33817399]

[21]    McDougald LR. Intestinal protozoa important to poultry. Poult Sci 1998; 77(8): 1156-8.
[http://dx.doi.org/10.1093/ps/77.8.1156] [PMID: 9706082]

[22]    Elbestawy AR, Ellakany HF, Abd El-Hamid HS, *et al. Leucocytozoon caulleryi* in Broiler chicken flocks: Clinical, hematologic, histopathologic, and molecular detection. Avian Dis 2021; 65(3): 407-13.
[http://dx.doi.org/10.1637/0005-2086-65.3.407] [PMID: 34427415]

[23]    Pohuang T, Jittimanee S, Junnu S. Pathology and molecular characterization of *Leucocytozoon caulleryi* from backyard chickens in Khon Kaen Province, Thailand. Vet World 2021; 14(10): 2634-9.

[http://dx.doi.org/10.14202/vetworld.2021.2634-2639] [PMID: 34903919]

[24]   Chiang YH, Lin YC, Wang SY, Lee YP, Chen CF. Effects of *Artemisia annua* on experimentally induced leucocytozoonosis in chickens. Poult Sci 2022; 101(4): 101690.
[http://dx.doi.org/10.1016/j.psj.2021.101690] [PMID: 35149282]

[25]   Nakata K, Watarai S, Kodama H, Gotanda T, Ito A, Kume K. Cellular immune responses in chickens induced by recombinant R7 *Leucocytozoon caulleryi* vaccine. J Parasitol 2003; 89(2): 419-22.
[http://dx.doi.org/10.1645/0022-3395(2003)089[0419:CIRICI]2.0.CO;2] [PMID: 12760672]

[26]   Itoh A, Gotanda T. The correlation of protective effects and antibody production in immunized chickens with recombinant R7 vaccine against *Leucocytozoon caulleryi*. J Vet Med Sci 2002; 64(5): 405-11.
[http://dx.doi.org/10.1292/jvms.64.405] [PMID: 12069072]

[27]   Schiavone A, Pugliese N, Otranto D, *et al*. *Dermanyssus gallinae*: the long journey of the poultry red mite to become a vector. Parasit Vectors 2022; 15(1): 29.
[http://dx.doi.org/10.1186/s13071-021-05142-1] [PMID: 35057849]

[28]   Fujisawa S, Murata S, Isezaki M, *et al*. Suppressive modulation of host immune responses by *Dermanyssus gallinae* infestation. Poult Sci 2023; 102(4): 102532.
[http://dx.doi.org/10.1016/j.psj.2023.102532] [PMID: 36796246]

[29]   Price DRG, Küster T, Øines Ø, *et al*. Evaluation of vaccine delivery systems for inducing long-lived antibody responses to *Dermanyssus gallinae* antigen in laying hens. Avian Pathol 2019; 48(sup1): S60-74.
[http://dx.doi.org/10.1080/03079457.2019.1612514]

[30]   Fujisawa S, Murata S, Takehara M, *et al*. *In vitro* characterization of adipocyte plasma membrane-associated protein from poultry red mites, *Dermanyssus gallinae*, as a vaccine antigen for chickens. Vaccine 2021; 39(41): 6057-66.
[http://dx.doi.org/10.1016/j.vaccine.2021.08.104] [PMID: 34509323]

[31]   Xu X, Wang C, Huang Y, *et al*. Evaluation of the vaccine efficacy of three digestive protease antigens from *Dermanyssus gallinae* using an *in vivo* rearing system. Vaccine 2020; 38(49): 7842-9.
[http://dx.doi.org/10.1016/j.vaccine.2020.10.010] [PMID: 33164806]

[32]   Bartley K, Turnbull F, Wright HW, *et al*. Field evaluation of poultry red mite (*Dermanyssus gallinae*) native and recombinant prototype vaccines. Vet Parasitol 2017; 244: 25-34.
[http://dx.doi.org/10.1016/j.vetpar.2017.06.020] [PMID: 28917313]

[33]   Zaheer T, Abbas RZ, Imran M, *et al*. Vaccines against chicken coccidiosis with particular reference to previous decade: progress, challenges, and opportunities. Parasitol Res 2022; 121(10): 2749-63.
[http://dx.doi.org/10.1007/s00436-022-07612-6] [PMID: 35925452]

[34]   Ravikumar R, Chan J, Prabakaran M. Vaccines against major poultry viral diseases: Strategies to improve the breadth and protective efficacy Viruses 2022; 14(6): 1195-5.
[http://dx.doi.org/10.3390/v14061195] [PMID: 35746665] [PMCID: PMC9230070]

[35]   Vermeulen AN. Progress in recombinant vaccine development against coccidiosis. A review and prospects into the next millennium Int J Parasitol 1998; 28(7): 1121-30.
[http://dx.doi.org/10.1016/s0020-7519(98)00080-0] [PMID: 9724883]

[36]   Britez JD, Rodriguez AE, Di Ciaccio L, Marugán-Hernandez V, Tomazic ML. What do we know about surface proteins of chicken parasites *Eimeria?*. Life (Basel) 2023; 13(6): 1295.
[http://dx.doi.org/10.3390/life13061295] [PMID: 37374079]

[37]   Juarez-Estrada MA, Graham D, Hernandez-Velasco X, Tellez-Isaias G. Editorial: Parasitism: the good, the bad and the ugly. Front Vet Sci 2023; 10: 1304206.
[http://dx.doi.org/10.3389/fvets.2023.1304206] [PMID: 37915945]

[38] Grabowski Ł, Pierzynowska K, Gaffke L, Cyske Z, Mincewicz G, Węgrzyn G. The use of phage display systems to combat infcctious diseases in poultry: diagnostic, vaccine, and therapeutic approaches. J Appl Microbiol 2023; 134(1): lxac012.
[http://dx.doi.org/10.1093/jambio/lxac012] [PMID: 36626750]

# CHAPTER 9

# Therapeutics, Prevention, and Control of Parasitic Diseases

**Kamlesh A. Sadariya[1,*], Tamanna H. Solanki[1], Vaidehi N. Sarvaiya[1]** and **Shailesh K. Bhavsar[1]**

[1] *Department of Veterinary Pharmacology and Toxicology, College of Veterinary Science and Animal Husbandry, Kamdhenu University, Anand, Gujarat, India*

**Abstract:** Poultry disease prevention and control are more important in maintaining flock health than the therapy of the disease. Poultry products are a major global protein source, with commercial poultry production especially showing steady expansion over the last decade. The poultry business faces substantial managerial, nutritional, and disease constraints as a result of the high number of parasite infections and infestations, which cause a variety of diseases and significantly reduce chicken productivity and growth. Poultry parasites encompass helminths, protozoa, ectoparasites, and haemoparasites. Several of these parasites are recognized as highly pathogenic leading to substantial production losses and mortality in poultry. Parasitic illnesses spread from poultry to poultry, from human/ intermediate host to poultry, or *vice versa via* contact or ingestion of infective larvae or oocysts in polluted water, soil, and food or through chicken products. Parasites live inside or outside their hosts and consume host nourishment and blood, reducing productivity and resulting in financial losses owing to control, treatment, and mortality costs. Parasitic diseases can limit and restrict the economic benefits of poultry farming. Endemic parasites are a major cause of economic loss in animal husbandry, particularly in tropical regions and underdeveloped countries. Parasitic disease controls are the husbandry practices utilized by the individuals involved in poultry farms that prevent diseases of poultry. This chapter will be helpful and valuable to veterinarians and other poultry personnel to refresh and update their knowledge on parasite infection prevention and control.

**Keywords:** Blood parasites, Coccidia, Control, Deworming, Ectoparasites, Flies, General principles, Helminths, Parasitic control, Parasitic disease, Poultry, Prevention.

* **Corresponding author Kamlesh A. Sadariya:** Department of Veterinary Pharmacology and Toxicology, College of Veterinary Science and Animal Husbandry, Kamdhenu University, Anand, Gujarat, India; E-mail: kasadariya@kamdhenuuni.edu.in

**Tanmoy Rana (Ed.)**

## INTRODUCTION

Poultry encompasses domestic birds raised for human consumption *i.e.* eggs and meat, comprising chickens, pigeons, turkeys, geese, ostriches, ducks, guinea fowl, and doves. Poultry parasites range from single-celled protozoans that develop either intracellularly or extracellularly to multicellular helminths (nematodes, trematodes, and cestodes), blood parasites, and ectoparasites as depicted in Fig. (1). Mostly seen parasitic infestation in poultry includes nematodes, cestodes, and coccidia, which can lead to significant harm and economic losses within the industry. Parasitic infestations result in malnutrition, reduced weight loss, feed conversion ratios, egg production, and fatalities among birds [1, 2]. Moreover, parasitic infections reduce the ability of the flock to fight against diseases and worsen existing health conditions [3, 4]. Parasitic life cycles may be direct or complex indirect cycles requiring various arthropod or animal hosts. Some species of parasites can infect nearly every organ system, although individual genera will affect specific organs or tissues (Fig. 1) [5].

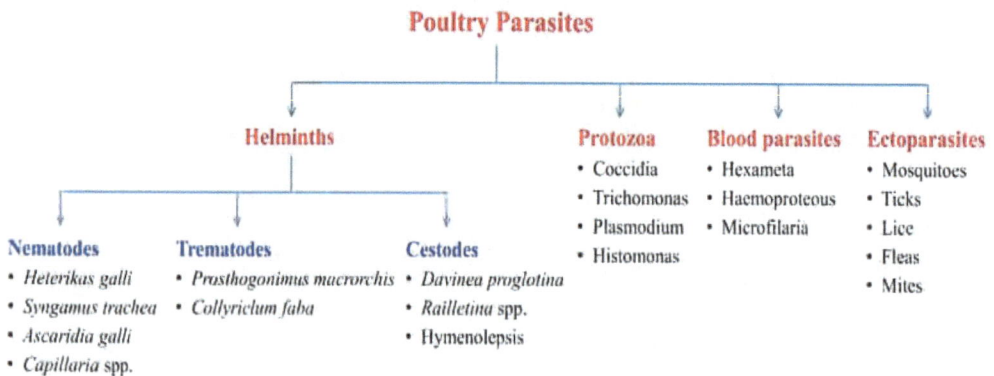

**Fig. (1).** Common poultry parasites.

Poultry diseases like coccidiosis and helminth infections lead to economic losses due to bird deaths, lower body weight, and increased expenses for prevention and treatment. These issues are common in modern poultry farming, especially in confined spaces [6, 7]. Parasitic infections can interfere with bird metabolism, causing poor feed use, slow growth, and delayed maturity. When multiple parasites affect birds, especially those in the gut, they increase the risk of chick deaths and reduce productivity in adults [8]. Treating these infections strategically with anthelmintics can help poultry owners minimize losses and boost productivity in backyard farming setups [4]. There are many parasites causing infections and infestation in poultry in various farms and different rearing systems.

## CONTROL AND PREVENTION OF POULTRY PARASITES

In commercial indoor production systems, the extent of parasitism is largely influenced by management practices. For instance, the adoption of total enclosure principles, enhancements in cleaning and disinfection procedures, and the implementation of production based on the "all in- all out" principle seem to have diminished the significance of parasitism. The ban on battery cages in several countries has led to the emergence of new intensive free-range systems. However, preventing parasitic infections in these systems has proven challenging. The utilization of outdoor areas, where parasite eggs can endure in the environment for extended periods, has heightened the risk of infections [7].

## GENERAL PRINCIPLES OF PARASITIC CONTROL

The main goal of a parasite control strategy is to minimize parasitic challenges in young birds, preventing symptoms and reducing production losses. Complete eradication of most parasites is uncertain due to the large number of eggs released, their environmental persistence, and transmission *via* feces. Before starting a control program, it is crucial to understand the parasitic infections in the population, including species present, prevalence, and transmission patterns, which may vary by region. If this knowledge is limited, an investigation should be conducted first before starting any control program.

Backyard poultry can host all parasite species, but commercial free-range systems often eliminate parasites requiring intermediate hosts. Most helminths with indirect life cycles are nearly eradicated, except *Raillietina* spp., transmitted by flies as production shifts from backyard to commercial systems, parasites with direct life cycles, such as *Ascaridia, Heterakis, Capillaria,* and *Eimeria* spp. tend to decrease. The best way to control poultry parasites is by improving flock management and hygiene. This can eliminate some parasites and reduce others to acceptable levels. Complete eradication through routine treatment is impossible, so control programs typically combine management improvements with antiparasitic drugs.

### Density of Birds

Maintaining an appropriate density of birds in any poultry production system is crucial. The density of birds (stocking rate) is crucial in any poultry production system. Excessive stocking can cause birds to come into closer contact with feces, increasing the risk of ingesting more infective parasitic eggs.

**Flock Size and Composition**

Research indicates that the susceptibility and incidence of parasitic diseases differ among poultry age groups. Older birds may carry various parasitic diseases, such as *Eimeria spp.*, *Ascaridia spp.*, and *Tetrameres spp.*, without showing clinical signs. Therefore, segregating age groups according to the "all in, all out" principle could be beneficial.

**Pen Utilization Alternatives**

Given that poultry share few parasites with other livestock, management practices may involve the combined use of pens (*e.g.*, poultry scavenging alongside other livestock) or the rotational use of pens (alternating poultry with other livestock in the same pen). However, when chickens scavenge in areas contaminated by pig parasites, there is a risk of liver and lung lesions caused by migrating *Ascaris suum* larvae. Some parasitic species with indirect life cycles and flukes may be effectively controlled by simply avoiding contact with freshwater habitats where intermediate hosts reside.

Pens can also be managed by incorporating crop rotation with poultry production, significantly reducing field contamination. It is important to acknowledge that infectious eggs, particularly those of nematodes, may survive for years in suitable environments. Developing such rotation programs necessitates a comprehensive understanding of the seasonal development and survival patterns of parasites in the specific area. For instance, in temperate regions, the eggs of *Eimeria* spp., *Ascaridia* spp., *Heterakis* spp. and *Capillaria* spp. cannot undergo embryonation and become infective during winter (*i.e.*, below 10-15°C).

**Cleaning of Pen**

In the upkeep of concrete pens, whether located outdoors or indoors, it is imperative to regularly remove the litter (weekly or more frequently) to significantly diminish the presence of parasitic eggs before they reach the infective stage. Additionally, efforts should be made to keep the floor as dry as possible, as external stages of parasites require nearly 100% humidity for development. The drainage capacity, which affects the dry microenvironment at the floor level, maybe a key factor in the effectiveness of slatted floors in reducing indoor parasitic transmission in intensive systems.

While washing concrete floors with high-pressure cleaners or steam cleaners is often recommended, this practice is debatable. Water use may improve conditions for egg and larval development, making it nearly impossible to eliminate all eggs, and could spread infective stages from sheltered crevices throughout the pens.

Alternatively, high temperatures, like those generated by a flame-thrower (gas), could be considered, though caution must be exercised due to the associated fire hazard. Disinfectants, while not particularly effective against parasite eggs, should still be included in overall actions to reduce viral and bacterial infections.

It is advised to apply lime wash and let it dry after the mechanical removal of trash and disinfection (Utilizing steam, combustion, and chemical cleaners). There are two objectives to this procedure: The two main ways that lime inhibits the survival of parasite eggs are: 1) Through its drying impact, and 2) By raising the pH level over 8. After applying lime, the house should be empty for two to four weeks before adding more animals.

## Regular Deworming

Frequently, farmers opt for routine deworming programs due to their convenience, often making worm treatments the primary control measure. However, the impact of each treatment tends to be short-lived when poultry are repeatedly re-infected. On the contrary, the effect is significantly prolonged when the transmission rate is low. It is crucial to recognize that each round of drug treatment increases selection pressure on the helminth population, fostering the development of anthelmintic resistance. Therefore, parasitic control programs should aim to minimize the number of treatments and instead emphasize other control measures. Despite this, certain routine anthelmintic treatments play a role in nematode control across various management systems.

Numerous deworming regimens have been developed; these are usually customized based on the age or stage of the poultry's reproductive cycle. Conventional procedures include treating hens just before they start laying, and then they are moved to a hygienic stable. The intention is to rid the chickens of worms in order to minimize production losses and avoid contaminating the environment.

When choosing a drug, consider the species of worms present. Some drugs exhibit a wider range of efficacy compared to others, and specific nematodes may be susceptible only to particular drugs. Additionally, factors such as cost and potential resistance development should be taken into account. It is essential to alternate between drugs with different modes of action to minimize the risk of anthelmintic resistance and avoid drugs to which resistance has already developed.

## Sufficient Nutritional Levels

Maintaining an appropriate nutritional level, particularly in terms of protein intake, can contribute to diminishing the overall impact of helminth infections. However, it is crucial to note that adequate nutrition should not serve as a replacement for a robust parasite control program. Interestingly, limited research suggests that protein levels above 14-16% may stimulate the growth of particular nematodes in the gut.

## CONTROL AND PREVENTION OF HELMINTHS IN POULTRY

In general, worm life cycles can be disrupted by resting the ground and changing trash between flocks. The most effective way to control parasites is to disrupt their life cycles. The approach used will depend on the parasite and the poultry system. Internal parasites are often not an issue for ranging chickens when the range is properly rested and rotated. Mobile housing-based systems provide far more flexibility in guaranteeing frequent rotation of ranging paddocks. If a post-mortem investigation of any bird is performed, the opportunity should be seized to determine the level of infestation and, if necessary, create appropriate control strategies. Occasional faecal egg counts may also be recommended for layers [9]. According to scientists, birds should not be kept in a paddock for more than 2-3 months and should be rotated around four farms surrounding a central residence. Some parasites multiply in damp litter, and a buildup may form when the litter is reused. This is best avoided, especially for layers. Meat-producing birds, with shorter lives, are less at risk.

Keeping grass short aids in parasite control. Worm larvae appear to be killed by UV radiation. Ground harrowing is another effective control method. If there is a build-up in fixed housing systems in the areas immediately outside the house, it may be necessary to physically remove the top 5 cm of soil on an intermittent basis.

Grouping birds of different ages can lead to the spread of parasites across groups, hence it should always be avoided. Furthermore, and maybe most significantly, different bird species should not be housed together. Keeping poultry on free-draining soil, free of excessive shadowing, and away from wet or water-logged places will also assist in minimizing the amount of potential intermediate hosts that are common in the life-cycle of many parasites (Table 1). Management systems have a significant impact on parasitic transmission success. In Table 1, a preliminary overview of parasitic occurrence in different production systems is given.

**Table 1. Common helminth infections affecting poultry [10, 11].**

| Parasite | Intermediate host or life cycle | Organ infected | Host |
|---|---|---|---|
| **Nematodes** | | | |
| *Ascaridia galli* | Direct | Small intestine | Chicken, duck, quail, turkey |
| *Capillaria caudinflata* | Earthworms | Small intestine | Chicken, duck, pigeon, game birds, turkey |
| *Capillaria contorta* | None or earthworms | Mouth, esophagus, crop | Chicken, duck, game birds, turkey |
| *Capillaria obsignata* | Direct | Small intestine, ceca | Chicken, pigeon, goose, quail turkey |
| *Heterakis gallinarum* | Direct | Ceca | Chicken, game birds, duck, turkey |
| *Oxyspirura mansoni* | Cockroaches | Eye | Chicken, quail, guinea fowl, turkey |
| *Strongyloides avium* | Direct | Ceca | Chicken, quail, goose, turkey |
| *Syngamus trachea* | None or earthworm | Trachea | Chicken, quail, pheasant, turkey |
| *Tetrameres americana* | Grass-hoppers, cockroaches | Proventriculus | Chicken, pigeon, duck, game birds, turkey |
| *Trichostrongylus tenuis* | Direct | Ceca | Chicken, pigeon, duck, turkey |
| **Cestodes** | | | |
| *Choanotaenia infundibulum* | House flies | Upper intestine | Chicken |
| *Davainea proglottata* | Slugs, snails | Duodenum | Chicken |
| *Raillietina cesticillus* | Beetles | Duodenum, jejunum | Chicken |
| *Raillietina echinobothrida* | Ants | Lower intestine | Chicken |
| *Raillietina tetragona* | Ants | Lower intestine | Chicken |

## CONTROL OF NEMATODES

Nematodes stand out as the most prevalent helminths in poultry, exhibiting both direct and indirect life cycles. In addition to the positive outcomes associated with enhanced management practices, the control of nematodes can be effectively accomplished through the administration of anthelmintic drugs.

Worms can cause problems for birds when they live in overcrowded conditions and do not get enough nutrients, especially Vitamin A. This deficiency makes birds more vulnerable to worms. The best way to protect birds from worms is by practicing good management and providing balanced food. The continuous presence of worm infestations can be effectively controlled by interrupting their life cycle. Eggs of worms are directly eaten by birds or by intermediary hosts. For a significant reduction in infestation, it is important to prevent direct exposure between birds and dropping. This can be achieved by keeping birds on wire. Implementing a rotational system for poultry runs can also help. By regularly changing the area where birds roam, the number of viable eggs in the soil decreases. If a run is left empty for around 8 months, few viable eggs will remain in the soil, reducing the risk of infestation [12].

**Steps for Effective Control and Prevention of Worm Infections in Birds**

1. **Annual Treatment or After Heavy Infestation**: Conduct an annual treatment or address severe worm problems by relocating the birds from their living area (run). Spreading of quicklime @ 0.5 kg per square meter over the ground will be helpful. Again three weeks afterward, thoroughly dig over the entire area to ensure the destruction of worm eggs.
2. **Preventing Ideal Conditions for Worm Survival**: Regularly inspect the shed and run for damp, dark spots where worm eggs can persist. Pay special attention to areas around water troughs, as they pose a higher risk. Modify these areas to make them unsuitable for worms to survive and cause infectious.
3. **Excluding Wild Birds**: To effectively control worms, prevent wild birds from entering the bird's living area. Wild birds can introduce worms into an otherwise clean pen.
4. **Intermediate Hosts:** Although challenging, reducing contact between birds and the intermediate hosts of parasites is essential. Eliminate breeding grounds for house flies, as they can carry worm eggs, thus lowering the risk of infestation.
5. **Be Careful with Insecticides:** Be cautious when using insecticides to control flies, ants, or termites. These chemicals may be ingested by the birds, potentially causing poisoning or leaving harmful residues in eggs and meat. Use these products judiciously to minimize any adverse effects on the birds.

**Treatment of Nematodes**

The treatment for nematodes in poultry involves various drugs, each with its recommended administration method and efficacy. Piperazine, Ivermectin (in drinking water) Levamisole and Fenbendazole (in feed) are among the options [13]. In free-range systems, where ascaridiosis poses a challenge, segregating and rearing young birds on the previously unused ground can be beneficial. For deep litter houses, feeding and watering systems that minimize fecal contamination are recommended. Levamisole, benzimidazoles like flubendazole, or piperazine salts can be given through drinking water or feed [14].

For *Ascaridia galli*, piperazine is the chosen treatment. Continuous hygromycin B administration in the diet is also frequent. Piperazine can be given in feed (0.2-0.4%), water (0.1-2%), or as a single treatment (50-100 mg/bird). Tetramisole, albendazole, and levamisole are effective treatments for chickens of various ages [15]. Fenbendazole is very effective at recommended doses and ivermectin has demonstrated effectiveness against immature and adult worms [15]

Traditional deworming compounds, such as piperazine and hygromycin, are typically used in feed or water. Hygromycin is applied at around 750 g/ton of feed, while piperazine use is at 2-3 kg/ton of feed. Individual treatment is also an option, with about 100 mg of piperazine per bird. These traditional dewormers act as narcotics that paralyze the worms without killing them. To effectively cure deworming, it is recommended to administer two or three doses spaced 7-10 days apart. This allows the worms to lose their attachment and exit through feces. It is essential to follow recommended dosages and intervals to ensure efficacy.

By adopting strategies like segregating young birds, managing deep litter setups, and implementing appropriate treatments at recommended intervals, effective control, and management of Ascaridiosis in free-range poultry systems will be helpful [16].

## CONTROL OF CESTODES

The shift from free-range to commercial indoor poultry production system has reduced tapeworm prevalence due to limited access to intermediate hosts, requiring effective prevention strategies. Upon identifying the tapeworm species present in a flock, specific preventive measures can be recommended. Controlling beetles, ants, or houseflies can limit the infection of *Raillietina* spp. in cage systems. Flies and ants in the facility can be controlled with insecticides. However, for beetles, when control is an issue, using alternating pens might be a useful method. It is worth remembering that Anthelmintic therapy can be used to control it, however, it is critical to note that therapy alone is ineffective unless the intermediary hosts are addressed.

### Treatment of Cestodes

To effectively control tapeworm infections, it is important to disrupt the tapeworm's reproduction cycle by killing intermediate hosts. Applying metaldehyde-based slug and snail bait around the house's perimeter is vital in this procedure. The goal is to target and diminish the population of intermediary hosts, thus ending the transmission cycle.

Chemical therapies for infected birds are another option, however, some may involve a 24-hour period of hunger for the bird. However, mature birds' egg production can be naturally disrupted. Products like praziquantel have shown efficacy against tapeworms, although many popular chemical therapies used for roundworms may be ineffective [16]. Niclosamide administration in feed is advised as a therapeutic option [13].

*Raillietina* and *Davainea* like tapeworms can be controlled by treatment of birds with anthelmintics butynorate and niclosamide. Simultaneously, efforts should be made to destroy slugs and snails whenever possible to limit the intermediate hosts [14]. This comprehensive approach will help disrupt the life cycle of the tapeworm, mitigating the risk of infection in poultry.

## CONTROL OF TREMATODES

Flukes that infect poultry, such as *Echinostoma revolutum* and *Prosthogonimus* spp., may involve freshwater snails or dragonflies in their life cycles. Controlling these infections can be made possible by avoiding contact between poultry and freshwater reservoirs, including even small ponds and temporary pools. Unlike with nematodes, there are currently no anthelmintic drugs specifically available for the prevention or control of trematodes (flukes) in poultry. Therefore, focusing on environmental management and preventing contact with potential intermediate hosts remains a key strategy in managing fluke infections in poultry. Regular monitoring and appropriate biosecurity measures are essential in preventing and minimizing the impact of these parasitic infections.

## COMMONLY USED DRUGS FOR THE CONTROL OF HELMINTHS IN POULTRY

The commonly used drugs for control of helminths in poultry are depicted in Table **2**. Fenbendazole, a benzimidazole anthelmintic, is licensed in the United States for use in hens against *A. galli* and *H. gallinarum* (1 mg/kg, PO in drinking water, every 24 hours for 5 days). Fenbendazole has also been demonstrated to be effective against *Ascaris* spp. when given once at 10-50 mg/kg; if necessary, the treatment can be repeated after 10 days (extra-label usage in the United States). Fenbendazole, at 10-50 mg/kg, is effective against *Capillaria spp.* when given daily for 5 days.

Table 2. Common drugs used for the control of helminths in poultry [17].

| Drug | Administration | Indications |
|---|---|---|
| Fenbendazole | In feed | *Ascaridia galli, Capillaria* spp., *Syngamus trachea* |
| Flubendazole | In feed | Intestinal nematodes and cestodes in chickens |
| Hygromycin | In feed | Intestinal nematodes (*Ascaridia galli*) |
| Levamisole | In feed | *Ascaridia galli, Heterakis gallinarum, Capillaria* spp., *Syngamus trachea* |
| Mebendazole | In feed | Intestinal nematodes, *Syngamus trachea*, cestodes |
| Piperazine | In feed or drinking water | *Ascaridia galli, Tetrameres* spp. |
| Thiabendazole | In feed | *Syngamus trachea* |

Fenbendazole is also effective against other nematodes when delivered at 10-50 mg/kg every 24 hours for 3-5 days, as a single dose of 20-100 mg/kg, or when added to drinking water at 125 mg/L for 5 days or to feed at 100 mg/kg (all off-label dosages in the United States). Fenbendazole should not be administered during molt, because it may interfere with feather re-growth. Flubendazole (1.43 mg/kg) is used widely in Europe against *Ascaridia* spp. and *H. gallinarum* [11]. Pyrantel tartrate was more effective than pyrantel pamoate against the adult stage of *A. galli* and slightly effective against *Capillaria* spp. when taken at 15-25 mg/kg (extra-label use in the United States). Poultry breeders looking to treat tapeworm infections should be aware that the expulsion of the parasite will only be a temporary solution if the scolex is not removed or the intermediate host is not eradicated as a source of re-infestation. Butynorate has demonstrated some efficacy as a feed additive when combined with piperazine and phenothiazine, as well as when taken individually (Table **2**).

## CONTROL OF COCCIDIA

Coccidiosis stands as the most common parasitic disease in poultry, characterized by a direct life cycle with a very short prepatent time. Controlling coccidiosis can be achieved through various methods:

1. **Improvement of Management**: Management strategies play a crucial role in preventing coccidiosis in poultry flocks. However, in commercial systems, these strategies may encounter challenges due to frequent failures and the high resistance of coccidial oocysts to disinfectants.
2. **Prevention and Control through Vaccination Programs**: Recent developments in research have led to the availability of commercially viable vaccines. These vaccines are usually based on live, attenuated coccidia strains. Vaccination is particularly convenient for large-scale commercial production

but may have limited applicability in backyard or smaller-scale production systems.

3. **Control through Chemotherapy:** Chemotherapy programs for poultry against coccidiosis may follow different approaches. Some programs are based on treating clinical outbreaks of coccidiosis, addressing the disease as it occurs.
4. Others adopt a preventive medication strategy to curb the potential development of coccidiosis.

A comprehensive approach to coccidiosis control involves a combination of improved management practices, vaccination programs (especially in commercial settings), and strategic chemotherapy. The choice of strategy often depends on the specific circumstances of the poultry production system.

The management of coccidiosis, especially in backyard and free-range systems, involves inducing strong immunity through controlled exposure and the use of broad-spectrum drugs during clinical outbreaks. Additionally, in broilers and breeders/ layers, various anticoccidial drug programs are employed to ensure optimal growth, prevent resistance, and manage outbreaks.

### For Clinical Outbreaks in Backyard and Free-Range Systems

- **Controlled Exposure for Natural Immunity**: Natural immunity can be achieved through controlled exposure, using either a commercial product or natural exposure to common coccidial species.
- **Treatment with Broad-Spectrum Drugs**: Using broad-spectrum drugs to treat clinical disease during outbreaks.
- **Consideration of Environmental Factors**: Managing outbreaks by considering factors such as management practices, climatic conditions, and seasonal variations.

### Programs for Anticoccidial Drug Use in Broilers

- **Continuous Feeding**: Using a single drug continuously from hatching to a week before slaughter.
- **Shuttle Programs**: Using one drug in the starter feed for the first 2-3 weeks and another in the grower feed to reduce the development of resistant coccidia strains.
- **Rotation Programs:** Regularly rotating drugs to prevent the development of resistant strains in the environment. Anticoccidial drug use programs for breeders and layers.

## Programs for Anticoccidial Drug Use in Breeders and Layers

- **Inducing Immunity**: Achieving natural immunity through controlled exposure or natural exposure.
- **Treatment with Broad-Spectrum Drugs**: Using broad-spectrum drugs to treat clinical disease during outbreaks.
- **Consideration of Environmental Factors**: Managing outbreaks by considering factors such as management practices, climatic conditions, and seasonal variations.

## Drug Resistance

Drug resistance can be reduced by using less intensive production systems, shuttle treatments, and frequent drug rotation. The overall strategy involves a combination of inducing natural immunity, treating clinical outbreaks with broad-spectrum drugs, and implementing programs that minimize the development of drug-resistant coccidia strains. The specific approach depends on the poultry production system and the goals of the operation.

## Drugs Used to Control Coccidia in Poultry

Sulfonamides are the most widely used drugs to control coccidia in poultry. They are recommended for three days in drinking water, with a two-day interval between treatments. Sulphaquinoxaline, sometimes combined with diaveridine or sulphadimidine, is preferred. When resistance occurs, mixtures of amprolium and ethopabate have proven effective [14]. Amprolium solution (0.024% in drinking water) for 3-5 days is effective. Sulfamethazine (0.1% for 2 days, 0.05% for 4 days) or commercial sulfa combinations are also recommended. Vitamin A and K supplements in water may aid in recovery [13]. Common drugs used to control coccidia in poultry are depicted in Table 3.

Table 3. Common drugs used to control coccidia in poultry [18].

| Type of compound | Generic name | Dosage |
|---|---|---|
| Benzeneacetonitriles | Diclazuril | Broiler: 1 ppm in feed. |
| Ionophorous antibiotics | Lasalocid | Broiler: 75-125 ppm in feed. |
| | Maduramicin | Broiler: 5 ppm in feed |
| | Monensin | Broiler: 100-125 ppm in feed. |
| | Narasin | Broilers: 70 ppm in feed. |
| | Salinomycin | Broilers: 60 ppm in feed. |

(Table 3) cont.....

| Type of compound | Generic name | Dosage |
|---|---|---|
| Quinolones | Decoquinate | Broilers: 30 ppm in feed. |
| | Methylbenzoquate | Chickens, Turkey: 8.35 ppm (with 100 ppm clopidol) in feed. |
| Sulfonamides | Sulfachloropyrazine | Chickens Turkey: 0.03% in water. |
| | Sulfadimethoxine | Broiler: 125 ppm in feed. |
| | Sulfadimethoxine + Amprolium | Chicken: 125+75 ppm in feed. |
| | Sulfadimethoxine + Ormetoprim | Chicken: 125+75 ppm in feed. |
| | Sulfaquinoxaline | Poultry: 125 ppm in feed for 8 wks. |
| | Sulfaquinoxaline + Pyrimethamine | Chicken: 0.005%+ 0.0015% in water. |
| Thiamine analogues | Amprolium | Chicken: 125-250 ppm in water |
| | Amprolium + Ethopabate | Layers: 125+4 to 40 ppm in feed. |
| Pyridones | Clopidol | Poultry: 125-250 ppm in feed. |
| Nitrobenzamides | Dinitolmide | Broiler: 125 ppm in feed. |
| Carbanilide | Nicarbazin | Broiler: 125 ppm in feed. |
| Febrifugine | Halofuginone | Chicken and Turkey: 3 ppm in feed. |
| Miscellaneous | Furazolidone | Chicken: 55 ppm in feed. |
| | Nitrofurazone | Chicken: 82 ppm in water for 5 days |
| | Toltrazuril | Broilers: 25 ppm in water. |
| | Furaltadone | 1 g/L of water. |

Prevention of avian coccidiosis is based on a combination of good management and the use of anticoccidial compounds in the feed or water. Thus, litter should always be kept dry and special attention should be given to litter near water fonts or feeding troughs [14]. Proper management, which limits litter saturation includes; appropriate installation and management of watering systems *e.g.* acceptable ventilation rate; nipple drinkers; providing adequate feeding space; maintaining recommended stocking density; inclusion of anticoccidials in feed at recommended levels that will prevent clinical infection; chemical and ionophoric anticoccidials for broilers; synthetic coccidiostats for breeders and floor-reared commercial egg production flocks that allow the development of premunity. It is necessary to replace roasters and breeding stock with anticoccidial vaccinations (Fig. **2**) [13].

## Managemental Aspects to Control the Illness in Poultry

• Coccidial oocysts are not destroyed by ordinary antiseptics and disinfectants like formalin, copper sulphate, phenol, sulphuric acid, potassium hydroxide, or potassium iodide. The oocysts are destroyed by ultraviolet light, heat or bacterial action in the absence of oxygen. Poultry houses are sealed and can be fumigated with ammonia or methyl bromide can be applied to the little or soil to kill the oocysts [20].

- Coccidiostats may be fed until the birds are 8-9 weeks old, after which they become immune. Rahman *et al.* found that levamisole enhanced the cell-mediated immunity, which has special value in preventing coccidiosis and observed 100% survivability in birds medicated with 2 mg of levamisole/chick on the 19th day of age [21].
- Shuttle and rotation programmes are being used to combat the development of drug resistance. This program consists of starting medication, incorporating one particular anticoccidial in feed, usually for the first three weeks of the growth followed by a change to another anticoccidial in the grower feed. For the finisher periods, anticoccidials are usually withdrawn from the feed to allow the excretion of drug residues before slaughter.
- Young chickens should be kept apart from older birds, which minimises infections.
- If birds are raised on the floor, place each new brood in a clean house with fresh litter. Keep the litter dry, stir it periodically, and remove it when damp.
- The waterer and feeder should be washed weekly with hot water and detergent.
- Waterers should be placed on wire platforms over floor drains and the feeders should be raised high enough to prevent their being fouled.
- Enough feeders must be used to prevent crowding.
- If raised on wires, wires should be cleaned regularly
- Flies, rats, and mice around the poultry houses should be eliminated as they carry coccidian mechanically.
- In the event of a coccidiosis outbreak, sick birds should be evacuated and fed, and watered in a separate enclosure. Healthy birds should be treated with coccidiostat.
- All dead birds and litter should be burnt.
- Special rubber shoes should be put on before entering pens and should be cleaned thoroughly after each use.

## Immunity and Vaccination

A species-specific immunity develops after natural infection, the extent largely depends on the severity of infection and the number of reinfections. Protective immunity is primarily a T-cell response. Chickens acquire immunity to coccidiosis by exposure and subsequent recovery from infection. Protective immunity is generally established after the accomplishment of 2-3 life cycles of *Eimeria*. Immunity to coccidiosis is specific for each species of coccidia and there is no cross-protection between various species of *Eimeria* in poultry. Protective immunity against coccidia is based mainly on cell-mediated immunity [22 - 25].

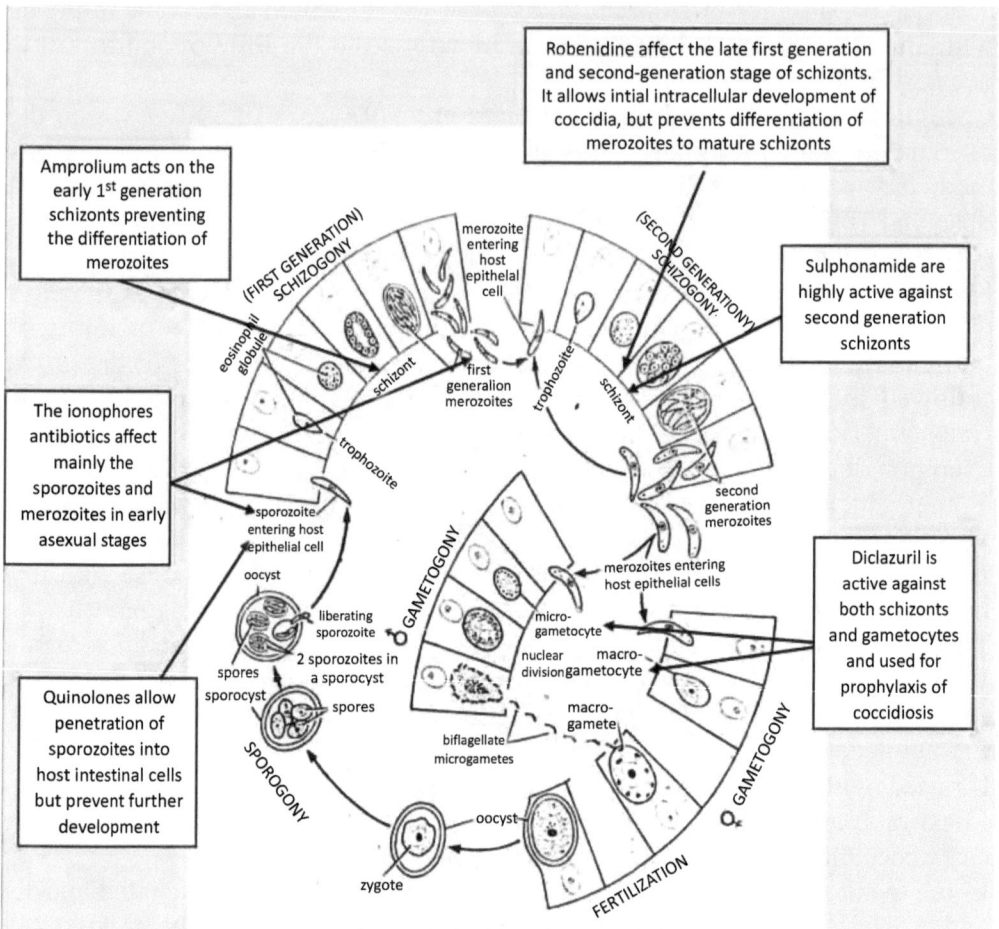

**Fig. (2).** Different stages of coccidia life cycle and effective anticoccidial drugs at different stages for coccidia [19]. (Source: Coccidia life cycle image- https://swarborno.com/life-cycle-of-eimeria-tenella with-diagram).

Commercial vaccines consist of live and sporulated oocysts of the various coccidial species, administered at low doses. Coccivac and cocivac-T are live vaccines and paracox-8 is a live attenuated vaccine used against coccidiosis. Anticoccidial vaccines should be given to day-old chicks, either at the hatchery or on the farm. Some vaccines sold in Europe and South America include attenuated lines of coccidia. Research has shown promise for vaccination in game birds.

## COMMON BLOOD PARASITES

Haemoparasites mainly found in poultry in tropical areas include *Plasmodium* spp., *Leucocytozoon* spp., *Haemoproteus* spp., *Aegytinella* spp., *Trypanosoma* spp. and micro filariasis of nematodes belonging to the suborder filariata [17]. Few of the blood parasites observed in the birds are of economic importance, for example, *Plasmodium* causes avian malaria and Leucocytozoonosis is pathogenic in younger birds (Table **4**).

Table 4. Common drugs used to control hemoparasites [17].

| Effective against | Drug and mode of application |
|---|---|
| Avian malaria | Chloroquine (1 mg/kg IM for 5 days) |
| | Chloroquine (2000 mg/L in water for 1 day) |
| | Quinacrine (1.6 mg/kg IM for 5 days) |
| | Primaquine (100 mg/kg PO for 1 day) |
| Prevention of Leucocytozonosis | Pyrimethamine (1 ppm) + Sulfadimethoxine (10 ppm) PO |
| Cure of Leucocytozonosis | Pyrimethamine (25 ppm) PO |
| *Aegyptinella* spp. | Tetracycline (15-30 mg/kg) PO |

## Control of Ectoparasites

To minimize the risk of transmitting ectoparasites from the wild to domestic birds, it is imperative to prevent any direct interaction between them. Erecting effective fencing becomes crucial to deter other birds from accessing the poultry environment.

### Ticks

Concerning ticks, both the nymphal and adult stages feed on hosts for a limited duration. Controlling ticks necessitates treating the surroundings, both indoors and outdoors, where the poultry reside. Following the mechanical cleaning of the stable, a high-pressure sprayer is employed to apply carbaryl, coumaphos, malathion, or stirofos to the entire structure, including walls, ceilings, cracks, and crevices. It is not advisable to use approved insecticides on outdoor facilities like feed troughs, woodpiles, and tree trunks due to environmental considerations.

### Mites

Management practices for controlling infections with chicken mites, tropical fowl mites, and northern fowl mites involve the use of acaricides such as carbaryl, coumaphos, malathion, stirofos, or a pyrethroid. It is essential to spray each bird and treat the entire stable, including all hiding places for the mites.

Prophylactic measures, including thorough cleaning and disinfection of the house, are highly advisable. Spraying all surfaces with insecticides, followed by a lime wash, is a recommended practice. Additionally, introducing new animals into a house immediately after cleaning and disinfection should be avoided.

For scaly leg mites, the control process should commence with the isolation or culling of affected birds. Subsequently, the house should undergo cleaning procedures similar to those recommended for other mites. Individual animals with affected legs can be treated by dipping the legs in kerosene, linseed, or mineral oil or by coating them with Vaseline. Treatments should be administered twice with a 10-day interval. Acaricides may also be used to treat infections.

It is imperative to examine animals before introducing them into an existing flock and preventive measures combined with proper cleaning and treatment protocols play a vital role in managing and preventing mite infestations.

*Fleas*

The most effective way to control infections with fleas is to remove litter and subsequently treat the house with insecticides such as permethrin. Prophylactic measures, as mentioned earlier, are highly recommended to prevent flea infestations.

**Control of Flies in Poultry House**

Several different species of flies may be found around broiler farms and laying houses and the most common of these species are the little house fly (*Fannia* spp.) and the house fly (*Musca domestica*). In caged layer houses, the manure is a very good location for breeding. In houses where sanitation is poor and where water spills keep the manure moist, fly breeding may especially be a problem. The house fly prefers sunlight and is a very active fly, which crawls over filth, people, and food. Because of these habits, it is the most important species from the standpoint of spreading human and poultry diseases and fly-specking eggs. Managing poultry manure in such a way that it becomes unattractive as a breeding site is an effective way to keep the fly population under control [23 - 25].

Fly control should be an integral part of every poultry producer's management program. Effective fly control is achieved by utilizing both chemical and non-chemical methods. Fly control inside the poultry house is an easier problem to handle if flies are prevented from entering. Through the proper use of screens for doors, windows, and curtain openings, the number of flies that enter the house can be minimized. As a last alternative to good management and sanitation programs, insecticides can be used effectively to complete the task of fly control. It must be re-emphasized that insecticides should not be used, instead of good management. Several methods of application including residual sprays, space sprays, vapor strips, fly baits, and larvicides can be considered for poultry farm use [24, 25]. Control of flies in poultry houses by insecticides is depicted in Table **5**.

Table 5. Control of flies in poultry house by insecticides [17].

| Name | Formulation |
|---|---|
| Bomyl (1%) | Bait |
| Dibrom | Bait |
| Dibrom (0.25%) | Spray |
| Dichlorvos (0.5%) | Spray |
| Dichlorvos (1%) | Bait |
| Permethrin (0.25%) | Spray |
| Stirofos (1%) | Spray |
| Tetrachlorvinfos (1%) | Spray |
| Trichlorfon (1%) | Bait |

## CONCLUDING REMARKS

Internal and external parasites in poultry pose a significant economic threat to the global poultry industry. Poultry production is experiencing rapid growth due to its cost-effectiveness and efficiency in converting nutrients into animal protein. Parasites significantly hinder poultry production in developing countries and their impact on productivity and health is limited. Various parasitic infestations can occur in poultry which generally include, helminths, protozoal infection, and ectoparasites. Parasites have a huge effect on poultry health and production. External parasites can also cause severe clinical symptoms in birds and negatively impact poultry egg or meat production, necessitating timely control and treatment monitoring. Insecticides should be considered a supplement to sanitation and management measures aimed at preventing fly and other insects from breeding.

Poultry health is significantly impacted by parasites like nematodes, cestodes, and coccidiosis, necessitating the implementation of control and prevention methods to boost poultry production. Parasitic infections can lead to malnutrition, decreased feed conversion ratios, egg production, weight loss, and mortality in poultry. Additionally, parasites make flocks more infective and aggravate the existing disease condition, which necessitates further research to increase poultry production. Among the various disease constraints, parasitic diseases pose a significant limitation to the effectiveness and ongoing development of poultry production in developing countries. Research is also needed to understand the various poultry parasites that are highly pathogenic and cause significant production losses and mortality along with their preventive and control measures. Thus, appropriate preventive measures should be applied to improve poultry production and keep poultry flocks healthy, productive, and profitable.

# REFERENCES

[1]     Puttalakshmamma G, Ananda K, Prathiush P, Mamatha G, Rao S. Prevalence of gastrointestinal parasites of poultry in and around Banglore. Vet World 2008; 2(2): 201.
[http://dx.doi.org/10.5455/vetworld.2008.201-202]

[2]     Attree E, Sanchez-Arsuaga G, Jones M, *et al.* Controlling the causative agents of coccidiosis in domestic chickens; an eye on the past and considerations for the future. CABI Agric Biosci 2021; 2(1): 37.
[http://dx.doi.org/10.1186/s43170-021-00056-5] [PMID: 34604790]

[3]     Gary DB, Richard DM. Intestinal parasites in backyard chicken flocks: Cooperative extension service. Gainesville: Institute of Food and Agricultural Sciences, University of Florida 2012; p. 32611.

[4]     Katoch R, Yadav A, Godara R, Khajuria JK, Borkataki S, Sodhi SS. Prevalence and impact of gastrointestinal helminths on body weight gain in backyard chickens in subtropical and humid zone of Jammu, India. J Parasit Dis 2012; 36(1): 49-52.
[http://dx.doi.org/10.1007/s12639-011-0090-z] [PMID: 23543701]

[5]     Ritchie BW, Harrison GJ, Harrison LR. Avian medicine: principles and application. Florida, USA: Wingers Publishing Incorporated 1994; p. 1384.

[6]     Amare A, Worku W, Negussie H. Coccidiosis prevailing in parent stocks: A comparative study between growers and adult layers in Kombolcha poultry breeding and multiplication center, Ethiopia. Glob Vet 2012; 8(3): 285-91.

[7]     Blake DP, Knox J, Dehaeck B, *et al.* Re-calculating the cost of coccidiosis in chickens. Vet Res 2020; 51(1): 115.
[http://dx.doi.org/10.1186/s13567-020-00837-2] [PMID: 32928271]

[8]     Ybañez RHD, Resuelo KJG, Kintanar APM, Ybañez AP. Detection of gastrointestinal parasites in small-scale poultry layer farms in Leyte, Philippines. Vet World 2018; 11(11): 1587-91.
[http://dx.doi.org/10.14202/vetworld.2018.1587-1591] [PMID: 30587893]

[9]     Shifaw A, Feyera T, Walkden-Brown SW, Sharpe B, Elliott T, Ruhnke I. Global and regional prevalence of helminth infection in chickens over time: a systematic review and meta-analysis. Poult Sci 2021; 100(5): 101082.
[http://dx.doi.org/10.1016/j.psj.2021.101082] [PMID: 33813325]

[10]    Kenneth S. Overview of Helminthiasis in Poultry, the merk veterinary manual 2013. Available from: http://www.mercmanuals.com/vet/nematode_and_cestode_infection/overview-of-helminthosis-in-poultry.html

[11]    Zirintunda G, Biryomumaisho S, Kasozi KI, *et al.* Emerging anthelmintic resistance in poultry: can ethnopharmacological approaches offer a solution?. Front Pharmacol 2022; 12: 774896.
[http://dx.doi.org/10.3389/fphar.2021.774896] [PMID: 35237147]

[12]    Lois S. Internal Parasites (Worms) of Poultry 1996. Available from: http://www.primaryindustry.nt.gov.au

[13]    Simon MS. Enteric diseases: ASA handbook on poultry diseases. 2nd ed. American Soybean Association 2005; pp. 133-43.

[14]    Urquhart GM, Armour J, Duncan JL, Dunn AM, Jennings FW. Veterinary Parasitology. 2nd ed. Oxford: Blackwell Science Ltd. 1996; pp. 224-34.

[15]    Sharma RL, Bhat TK, Hemaprasanth . Anthelmintic activity of ivermectin against experimental Ascaridia galli infection in chickens. Vet Parasitol 1990; 37(3-4): 307-14.

[http://dx.doi.org/10.1016/0304-4017(90)90014-3] [PMID: 2267731]

[16]    Leeson S, Summer JD. Internal Parasites: Broiler Breeder Production, 1ˢᵗ Published by Nottingham University Press in 2000 and Digitally reprinted in 2009 from Broiler Breeder Production.

[17]    Permin A, Hansen JW. Epidemiology, diagnosis and control of poultry Parasites. Food and agriculture organization of the united nations 1998.

[18]    Chakrabarti A. A textbook of preventive veterinary medicine. New Delhi: Kalyani publishers 2017.

[19]    Sandhu HS. Essentials of veterinary pharmacology and therapeutics. 2ⁿᵈ ed., Kalyani publishers 2017.

[20]    Horton-Smith C, Taylor EL, Turtle EE. Ammonia fumigation for coccidial disinfection. Vet Rec 1940; 52: 829-32.

[21]    Gholami MH, Rassouli A, Mirzaei S, Hashemi F. The potential immunomodulatory effect of levamisole in humans and farm animals. J Adv Vet Anim Res. 2023 Dec 31;10(4):620-629.
        [http://dx.doi.org/10.5455/javar.2023.j717. ]

[22]    Hauck R, Macklin KS. Vaccination against poultry parasites. Avian Dis 2024; 67(4): 441-9.
        [PMID: 38300662]

[23]    Berry JG. Fly control in the poultry house 2003. Available from: http://osufacts.oksatate.edu

[24]    Townsend LH Jr. The synthetic pyrethroid Ectiban permethrin as a treatment in the pest management of flies in caged-layer poultry houses. Virginia Polytechnic Institute and State University 1977. Available from: https://www.uky.edu/Ag/PAT/recs/livestk/recpou/poufly.htm

[25]    Jilo SA, Abadula TA, Abadura SZ, Gobana RH, Hasan LA, Nair SP. Review on epidemiology, pathogenesis, treatment, control and prevention of gastrointestinal parasite of poultry. Int J Vet Sci Anim Husb 2022; 7(5): 26-34.
        [http://dx.doi.org/10.22271/veterinary.2022.v7.i5a.439]

CHAPTER 10

# Fluke Parasites in Poultry

**R.S. Ghasura[1,*], Tanmoy Rana[2], S.T. Parmar[3], S.V. Mavadiya[4] and Vandeep Chahuan[1]**

*[1] College of Veterinary Science & A.H -Anand, Kamdhenu University, Anand, Gujarat, India*

*[2] Department of Veterinary Clinical Complex, West Bengal University of Animal & Fishery Sciences, Kolkata, India*

*[3] College of Veterinary Science & A.H -Navsari, Kamdhenu University, Anand, Gujarat, India*

*[4] College of Veterinary Science & A.H -Junagadh, Kamdhenu University, Anand, Gujarat, India*

**Abstract:** Although rarely in commercial settings, flea infections in poultry present serious health hazards in backyard and free-range habitats, particularly among warmer, wetter areas. The three main fluke species that plague poultry are investigated in this chapter: *Collyriclum faba* (subcutaneous cysts), *Philophthalmus gralli* (eye fluke) and *Prosthogonimus macrorchis* (oviduct fluke). Insects and snails are the intermediate hosts that these parasites need. Clinical symptoms include cysts, decreased egg production, weight loss, and eye problems. Since adult flukes are usually seen at lesion sites, diagnosing fluke infections is difficult since eggs are not always present in feces. Since few and frequently poor treatment options exist, such as praziquantel and fenbendazole, preventive efforts concentrate on environmental control to avoid intermediate hosts. Keeping chickens in areas free of flukes is essential for their well-being and output.

**Keywords:** Diseases, Fluke, Infection, Infestation, Poultry parasites.

## INTRODUCTION

Over the past few decades, there has been a significant increase in the number of widely and intensively housed chickens due to the growing demand for poultry products for human consumption [1, 2]. While rare in commercial poultry operations, fluke diseases pose a serious health issue in backyard and free-range environments, especially in warmer, wetter regions. The fluke life cycle, which needs intermediate hosts like snails and insects like mayflies and dragonflies, is aided by these habitats. Poultry raised in backyards and on farms have a higher chance of coming into touch with these hosts, which increases the risk of

*Corresponding author R.S.Ghasura: College of Veterinary Science and Animal Husbandry – Anand, Kamdhenu University, Anand, Gujarat, India; E-mail: rghasura21@kamdhenuuni.edu.in

infection. In the fields of veterinary medicine and poultry farming, parasites and parasitic illnesses pose a serious threat. These illnesses not only harm the well-being and output of chickens but also provide significant financial difficulties for the sector. It is essential to comprehend the biology, life cycles, and epidemiology of these parasites to develop management and control plans that are effective. A variety of parasite illnesses can affect poultry, which includes chickens, turkeys, ducks, and other birds kept for meat, eggs, or breeding. It is known that poultry can contract oviduct flukes from over 24 species across two genera. Three species have been identified in chickens: *Prosthogonimus ovatus, P. macrorchis,* and *P. pellucidus* [3].

*Collyriclum faba, Philophthalmus gralli,* and *Prosthogonimus macrorchis* are the three primary fluke species that infect poultry. The oviduct fluke, *Prosthogonimus macrorchis*, is especially dangerous since it can seriously impair a bird's ability to reproduce. The symptoms of infection in birds include cloacal discharge, decreased egg production, and weight loss. These flukes can induce lesions that range in severity from minor oviduct rupture to severe inflammation. Conversely, birds who have *Philophthalmus gralli* in their eyes may go blind as a result of this infection. This impairs the bird's capacity to forage and makes it more vulnerable to environmental dangers and predators [4].

Subcutaneous cysts caused by *Collyriclum faba* have the potential to cause subsequent bacterial infections. These cysts, which are frequently located close to the vent, can make heavily afflicted birds unable to move and unappetizing.

Reducing poultry contact with intermediate hosts is key to preventing fluke infections. This can be accomplished by preventing chickens from entering regions with water and places where aquatic insects and snails are common. However, there aren't many choices for treatment after the infection has set in. Although some medications, such as fenbendazole and praziquantel, have had some effectiveness, there are currently no approved medicines that are consistently beneficial for use in poultry. Furthermore, a number of parasite illnesses are zoonotic, which means that humans may contract them from chickens and hence be in danger to public health. This book chapter explores the several parasites that impact poultry, looking at their life cycles, means of transmission, symptoms, and techniques for diagnosis. Additionally, it examines new and existing methods for treating, managing, and preventing parasite infections in chickens (poultry), while highlighting the significance of integrated management practices. Poultry producers, veterinarians and researchers can improve poultry health and productivity by safeguarding poultry chicks against parasite illnesses by thoroughly comprehending these factors [5].

# TYPES OF FLUKE PARASITES IN POULTRY

In poultry farming, parasitic infections are a serious problem that has a big impact on the health and welfare of the birds as well as the operations' ability to make money. *Prosthogonimus* is a genus of trematodes belonging to the family *Prosthogonimidae* and includes several species. These flatworms infect the bursa Fabricius, the oviduct, and the posterior intestine of various poultry and wild bird species, including chicken, ducks, geese, and other birds. The genus *Prosthogonimus* is widespread and has been reported in many regions worldwide, including Africa, Asia, Europe, North and South America [6]. The prevalence of helminth infections can be influenced by many factors such as the climatic conditions and agro-ecological zones, the accumulation of infective stages of larvae or eggs in the environment, the presence of intermediate hosts, and the individual susceptibility of the final host [7]. These illnesses, which can result in significant financial losses and jeopardize the safety and quality of chicken products, are brought on by a diverse range of endoparasites (such as nematodes, cestodes, trematodes, and protozoa) and ectoparasites (such as mites, lice, and fleas) (Fig **1**) [8].

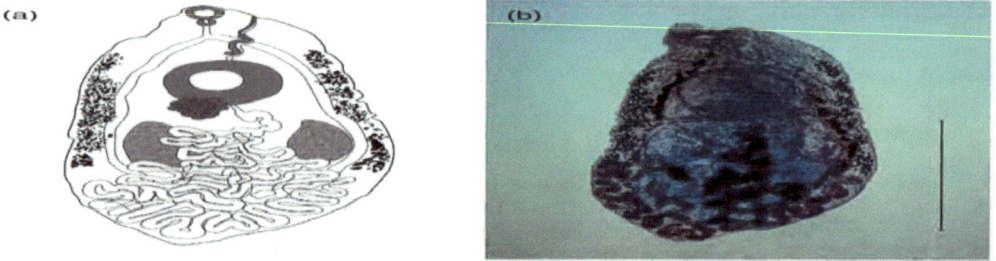

**Fig. (1).** *Prosthogonimus cuneatus* was recovered in *Erithacus rubecula*. They were drawn with Adobe Illustrator 2020 (**a**) and coloured with Semichon's carmine (**b**) Bar: 1000 $\mu$m [6].

## *Prosthogonimus macrorchis*

*Prosthogonimus macrorchis*, commonly known as the oviduct fluke, primarily infects poultry through the ingestion of metacercariae found in dragonflies, which serve as the secondary host. This fluke localizes in the oviduct of birds, causing significant reproductive issues. Symptoms of infection include inappetence, droopiness, weight loss, and decreased egg production, often leading to an increase in the number of soft-shelled eggs. Severe cases can result in lesions ranging from mild inflammation to oviduct distention or rupture, potentially leading to the bird's death. Due to the specific nature of its lifecycle, involving both snail and dragonfly hosts, controlling the environment to limit bird exposure to these intermediates is crucial for prevention (Figs. **2** and **3**).

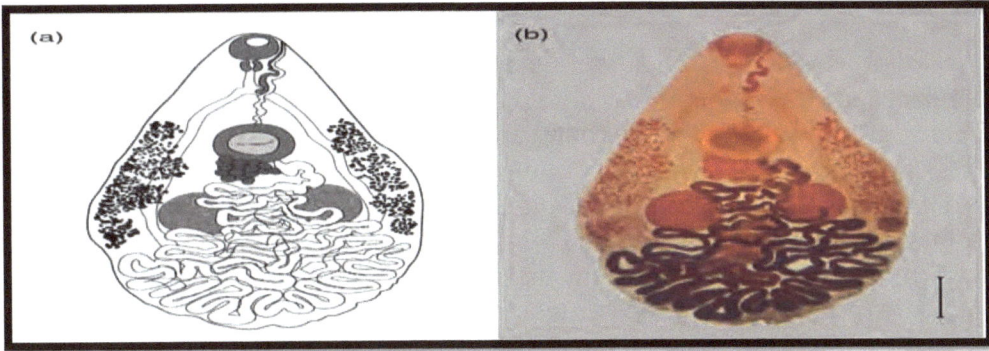

**Fig. (2).** *Prosthogonimus macrorchis* was recovered in *Ciconia ciconia*. They were drawn using Adobe Illustrator 2020 (**a**) and coloured with Semichon's carmine (**b**) Bar: 1000 $\mu$m [6].

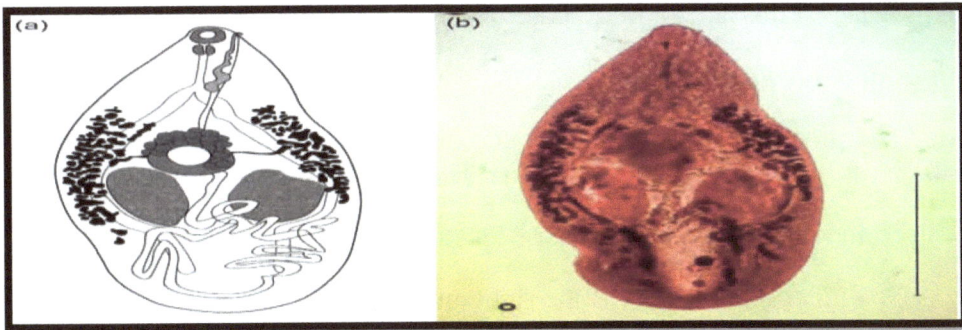

**Fig. (3).** *Prosthogonimus ovatus* was recovered in *Turdus philomelos*. They were drawn using Adobe Illustrator 2020 (**a**) and coloured with Semichon's carmine (**b**) Bar: 1000 $\mu$m (Öztürk, M., & *Kumar* S) [6].

## *Philophthalmus gralli*

*Philophthalmus gralli* is another significant fluke parasite known to infect the eyes of birds. This fluke is particularly dangerous as it can lead to blindness, severely affecting the bird's ability to feed and navigate its environment. Infected birds may show signs of ocular discharge, swelling, and irritation. Blindness not only reduces feed intake but also increases vulnerability to predators and environmental hazards. Similar to *Prosthogonimus macrorchis, Philophthalmus gralli* requires an intermediate host, typically snails, making environmental management a key preventive measure. While some treatments have been attempted, such as the use of praziquantel, results have been inconsistent, emphasizing the importance of prevention.

## *Collyriclum faba*

*Collyriclum faba* forms subcutaneous cysts in infected birds, which can lead to secondary bacterial infections. These cysts, typically 4–6 mm in diameter, often appear near the vent but can be found anywhere on the body. They contain adult flukes and can ooze exudates, attracting flies and increasing the risk of infection. In young birds, heavy infections may cause locomotor difficulties, inappetence, and even death. The lifecycle of *Collyriclum faba* is not well understood but likely involves snails and aquatic insects. Surgical removal of the cysts is a common treatment, though preventive measures focusing on limiting access to potential intermediate hosts remain the best strategy.

Understanding these fluke parasites and their lifecycles is essential for managing and preventing infections in poultry, especially in backyard and free-range settings where birds are more exposed to intermediate hosts.

## *Echinostoma revolutum*

**Hosts:** The principal hosts are ducks and geese, the parasite may occur in other aquatic birds, pigeons, fowl, and humans. The parasite is seen worldwide.

**Predilection site:** The adult worms are located in the rectum and caeca.

**Life cycle and epidemiology:** If the right circumstances are present, such as high humidity and high temperatures, *E. revolutum* eggs pass through the feces and mature in three weeks. A snail (*Lymnaea spp., Sta gnicola palustris, Helisoma trivolvis, Physa spp., or Planorbis tenuis*) serves as the intermediary host for the miracidium's penetration. However, other possible intermediate hosts include *Bulinus, Biomphalaria, Succinea, Pseudosuccinea,* and *Corbiculina.* Within two to three weeks, cercariae in snails can either encyst or escape and infect another snail. When birds eat infected snails, they contract the infection. The 15–19 day prepatent period is in effect.

**Clinical signs and pathogenicity:** Heavy infections with *E. revolutum* may cause emaciation and catarrhal enteritis. Death may occur in young animals [4].

## LIFE CYCLE AND TRANSMISSION OF FLUKE PARASITES IN POULTRY

Fluke parasites have complex lifecycles that typically involve multiple hosts, including snails and insects such as dragonflies or mayflies, as intermediate hosts. The lifecycle begins when fluke eggs are excreted in the feces of an infected bird. These eggs hatch in water, releasing larvae that infect snails. Within the snails, the larvae undergo several developmental stages before emerging as free-swimming cercariae. These cercariae then infect a secondary host, such as a dragonfly or mayfly, by encysting as metacercariae. Birds become infected by ingesting these infected insects. Once inside the bird, the metacercariae migrate to specific organs, such as the oviduct, eyes, or subcutaneous tissues, where they mature into adult flukes and continue the cycle. Preventing exposure to these intermediate hosts is crucial in managing fluke infections in poultry [6].

## CLINICAL SIGNS AND DIAGNOSIS OF FLUKE PARASITES IN POULTRY

### *Prosthogonimus macrorchis*

Infections with *Prosthogonimus macrorchis* can be particularly severe in poultry. Heavy infections often result in significant weight loss, decreased egg production, and cloacal discharge. Lesions caused by this fluke may lead to inflammation and in severe cases, rupture of the oviduct. The infection process can severely impact the bird's reproductive system, leading to an increase in soft-shelled eggs and overall poor health. These clinical signs are indicative of the parasite's detrimental effect on the bird's physiology.

### *Philophthalmus gralli*

*Philophthalmus gralli* primarily infects the eyes of birds, leading to potential blindness. This condition severely affects the bird's ability to feed and navigate its environment, making it more vulnerable to predators and environmental challenges. Clinical signs include ocular discharge, swelling, and irritation. The impact on the bird's vision is particularly concerning as it directly influences its ability to survive and thrive.

### *Collyriclum faba*

Infections with *Collyriclum faba* are characterized by the presence of subcutaneous cysts. These cysts, often 4-6 mm in diameter, can cause significant discomfort and lead to secondary bacterial infections due to the exudate they produce. In young birds, these cysts can result in locomotor difficulties and inappetence, severely affecting their growth and development. In severe cases, heavy infections may lead to death [6].

### *E. revolutum*

**Clinical signs and pathogenicity:** Heavy infections with *E. revolutum* may cause emaciation and catarrhal enteritis. Death may occur in young animals.

# DIAGNOSIS

Diagnosing fluke infections in poultry is challenging due to the inconsistent presence of fluke eggs in fecal samples. Traditional fecal examinations often fail to detect the parasites. Adult flukes are typically observed at the site of lesions during necropsy or post-mortem examinations. This direct observation remains the most reliable method for confirming fluke infections, although it is not practical for early detection. Advanced diagnostic methods, such as molecular techniques, may offer more reliable detection but are not commonly used in routine poultry management. Therefore, preventing exposure to intermediate hosts remains a crucial strategy for managing fluke infections in poultry.

## PREVENTION AND CONTROL OF FLUKE INFECTIONS IN POULTRY

Preventing fluke infections in poultry hinges on minimizing birds' exposure to the intermediate hosts necessary for the fluke lifecycle. Intermediate hosts such as snails and insects like dragonflies or mayflies thrive in bodies of water and areas with high insect activity. Therefore, restricting poultry access to these environments is critical. This can be achieved by:

- **Enclosing Poultry Areas**: Use physical barriers to prevent birds from accessing water bodies and damp areas where intermediate hosts are prevalent.
- **Environmental Management**: Modify the environment to reduce standing water and other habitats that support the lifecycle of snails and insects.
- **Regular Monitoring**: Regularly inspect poultry areas for the presence of intermediate hosts and take appropriate measures to eliminate them if found.

## TREATMENT

Effective treatments for fluke infections in poultry are currently limited. Some drugs, such as praziquantel and fenbendazole, have been used with varying degrees of success. However, these treatments are not universally effective and are not specifically approved for use in poultry. Carbon tetrachloride has also been used, but it is highly toxic to poultry and not a recommended treatment option.

Given these limitations, the primary focus remains on preventive measures. When an infection is suspected or confirmed, managing the health of the affected birds and reducing the spread to others becomes paramount. This includes isolating infected birds and ensuring they receive supportive care to mitigate the impact of the infection.

# CONCLUDING REMARKS

Management of fluke infections in poultry relies heavily on preventive strategies due to the limited and often ineffective treatment options available. Maintaining a fluke-free environment is essential for the health and productivity of poultry, particularly in backyard and free-range settings where birds are more likely to come into contact with intermediate hosts. Environmental control measures, such as restricting access to potential habitats of intermediate hosts and modifying the landscape to reduce standing water, are critical components of an effective prevention strategy.

By focusing on these preventive measures, poultry producers can minimize the risk of fluke infections and ensure the overall well-being of their flocks. Continuous monitoring and adapting management practices based on the presence of intermediate hosts can help maintain a healthy poultry population, free from the debilitating effects of fluke infections.

# REFERENCES

[1] Das M, Laha R, Doley S. Gastrointestinal parasites in backyard poultry of subtropical hilly region of Meghalaya. J Entomol Zool Stud 2020; 8(5): 1301-5.

[2] Kigston N. Trematodes. Diseases of Poultry. 7th ed. Iowa: Iowa state Univ. Press 1978; pp. 777-81.

[3] Magwisha HB, Kassuku AA, Kyvsgaard NC, Permin A. A comparison of the prevalence and burdens of helminth infections in growers and adult free-range chickens. Trop Anim Health Prod 2002; 34(3): 205-14.
[http://dx.doi.org/10.1023/A:1015278524559] [PMID: 12094676]

[4] Muriu J. Impact of Parasites and Parasitic Diseases on Animal Health and Productivity. J Anim Health 2023; 3(1): 13-23.
[http://dx.doi.org/10.47604/jah.2100]

[5] Ola-Fadunsin S D, Uwabujo P I, Sanda I M, *et al.* Gastrointestinal helminths of intensively managed poultry in Kwara Central, Kwara State, Nigeria: its diversity, prevalence 2019.

[6] Öztürk M, Umur Ş. The oviduct fluke, *Prosthogonimus* species in wild birds, Türkiye. Vet Med Sci 2023; 9(5): 2329-35.
[http://dx.doi.org/10.1002/vms3.1209] [PMID: 37465979]

[7] Permin A, Hansen JW. Epidemiology, diagnosis and control of poultry parasites. FAO Animal Health Manual 4, Roma, Italy. 1998; pp. 1-160.

[8] Sharma N, Hunt PW, Hine BC, Ruhnke I. The impacts of *Ascaridia galli* on performance, health, and immune responses of laying hens: new insights into an old problem. Poult Sci 2019; 98(12): 6517-26.
[http://dx.doi.org/10.3382/ps/pez422] [PMID: 31504894]

# CHAPTER 11

# Round Worm Infection

**Jayalakshmi Jaliparthi[1,*] and P. Ramadevi[2]**

[1] *Department of Veterinary Parasitology, SKPP AHP, S.V.V.U, Ramachandrapuram, Andhra Pradesh, India*

[2] *Department of Veterinary Parasitology, C.V.Sc, S.V.V.U, Garividi, Andhra Pradesh, India*

**Abstract:** Diseases caused by nematode infestations pose a significant challenge to poultry production, impacting economic viability and overall bird health. Over 50 nematode species, including large roundworms (*Ascaris* sp.), small roundworms (*Capillaria* sp.), and cecal worms (*Heterakis gallinarum*), inflict pathological harm on poultry, waterfowl, and wild birds. The resulting economic losses include malnutrition, reduced feed conversion, weight loss, diminished egg production, and increased mortality in young birds. Concurrent infestations with multiple gastrointestinal-preferring parasites contribute to early chick mortality and productivity losses in adult birds. Nematode infestations extend beyond direct losses, increasing susceptibility to other diseases and worsening existing health conditions. Efficient and prompt diagnosis is crucial for controlling parasitic infections. Diagnosis methods include fecal sample analysis through flotation techniques, necropsy examination, ELISA technique, and a loop-mediated isothermal amplification assay with lateral flow dipstick for visual detection of parasitic eggs. The preferred drug for treating roundworms is piperazine, though recent medications like albendazole and levamisole have shown high success rates. Flubendazole, pyrantel tartrate, and ivermectin are also effective treatments. Poultry commonly harbors six species of *Capillaria* sp., necessitating specific diagnosis and treatment approaches. Preventive measures include rigorous cleanliness, optimal ventilation, moisture control, and avoiding overcrowding. Regular deworming, age-specific bird separation, and litter replacement are essential for controlling parasitic infections. The use of insecticides to eliminate intermediate hosts is discouraged due to environmental concerns. A comprehensive and proactive approach is vital for sustaining the health and productivity of poultry in the face of nematode challenges.

**Keywords:** *Ascaridia galli, Capillaria, Heterakis gallinarum, Oxyspirura mansoni,* Poultry Nematodes, Roundworms, *Subulura brumpti, Syngamus trachea, Tetrameres* sp.

---

* **Corresponding author Jayalakshmi Jaliparthi:** Department of Veterinary Parasitology, SKPP AHP, S.V.V.U, Ramachandrapuram, Andhra Pradesh, India; E-mail: raghava.plr@gmail.com

**Tanmoy Rana (Ed.)**

# INTRODUCTION

The disease poses a significant challenge to poultry production, with nematodes emerging as the predominant and crucial helminth species affecting poultry, waterfowl, and wild birds. There are over 50 identified nematode species impacting poultry, including large roundworms (*Ascaris* sp. or ascarids), small roundworms (*Capillaria* sp. or capillary/threadworms), and cecal worms (*Heterakis gallinarum*). These nematodes, particularly the majority among them, inflict pathological harm on the host, resulting in substantial economic losses for the poultry industry. The damage caused includes malnutrition, reduced feed conversion ratio, weight loss, diminished egg production, and mortality in young birds [1]. Additionally, parasitic infestations can increase the susceptibility of poultry to other diseases and worsen existing health conditions [2, 3].

Concurrent infestations with multiple parasites, especially those with a gastrointestinal preference, play a significant role in early chick mortality and contribute to productivity losses in adult birds [4]. The overall impact of nematode infestations extends beyond direct losses, affecting the overall health and productivity of poultry in the industry. Nematodes, belonging to the phylum Nemathelminthes and the class Nematoda, are parasitic worms affecting poultry. These worms are unsegmented and typically display a cylindrical and elongated shape. The cuticle of nematodes may exhibit various features such as circular annulations, smooth surfaces, longitudinal striations, or ornamentations like cuticular plaques or spines. All nematodes possess an alimentary tract, and they exhibit separate sexes. The life cycle of these worms can be either direct or indirect, involving an intermediate host [5]. Furthermore, mechanical transmission by earthworms or cockroaches is noteworthy [6]. It is important to emphasize that there is no development of the larval stage within these carriers (Table **1**).

**Table 1. Common roundworms of poultry.**

| Roundworm | Definitive host | Intermediate host | Site of predilection |
|---|---|---|---|
| *Capillaria annulata* | Fowl, turkey | earthworms | Esophagus and crop |
| *Capillaria caudinflata* | Fowl, pigeons, wild birds | earthworms | Duodenum and Ileum |
| *Capillaria. obsignata* | Chickens, turkeys, partridges, pigeons, guinea fowl, and quail | Direct | Small intestine |
| *Capillaria anatis* | Fowl, anatine birds | Direct | Caeca |
| *Ascaridiagalli* | Fowl, guinea fowl, turkey, goose, wild birds | Direct | Small intestine |
| *Subulura brumpti* | Chickens, turkeys, guineafowls, ducks, pheasants, grouse, quails | Beetles, cockroach | Caeca |

*(Table 1) cont.....*

| Roundworm | Definitive host | Intermediate host | Site of predilection |
|---|---|---|---|
| *Oxyspirura mansoni* | Fowl, turkey | cockroaches | Eye (nictitating membrane) |
| *Syngamus trachea* | Chickens, pheasants, turkeys, and peacocks | Direct | trachea and lungs |
| *Tetrameres americana* | Fowl, Turkey, duck, pigeon | Grasshoppers, cockroaches | Proventriculus |
| *Heterakis gallinarum* | Chickens, Turkey, duck, game birds | Direct | Caeca |
| *Cheilospirura hamulosa* | Goose, chickens, turkeys | Beetles, grasshoppers | Gizzard |
| *Dispharynx spiralis* | Turkeys, pigeon, guinea fowl, pheasants | Beetles, grasshoppers | Proventriculus and Oesophagus |
| *Amidostomum* | Waterfowl, wild geese, ducks, parakeets. | Direct | Gizzard sometimes proventriculus and esophagus |

### *Ascaridia galli*

**Order**: Ascaridida

**Super family:** Ascaridoidea

**Family:** Ascarididae

**Genus:** *Ascaridia*

*Ascaridia galli*, the roundworm species, is highly prevalent and pathogenic, particularly in domestic fowl such as *Gallus domesticus*. This species is known for its widespread occurrence and significant impact on domestic poultry [7]. It can also infest other species of poultry, including turkeys, geese, and wild birds. The parasitic nature of *Ascaridia galli* makes it a notable concern in various poultry populations, causing potential harm and health issues in affected birds (Fig. **1**).

The largest nematode, *Ascaridia galli* is a semitransparent, creamy-white, cylindrical-bodied nematode. At its anterior end lies a distinctive mouth surrounded by three prominent tri-lobed lips, with the dorsal lip wider than the subventral ones. The lip edges are furnished with teeth-like denticles (Fig. **2**) [8]. The entire body is enveloped in a robust proteinaceous cuticle, exhibiting transverse striations and featuring a pair of faintly developed cuticular alae. Notably, two conspicuous papillae are present on the dorsal lip, and each subventral lip hosts one. The esophagus lacks a posterior bulb, and these papillae serve as the nematode's sensory organs. *Ascaridia galli* shows clear sexual dimorphism [9].

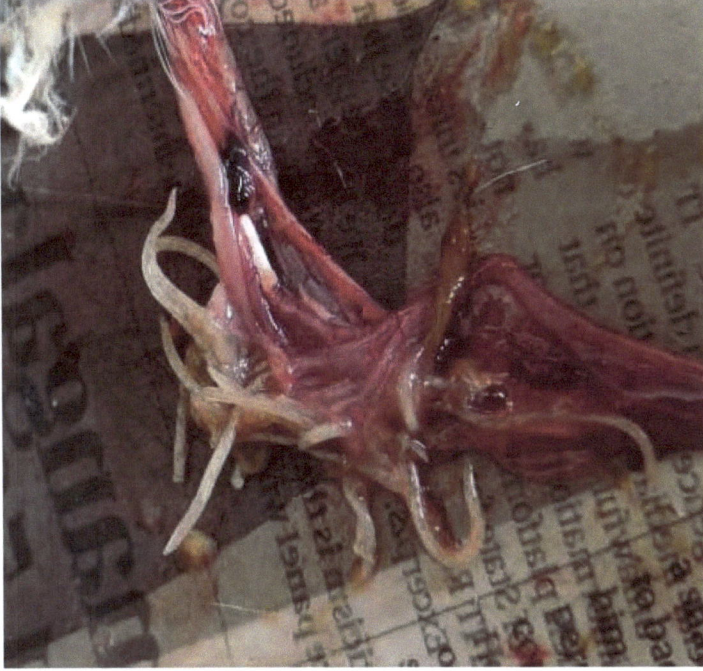

**Fig. (1).** Obstruction of poultry intestine with adult *A. galli* worms.

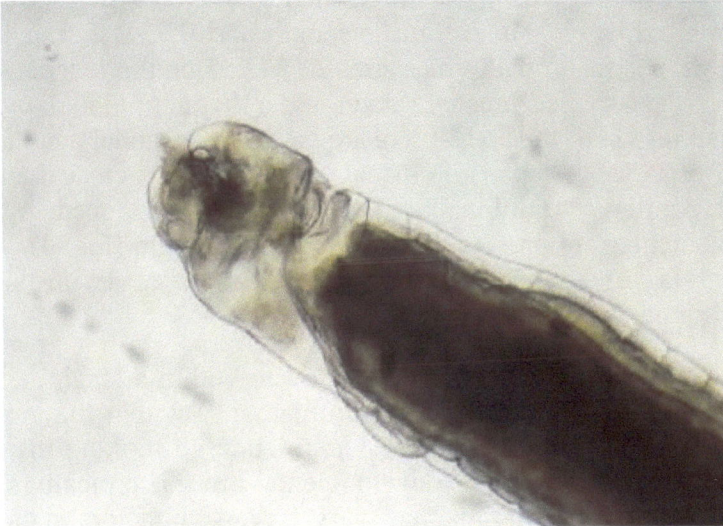

**Fig. (2).** Anterior end of *A. galli*.

Females are markedly larger and more robust, measuring between 72 to 102 in length and 2.8 to 5.2 in breadth. Their vulva opening is positioned slightly posterior to the middle section, with the distance ranging from 18 to 33mm from the anterior end [10]. The tail end of females is characterized by a blunt and straight structure, featuring a caudal spine (Fig. **3**).

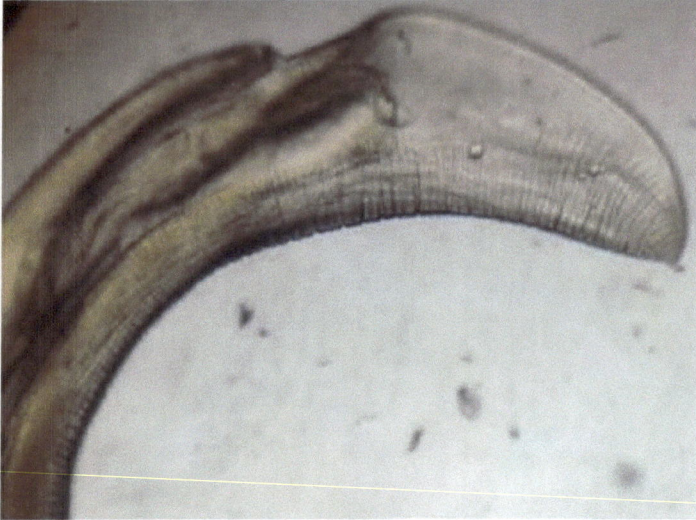

**Fig. (3).**  Tail end of female *A. galli.*

In contrast, males can be easily distinguished by their shorter and smaller size, measuring approximately 50–76 mm in length and 0.43–1.5 mm in maximum breadth. The esophagus of males measures 2.12–2.35 mm in length. Additionally, males have an oval-shaped preanal sucker and a distinct pointed and curved tail [11]. In the tail region of the body, there are ten pairs of caudal papillae, organized as 3 pairs of precloacal, 1 pair of cloacal, 3 pairs of post-cloacal and 3 pairs of sub-terminal papillae. Additionally, a pair of well-developed, approximately equal-length spicules are present, measuring 1.4–1.65 mm (Fig. **4**). The eggs are elliptical with a thick shell and measure 52-64 x 41-49 µm and are not embryonated upon deposition [11, 12].

**Life cycle**: *A. galli* undergoes a direct life cycle within a single host, requiring two main populations: the sexually mature parasites within the gastrointestinal tract and the infective stage (L2). The larvae undergo molting inside the eggs, progressing to the L3 stage. This developmental process typically spans around two weeks, though the duration may vary based on factors such as weather conditions. The life cycle finishes when new hosts eat the infective eggs, typically through contaminated water or feed. Earthworms, acting as transport hosts, are believed to contribute to the spread of *A. galli*. This is why birds that roam freely are more likely to get infected [13, 14].The L2-larvae-containing eggs are moved mechanically to the duodenum. Once ingested by a chicken, the infective eggs reach the proventriculus and hatch [13]. The larva, triggered by factors like temperature, carbon dioxide levels, and pH, then emerges from its egg. The larva subsequently burrows into the small intestine's mucosal lining, where it goes through two further molts at eight days and 14–15 days.

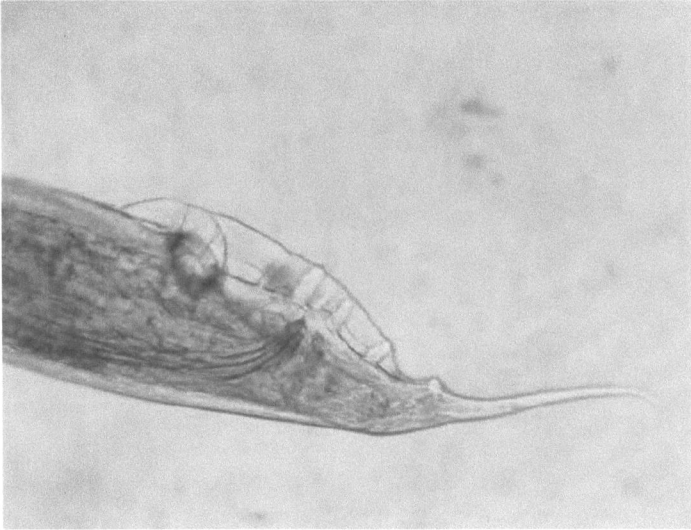

**Fig. (4).** Tail end of male *A.galli*.

During this stage of their life cycle, the worms inflict the greatest harm to their host. After that, they re-enter the small intestine and mature into adults, living their whole lives there, eating on the contents of the gut and excreting copious amounts of eggs that are subsequently expelled by a host and allowed to complete their life cycle. When the animal can generate an immune response to the larvae, particularly if there's pre-exposure, the larvae refrain from maturing into adults. Instead, they conceal themselves in the mucosa of the small intestine. This occurrence is frequent in infections of older birds.

**Pathogenesis**: *Ascaridia galli* can affect fowl across all age groups, with the most significant impact observed in young birds under 12 weeks old. Heavy infections are often associated with dietary deficiencies in essential elements such as vitamins (A, B, B12), minerals, and proteins. The primary manifestation occurs during the prepatent phase, where larvae residing in the mucosa induce catarrhal enteritis. In cases of severe infection, there is a higher risk of haemorrhagic enteritis [15]. Significant infestations play a pivotal role in causing weight depression and diminished egg production in poultry farming. In cases of severe infection, there is a risk of intestinal blockage, leading to symptoms such as unthriftiness, drooping wings, and bleaching of the head (Fig. **5**).

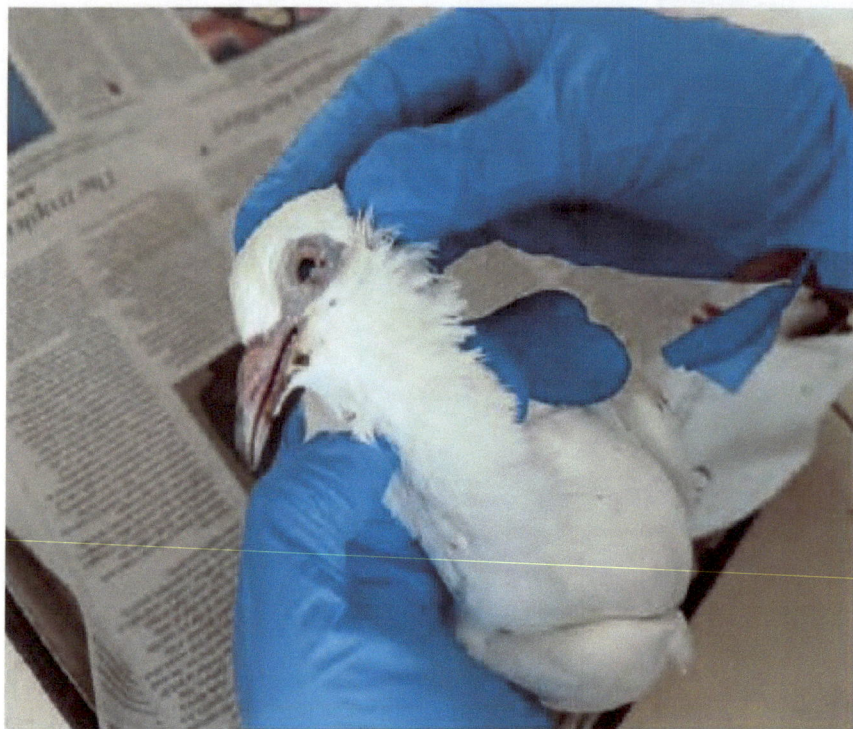

**Fig. (5).** Bird showing the symptoms of worm burden.

Moreover, it contributes to blood loss, decreased blood sugar levels, reduced thymus gland size, slowed growth, and a substantial rise in mortality rates.

In cases of intense infestation, mature worms can ascend the oviduct and potentially be discovered in the eggs of hens. Occasionally, these worms may also be present in the feces of the birds [16]. Widespread *A. galli* infections have the potential to decrease egg output in breeders and commercial layers kept in floor housing. Mortality can result from intestinal obstruction (Fig. **1**), particularly in birds with compromised immunity or those dealing with concurrent debilitating conditions [17].

**Diagnosis**: The basis for controlling parasitic infections lies in efficient and prompt diagnosis. Ascariasis can be routinely diagnosed by detecting the nematode's eggs in fecal samples, either through the floatation technique or by examining the intestine during necropsy [18]. An alternative non-invasive method involves utilizing the ELISA technique to identify *A. galli* coproantigen in poultry bird droppings, employing polyclonal antibodies [19]. A loop-mediated isothermal amplification assay coupled with a lateral flow dipstick (LAMP-LFD) test was devised (Panich *et al.*, 2023). This method specifically targets the internal transcribed spacer (ITS-2) and facilitates the visual detection of *A. galli* eggs in fecal samples.

**Treatment**: The preferred drug for treating *Ascaridia galli* is piperazine. It can be administered as 0.2-0.4% to chickens through feed, 0.1-0.2% through water, or as a single treatment (50-100 mg/bird). Notably, piperazine exhibits limited efficacy in young chickens. On the other hand, tetramisole, provided as a 10% solution in drinking water, proves to be 89-100% effective for chickens of different ages. Another common approach involves continuous medication through feed using hygromycin B at a dosage of 8 g/tonne of feed over an 8-week period. Additionally, phenothiazine can be employed with a dosage of up to 2200 mg/kg, although its effects can vary. Moreover, alternative drugs such as mebendazole at a dosage of 2 g in 28 kg of feed, haloxon at 30 g per 50 g of feed, and fenbendazole at 10–50 mg/kg (with the option of repeating the treatment after 10 days) have demonstrated effectiveness in successfully treating *Ascaridia* infections [20].

Recent medications, such as albendazole and levamisole, have proven to be highly successful in addressing *Ascaridia* infections. In Europe, the commonly employed treatment for *Ascaridia* spp. involves the use of flubendazole at a dosage of 1.43 mg/kg. Notably, pyrantel tartrate exhibits superior efficacy compared to pyrantel pamoate when targeting the adult stage of *A. galli*. Furthermore, studies indicate that Ivermectin boasts a 90% effectiveness rate against immature worms and a 95% effectiveness rate against adult worms.

## *Capillaria*

**Order:** Enoplida

**Super family:** Trichuroidea

**Family:** Capillariidae

**Genus:***Capillaria*

Poultry commonly harbors six species of *Capillaria: C. annulata, C. contorta, C. caudinflata, C. bursata, C. obsignata* (also known as *C. columbae*), and *C. anatis*. All six species are reported in both domesticated and wild birds, exhibiting a cosmopolitan distribution [21]. These *Capillaria* species inhabit various parts of the intestinal tract. *C. annulata* and *C. contorta* are located in the crop and esophagus. On the other hand, *C. caudinflata, C. bursata,* and *C. obsignata* parasitize the small intestine, while *C. anatis* is found in the caeca. The worms belonging to this genus are small, hair-like, and challenging to detect in the intestinal contents (Fig. **6**).

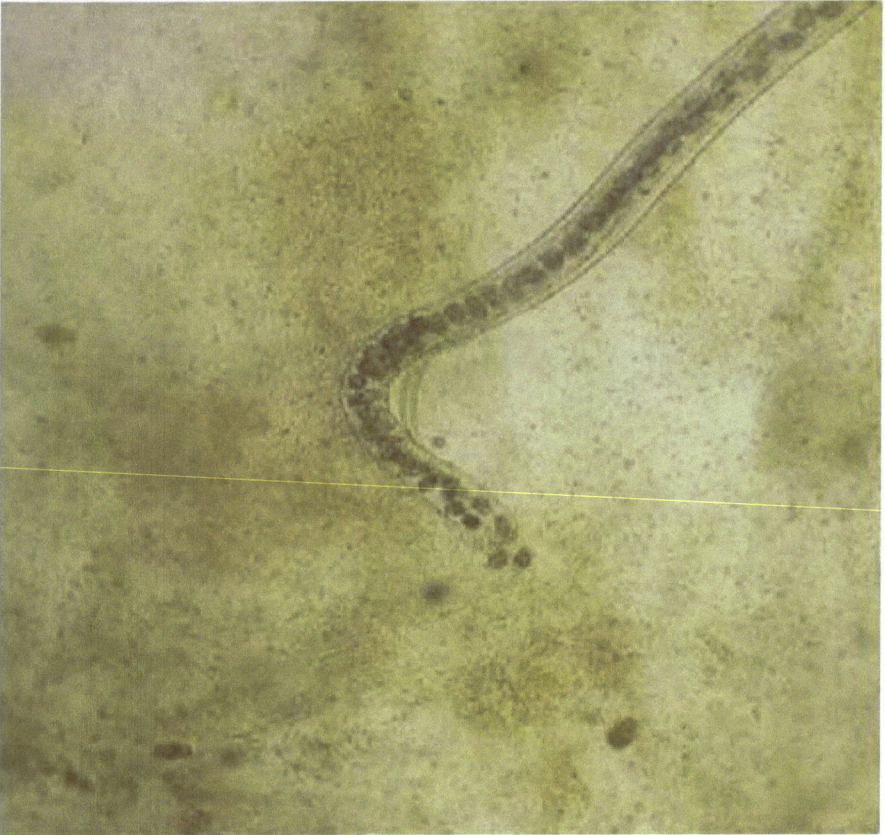

**Fig. (6).** Female adult *Capillaria* sp. in the intestinal scrapings of poultry.

## *C. annulata*

This widely distributed species infects the esophagus and crop of various birds, including fowl and turkeys. While prevalent in domestic turkeys, it can also cause a substantial disease in captive wild turkeys. *C. annulata* males typically range from 15 to 25 mm in length, and females measure between 37 and 80 mm. A distinctive feature of the species is the cuticle at the anterior end forming a notable swelling behind the head. The eggs exhibit characteristic bipolar plugs and have dimensions of 60 x 25 micrometers. Eggs, excreted in the feces of hosts, undergo environmental development for 11–12 days before being ingested and progressing through further development in earthworms. Essential intermediate hosts include *Allolobophora caliginosa*, *Allolobophora parva*, *Aporrectodea rosea*, *Eisenia foetida*, *Helodrilus caliginosus*, and *Lumbricus terrestris* [22, 23].

## *Capillaria caudinflata* (Hair worm)

These worms are predominantly found in the duodenum and ileum of both fowl and pigeons. They share a close relation to *Trichuris* species but are smaller and possess a hair-like appearance. Their structure is characterized by a gradual thickening from a thinner anterior to a thicker posterior end. Males measure 9-14 mm in length and have a single spicule, while females range from 14-25 mm, featuring a cylindrical tail. In males, the esophagus is half the length of the body, while in females, it is one-third the length of the body. Female worms are oviparous, and their eggs are colorless, barrel-shaped, with nearly parallel sides. In comparison to *Trichuris* species eggs, the bipolar plugs of these eggs do not project as far. The life cycle is similar to that of *C. annulata*, with a prepatent period lasting 21 days [24].

## *C. obsignata* (Synonym, *C. columbae*)

These thread-like worms, characterized by a whitish color and a cuticle with transverse striations, inhabit the small intestine. They primarily infest avian species such as chickens, turkeys, partridges, pigeons, guinea fowl, and quail. The male worms measure between 9.5 and 11.5 mm in length, with a width ranging from 0.035 to 0.04 mm. The esophagus spans a length of 5.31–9.98 mm. Additionally, their spicule, measuring 0.98–1.05 mm in length and 0.012 mm in width at the proximal end, expands into an open funnel shape. The spicule ends distally with a rounded tip. A thin, transversely striated sheath envelops the spicule, devoid of any spikes and upheld by two dorsolateral papillae, shaping a pseudo bursa. The cloacal opening is situated at the terminal end [25, 26]. The female shows dimensions of 10.5–14.5 mm in length and 0.048–0.09 mm in width. The esophagus extends from 4.54 to 98.69 mm. The vulva is positioned approximately halfway between the anterior end and features slightly swollen borders. The vagina is tiny and muscular. The anus is positioned subterminally. The eggs are oval-shaped, measuring 0.04–0.06 mm in length and 0.028–0.03 mm in diameter. The inner layer of the eggshell creates a small collar at the poles. The life cycle is direct; eggs expelled in the feces mature into the infective stage within 6–7 days [27].

## *C. anatis*

This species is found in the caeca of domesticated poultry and waterfowl. The males have elongated, thread-like morphology, measuring 10.5–12.9 mm in length and 0.06–0.09 mm in diameter. The length of the esophagus is about 4.23 to 6.25 mm. The spicule exhibits variable dimensions, with a length ranging from 1.0 to 1.02 mm and a width from 0.014 to 0.025 mm. It possesses three longitudinal thickenings and only slight proximal expansion. Two lateral lobes are present at the caudal end of the body, and the cloacal opening is situated terminally. The female nematode has a body length ranging from 14.3 to 18.5 mm and a diameter of 0.051–0.14 mm. The vulva is positioned at approximately one-third of the body length, lacking an appendage, while the vagina is elongated, measuring 0.025–0.65 mm. The body terminates bluntly at the caudal end, and the anus is situated subterminally. The eggs have dimensions of approximately 0.051–0.065 mm in length and 0.025–0.03 mm in width [28]. These eggs exhibit a distinctive thick, rugose outer shell layer. At the poles, the inner layer curls and shapes into a broad collar. The life cycle follows a direct pattern.

**Pathogenesis**: Clinical manifestations depend on the specific locations within a host where particular *Capillaria* species develop and the severity of the infection. Birds with a low parasite count may show no visible clinical signs [29, 30]. The majority of wild birds that are free-ranging have low-intensity infections, but those that pass away from capillary infections are typically found dead without showing any symptoms. Younger birds typically have the most severe infections, with older birds acting as carriers of the infection. Birds carrying high concentrations of *C. obsignata, C. annulatus,* or *C. caudinflata* may exhibit nonspecific symptoms such as reduced water intake, emaciation, diarrhea, and ruffled feathers. Additionally, birds may show signs of ataxia and weakness; if these are apparent, they often die [29]. Clinical symptoms are not usually a reliable predictor of illness. Heavy infections can cause hemorrhagic enteritis and bloody diarrhea. Pigeon infections with *C. obsignata* are highly pathogenic and can result in significant mortality rates. Generally, capillaria species that infect the upper gastrointestinal tract (oral cavity, esophagus, and crop) are more pathogenic than intestinal species because they can cause inflammation, dilatation of the crop or esophagus, thickening of the mucosa, ulceration, exudation, and fibrin necrotic plaques [31].

**Diagnosis:** Capillarid infection can be diagnosed by identifying eggs in fecal samples or mucosal scrapings. Alternatively, diagnosis can involve detecting eggs or adult worms in histologic sections of tissues. Capillarid eggs are easily identified by their distinctive bipolar plugs. Examining the vulvar region of female worms and thoroughly examining the posterior and anterior ends of adult worms of both sexes are necessary for the identification of *Capillaria* species.

**Treatment**: Methyridine (150 mg/kg), fenbendazole (8 mg/kg), levamisole (30 mg/kg), febantel, pyrantel tartrate (75 mg/kg), and hygromycin B (0.00088-

0.00132%) and febantel are very effective in treating capillariasis in a variety of bird species, such as partridges, pheasants, turkeys, and chickens. These medications have proven successful in the treatment of *C. obsignata* infection in pigeons and oral *Capillaria* infection in raptors [32]. Ivermectin administered subcutaneously to captive guinea fowls is effective in treating *C. caudinflata* infections [33]. The control of capillariasis infection in wild birds is usually impractical and unnecessary, given the limited pathogenic effects associated with most infections. To significantly reduce infection intensity and the risk of disease in captive birds, emphasis should be placed on maintaining proper sanitation in living quarters and raising birds in wire-bottom cages. This approach is effective because the transmission of capillaries relies on fecal contamination and exposure to either eggs or earthworms infected with the parasite.

### *Heterakis gallinarum*: **Caecal worm**

**Class:** Secernentea

**Order:** Ascaridida

**Superfamily:** Subuluroidea

**Family:** Heterakidae

**Genus:***Heterakis*

**Morphology:** These are small to medium-sized roundworms that inhabit the caeca of both domestic and wild birds, distributed worldwide. Other synonyms are *H. papillosa, H. vesicularis* and *H. gallinae.* The adult worms are whitish in colour, with males measuring about 7-13mm in length and females about 10-15mm. They possess three lips around the mouth, a small buccal cavity, and a pharynx. The oesophagus has a robust posterior bulb (Fig. 7).

The tail end of males is elongated and pointed, with unequal spicules - the right spicule being slender and long (2mm), and the left one short (0.65-0.7 mm) with broad alae. A large precloacal sucker and prominent caudal alae supported by 12 pairs of caudal papillae are present. Large lateral alae are found on the lateral aspect of the body. In females, the vulva opens behind the middle of the body (Fig. **8**). The eggs measure 65-80 x 35-46 µm, with thick and smooth shells, and are unsegmented when laid. Another species, *H. isolonche*, occurs in game birds, especially in pheasants [34].

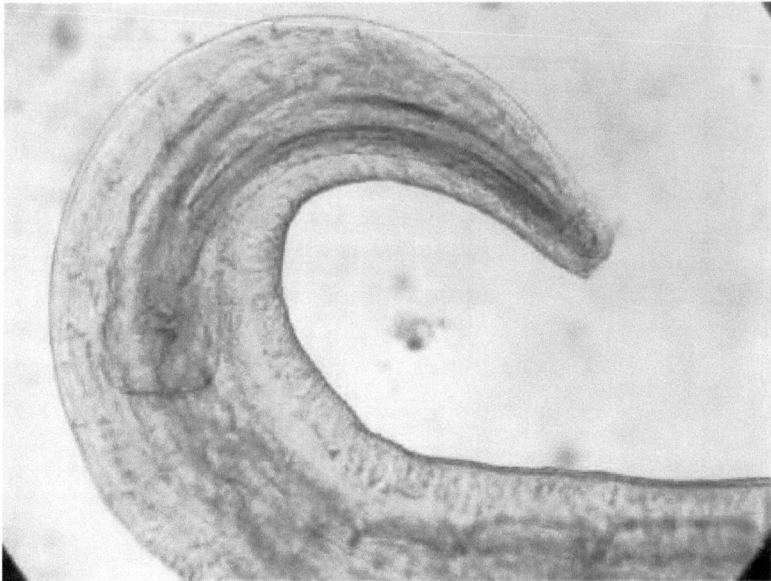

**Fig. (7).** Anterior end of *Heterakis gallinarum*.

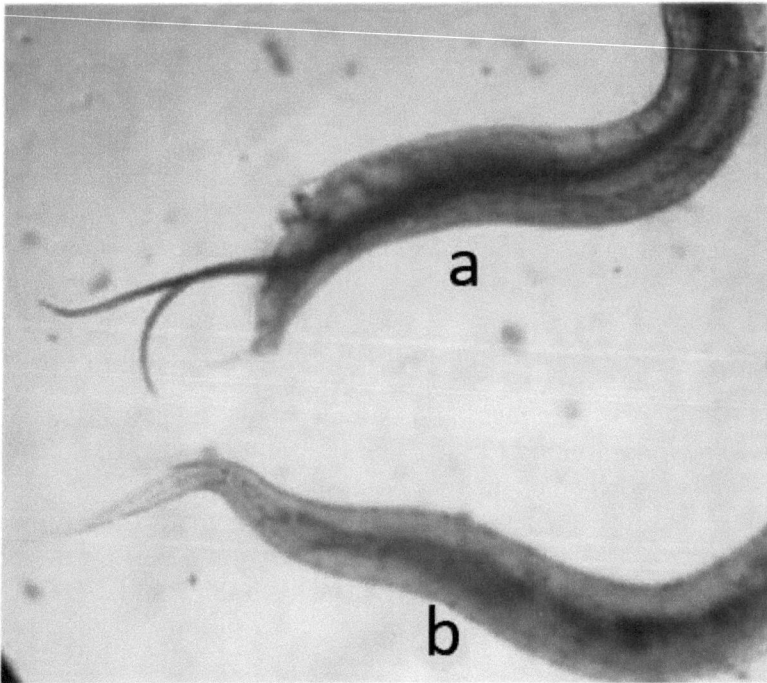

**Fig. (8).** Tail end of male and female *H. gallinarum*.

**Life cycle:** The eggs are passed out along with the faecal droppings of the fowl and become infective after two weeks on the ground, under optimum temperature conditions. After ingestion by the host, the infective larvae hatch in the intestine within one to two hours. By the 6th day, they molt to the third-stage larvae, and by the 10th day, to the fourth stage, and by the 15th day, to the fifth stage. The prepatent period is 24 to 30 days. Earthworms may act as transport hosts. Eggs, after being ingested by earthworms, pass through the gut and hatch. The L2 stage larvae migrate into the tissues of the earthworm and await ingestion by the fowl [35]. In the lumen of the fowl's caecum, the *H. gallinarum* larvae are released, undergo moulting, and mature into adults.

**Pathogenesis:** Adult worms in the caeca are less pathogenic, but heavy infections can cause thickening of the caecal mucosa with petechial haemorrhages on the surface. Another important aspect of caecal worms is that the eggs of *H. gallinarum* act as carriers for the protozoan parasite *Histomonas meleagidis*, the causative agent of blackhead disease in turkeys [36].

### *Subulura brumpti*

**Order:** Ascaridida

**Super family:** Subuluroidea

**Family:** Subuluridae

**Genus:** *Subulura*

The mature worms are found in the lumen of the caeca and are quite prevalent in chickens, turkeys, guineafowls, ducks, pheasants, grouse, and quails across North and South America, Africa, and Asia.

The mouth is encircled by six underdeveloped lips. Dorsally and ventrally, there are two pairs of larger papillae, accompanied by well-developed amphids situated laterally. The pharynx's walls create three "teeth". The cephalic alae exhibit transverse striations and extend to the anterior section of the intestine. The length of males ranges from 6.9 to 10.0 mm. The esophagus is club-shaped with a marked posterior bulb, and measures between 0.98 and 1.10 mm in length. The tail is curved ventrally and terminates in a prolongation. Caudal papillae include three pairs preanal, two pairs adanal, and five pairs postanal papillae. Near the third postanal papillae, two small structures resembling papillae project ventrally. The spicules are equal and similar, measuring between 1.22 and 1.31 mm in length. Female Length: 9 to 17.5 mm; length of the esophagus: 1.08 to 1.29 mm. Tail that is conical, straight, and ends in a sharp point. The vulva is positioned anterior to the middle of the body, ranging from 4.90 to 6.05 mm from the anterior end. The eggs are nearly spherical, possessing thin shells, and are fully embryonated upon deposition. The lifecycle is predominantly indirect, with various beetles serving as the intermediate hosts [11].

**Pathogenesis**: The overall health of birds infected with *S. brumpti* remained unaffected. However, in severe cases, there was a notable reduction in feed consumption and egg production, along with the observation of blood-tinged faecal droppings. Additionally, the affected birds exhibited signs of dullness and depression, characterized by ruffled feathers. Postmortem examinations of deceased birds revealed severe inflammation of the caecal mucosa, and the caecum was filled with hemorrhagic contents containing numerous tiny worms [12].

### *Oxyspirura mansoni*

**Order:** Spirurida

**Super family:** Spiruroidea

**Family:** Thelaziidae

**Genus:** *Oxyspirura*

*Oxyspirura mansoni* is found beneath the nictitating membrane in fowls and turkeys. The anterior end of the worms is rounded, while the posterior end is sharp. The pharynx is short, broader at its posterior end, and connects to a club-shaped esophagus, resembling an hourglass in shape. The male's body measured 10-16 mm in length and 275 μm in width. The male's body length was shorter compared to that of the female, with the testicles occupying a quarter of its body length. The posterior end is characterized by a sharp and concave structure, featuring two unequal spicules measuring 3-3.5 mm and 0.2-0.22 mm in length. Two, four pairs of post-cloacal and pre-cloacal papillae are present. The measurements for the female ranged from 12 to 19 mm in length. Females were distinguished by the presence of two uteri occupying the posterior part of their body. The posterior section of the female features a vulva measuring 50-65 x 45 μm. The eggs measured 55 μm x 40 μm and had a distinctive oval shape [15].

**Life cycle:** This nematode undergoes a digenetic biological cycle, and various wild and domestic avian species can act as the definitive host [14]. *Oxyspirura mansoni* eggs are laid in the eyes of chickens, travel through the nasolacrimal duct to reach the pharynx, get swallowed, expelled in the feces, and subsequently consumed by the Surinam cockroach (*Pycnoscelus surinamensis*). The larvae attain the infective stage within the cockroach. Upon consumption of infested intermediate hosts by chickens, liberated larvae move up the esophagus to the mouth and then travel through the nasolacrimal duct to the eye, completing the cycle. It's possible for other insect species to act as the intermediary host. Larvae develop into infectious stages in cockroaches. The cycle is finished when released larvae go up the esophagus, past the mouth, and into the eye after afflicted intermediate hosts are consumed by hens. It's possible for other insect species to act as the intermediary host.

**Pathogenesis:** Clinical symptoms like discomfort, ocular irritation, increased tear production, conjunctivitis, scratching of the eye, inflammation of the eye (ophthalmia), inflammation of the cornea (keratitis), cloudiness in the cornea (corneal opacity), and swelling of the nictitating membrane, potentially protruding beyond the eyelids [19]. At times, a clear discharge may develop, potentially leading to the closure of the eye as a result of adhesion to the eyelid. In extreme situations, the entire eye can be impacted, leading to thickening of the cornea and the eye cavity being filled with a white, cheesy exudate, and in some instances, the eyeball might be destroyed [18].

**Diagnosis and Treatment**: *O. mansoni* can be diagnosed by physical examination of the eye, detecting the eggs in lacrimal secretions, or by examining the eye during necropsy. Instill 1-2 drops of a 5% cresol solution into the lacrimal sac of the eye, and then flush the eye with sterile water to remove any remaining solution and debris. Alternatively, the use of either a 10% tetramisole solution as an eye wash or oral administration of 40mg/kg can be effective.

*Tetrameres*

**Order:** Spirurida

**Super family:** Spiruroidea

**Family:** Tetrameridae

**Genus:** *Tetrameres*

*Tetrameres*, primarily a proventricular parasite, predominantly infest both domestic and wild birds (Fig. **9**) (Table **2**).

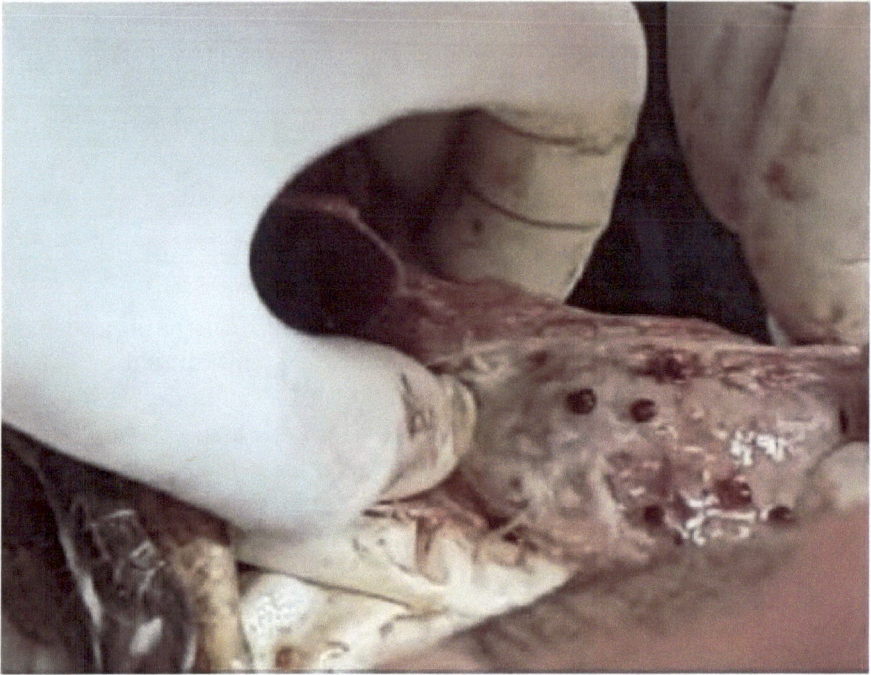

**Fig. (9).** Adult *Tetrameres* in the proventriculus of poultry.

**Table 2. Different *Tetramere* species present in birds.**

| Species name | Host | Intermediate host |
|---|---|---|
| *T. americana* | Fowl, Turkey in the USA, South Africa. | *Melanoplus femurrubrum, M.differentialis, Blatella germanica.* |
| *T. fissispina* | Duck, Pigeon, Fowl, Turkey, and wild aquatic birds | Water crustacea- *Daphnia pulex, Gammarus pulex* |
| *T. crami* | Domestic and wild ducks in North America. | Amphipods- *Gammarus fasciatus, Hyalella knickerbockeri* |
| *T. confusa* | Fowl, pigeon in Brazil | Water crustacea- *Daphnia pulex, Gammarus pulex* |
| *T. mohtedai* | Fowl in India | Grasshoppers, cockroaches- *Spathosternum prasiniferum, Oxya nitidula,* and *Setamorpha nutella.* |
| *T. pattersoni* | Quail | Grasshoppers, cockroaches. |

The males have a length of 5-5.5 mm, featuring a delicate and slender build, white coloration, and a cuticle armed with four rows of spines. Females, ranging from 3.5 to 4.5 mm in length, exhibit a globular or subspherical shape, displaying a bright red color, with four grooves along longitudinal lines on the body. Both anterior and posterior extremities resemble conical appendages. Typically, males are freely located in the gland's lumen, but during mating, they move into the female's glands, except for *T. fissispina*, where the female migrates first. The parasitic eggs have a thick-shelled and embryonated structure, measuring about 50-60 μm in length and 30 μm in width [12].

**Life Cycle and Epidemiology**: The female deposits eggs within the proventricular glands, and these eggs are subsequently expelled in the bird's droppings. Intermediate hosts, like grasshoppers (*Melanoplus femurrubrum or M. differentialis*) or cockroaches (*Blatella germanica*), ingest the eggs. Within the intermediate hosts, the larvae hatch from the eggs and progress to an infectious stage. Infection of the ultimate host occurs when the intermediate host, now carrying the infection, is consumed. Following ingestion, both males and females migrate to the proventriculus, where they embed themselves in the glands. After mating, the males exit the glands and perish.

**Clinical Signs and Pathogenicity:** The female worms feed on blood, resulting in significant irritation and inflammation. The movement of young worms within the host leads to the death of chicks. Infected birds exhibit symptoms such as anorexia, diarrhea, emaciation, weight loss, and anemia. In chickens with substantial infections (where more than 10 females are embedded in the glands), the proventriculus thickens and swells, with glandular necrosis, wall exfoliation, and partial obstruction of the lumen observed [17].

### *Amidostomum anseries*

**Order**: Strongylida

**Super family:** Strongyloidea

**Family:** Amidostomidae

**Genus:** *Amidostomum*

These are elongated, slender, coiled thread-like reddish-colored worms found just beneath the lining and grinding pads of the gizzard, occasionally in the proventriculus and esophagus of waterfowl, including wild geese, ducks, and parakeets. The male worm measures 10-17 mm in length, featuring two equal spicules each measuring 0.2-0.3 mm. Females are 20–21.15 mm long and 0.28–0.31 mm wide, with a transversely striated cuticle. The buccal capsule is sub-globular with a sharp tooth. The vulva is positioned 2.75–3.2 mm from the tail tip, and the anus is located about 0.31–0.35 mm from the tail. The eggs have dimensions of 100–110 × 50–60 μm.

**Life Cycle:** The life cycle is direct, with larvae ingested by birds entering the gizzard and burrowing into the surface lining. There, they undergo molting and develop into adults. Sexual maturity is reached by the adults approximately 10-15 days after the final molt. Once a bird is infected, it can host gizzard worms for an extended period, persisting for several years [11].

**Pathogenesis and Lesions**: Migratory birds initially encounter gizzard worms on their breeding sites. Gizzard worms can be fatal for birds, with a higher incidence of death observed in very young birds compared to adults, particularly during the fall and winter months. Mature worms migrate within the gizzard, feeding on blood in the mucosa, leading to hemorrhage, plasma protein leakage, and potential ischemia, resulting in erosions and ulcers [17]. The parasite releases toxins that contribute to the localized formation of ulcers and give rise to generalized symptoms such as depression, emaciation, dyspnea, and dysphagia [14]. Lesions include the sloughing off of the gizzard lining, inflammation, hemorrhage, and erosion of the grinding pads.

**Diagnosis and Treatment**: Ventricular nematodiosis is diagnosed by observing worms in the koilin lining and gizzard muscle or detecting eggs in the feces. Species identification necessitates the examination of both male and female adult worms. Modern anthelmintics, such as benzimidazole, levamisole (administered at 25 ml/kg in water), cambendazole (60-80 mg/kg), and pyrantel tartrate (50 mg/kg), have proven to be effective treatments.

### *Acuaria hamulosa* (Syn. *Cheilospirura hamulosa*)

**Order:** Spirurida

**Super family:** Spiruroidea

**Family:** Acuariidae

**Genus:** *Cheilospirura*

This gizzard worm is frequently found in the North American ruffed grouse. *A. hamulosa* is prevalent in chickens and turkeys across North and South America, Europe, Africa, and Asia. Additionally, this species affects partridges, quail, pheasants, and wild turkeys. The lips are triangular in shape and carry two conical papillae. The anterior portion of the cuticle is composed of cordons, organized in dual rows and configured as plaques. These extend from the front end to the point corresponding to the anterior end of the larger spicule in males and reach the vulva region in females.

The males have a length ranging from 10 to 14 mm and a breadth of 0.29 to 0.33 mm. The cuticle shows spaced striations, with cordons measuring between 7.56 and 7.98 mm in length. The esophagus is divided into an anterior muscular part and a posterior glandular part. The caudal end is coiled and features caudal alae. The spicules are unequal, with the larger spicule measuring 1.07 to 1.09 mm in length, while the smaller spicule is short and broad, approximately 0.28 to 0.29 mm long. There are 10 pairs of caudal papillae, with 3 pairs preanal, 1 pair adanal, and 6 pairs postanal. The females range in size from 16 to 29 mm in length and 0.35 to 0.55 mm in width. The cuticle exhibits distinct striations, with cordons measuring between 10.95 and 15.75 mm in length. The vulva is positioned at a distance of 9.15 to 10.35 mm. The tail is pointed, and the eggs are oval-shaped, possessing a thick embryonated shell, measuring 40 to 45 mm in length and 28 to 30 mm in width [12].

## *Acuaria spiralis* (*Dispharynx spiralis*)

**Order:** Spirurida

**Super family:** Spiruroidea

**Family:** Acuaridae

**Genus:** *Dispharynx*

This organism is found in the proventriculus and oesophagus, and occasionally in the intestine of chickens, turkeys, pigeons, guinea fowl, and pheasants across America, Africa, and Asia. *Acuaria spiralis* is identified by the presence of 'cordons,' which are cuticular ridges or grooves located in the anterior part of the body. These cordons may be both non-recurrent or recurrent, running down the body and curving back forward. The lips typically exhibit a small, triangular shape, while the pharynx is cylindrical (Fig. **10**). Males measure 7-8 mm in length, featuring lateral alae at the caudal end, a slender left spicule, and a boat-shaped right spicule. The posterior end of the female is blunt, with a length of 9-10 mm, and the vulva is situated in the posterior third of the body [19].

**Life Cycle:** The life cycles of these *Acuaria* species are characterized by an indirect process. Grasshoppers and beetles, including *Melanoplus, Oxya nitidula,* and *Spathosternum prasiniferum,* serve as intermediate hosts for *Acuaria hamulosa.* Isopods like *Porcellio leavis, P. scaber*, and *Armadillidum vulgare,* along with *Oxya nitidula* and *Spathosternum prasiniferum*, function as intermediate hosts for *Dispharynx spiralis.* Mature female worms deposit embryonated eggs in the host's intestinal tract, and these eggs are expelled through the feces. Intermediate hosts consume the eggs, and within 3 to 8 weeks, the eggs mature into infective L3 larvae, the duration varying based on the worm species and the host. Birds acquire infection by consuming contaminated beetles, grasshoppers, or other intermediate hosts. After digestion, the larvae are released and promptly migrate to the preferred organ, where they undergo full development into adult worms and initiate egg production [24].

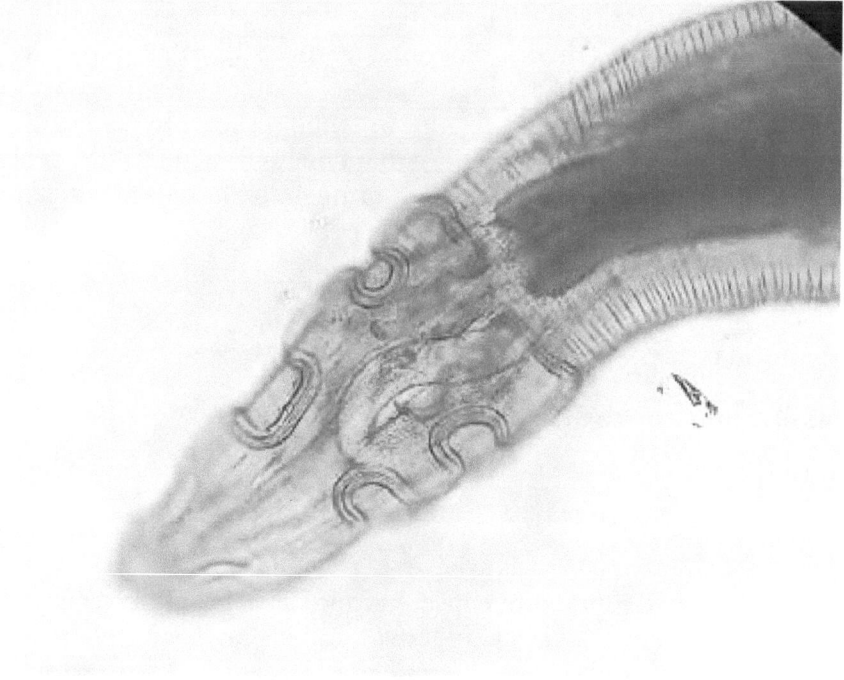

**Fig. (10).**  Anterior end of *Dyspharynx spiralis*.

**Pathogenesis**: Light infections are generally harmless, but heavy ones, especially involving *Acuaria spiralis*, can pose significant dangers, especially to young birds. These infections can deeply penetrate the affected organs, leading to the formation of nodules that severely impede swallowing and cause damage to the organ linings, such as ulcers, inflammation, and thickening. Additionally, there may be atrophy of the muscles in the crop and proventriculus, resulting in a loss of elasticity. Clinical signs of such infections include weakness, anemia, reduced appetite and weight, and decreased egg production in layers. *Acuaria hamulosa* infections can also lead to emaciation, weakness, and anemia, particularly in cases of severe infection.

**Diagnosis**: The detection method relies on finding characteristic eggs in the feces or identifying the worms in their preferred locations during a post-mortem examination.

**Treatment**: Many traditional broad-spectrum anthelmintic drugs can effectively combat *Acuaria* worms. Examples include various benzimidazoles such as albendazole, fenbendazole, flubendazole, mebendazole, oxfendazole, and others. Levamisole and macrocyclic lactones like ivermectin are also proven to be effective. Additionally, some compounds with a more specific spectrum, like piperazine derivatives and pyrantel, show efficacy against these worms.

### *Syngamus trachea*: **Gape worm**

**Synonyms:** Gape worm, red worm, and fork worm

**Order:** Strongylida

**Superfamily:** Strongyloidea

**Family** Syngamidae

**Genus:** *Syngamus*

Fully grown worms exhibit a vivid red hue and inhabit the respiratory passages of birds. They predominantly reside in the trachea, bronchi, and bronchioles of various avian species such as chickens, quails, turkeys, guinea fowl, geese, peafowl, and pheasants. Other avian groups prone to *Syngamus trachea* infections include Columbiformes and Psittaciformes, particularly cockatoos, birds of prey, and Passeriformes, with a notable prevalence in Corvidae and starlings [9]. Typically, *S. trachea* worms are discovered in pairs, with females and males permanently joined in copulation, forming a Y-shaped configuration.

**Morphology:** *Syngamus trachea*, a medium-sized species of worm, showcases males measuring up to 6mm in length and females up to 20mm, both displaying a reddish tint. Resembling other roundworms, their bodies are enveloped by a pliable yet durable cuticle. They possess a cup-shaped buccal capsule with 6 to 10 teeth. The tail end of the male is furnished with a bursa with short and stout rays. Spicules are equal and measure 53x82um. A notable characteristic of these worms is their ongoing copulatory activity, with the shorter male firmly adhering to the female, producing a Y-shaped arrangement reminiscent of a fork. The eggs of these worms are ellipsoid in shape, measuring roughly 70-100 by 43-46um. They exhibit a sturdy shell with plug-like thickenings at each pole and typically contain approximately 16 cells.

**Life cycle:** The eggs escape from under the bursa of the male worm and are transported up the trachea within excess mucus produced in response to infection. They are then swallowed and passed in the feces. Unlike other strongylids, the larvae develop within the egg and moults twice in the egg. Larvae may or may not hatch from the eggs. Chickens contract *S. trachea* infection through inadvertent ingestion of the egg of free infective larvae present in the surrounding environment, feed, or water, often due to contamination with feces from an infected bird or ingestion of a transport host containing the larvae. The common earthworm serves as the most prevalent transport host, although various other invertebrates such as slugs, snails, and beetles can also act as carriers. After entering the intestine of the final host, the larvae migrate to the lungs, possibly through the bloodstream, as they are found in the alveoli within 4-6 hours. Parasitic moults occur within the lungs within five days, the young worms migrate to the bronchi. Copulation typically takes place around day seven in the trachea or bronchi, followed by rapid female growth. The prepatent period spans 17-20 days.

**Pathogenesis:** The severity of the disease varies depending on the age of the birds and the extent of infection. Young and small birds are more vulnerable compared to adults due to their narrower tracheal openings. Turkeys exhibit higher susceptibility to the infection. The infection becomes more pathogenic in cases of heavy infestations, where larval migration within pulmonary tissues leads to ecchymoses, edema, and lobar pneumonia, resulting in respiratory distress. Adult worms attach to the tracheal mucosa, feeding on blood, causing catarrhal tracheitis and the secretion of mucus into the air passages. This can lead to air passage occlusion, manifesting characteristic signs of gapes such as dyspnea, asphyxia, head shaking, coughing, neck extension, and gaping movements. Deep embedding of adult male worms in the tracheal mucosa may induce nodule formation. Tracheal obstruction by adult worms in heavy infestations may cause birds to cease feeding. Death may occur due to asphyxia or progressive emaciation, anemia, and weakness. Postmortem examination may reveal worms in the posterior part of the trachea, with affected carcasses appearing emaciated and anemic.

**Prevention**: Ensuring rigorous cleanliness in poultry yards and housing is crucial to prevent parasitic infections. Special attention is necessary for young birds, especially in deep-litter systems where nematode infections are more common, particularly in damp conditions. It is also essential to maintain appropriate ventilation and moisture levels in the litter. It is recommended to stack the litter in the housing area for a few days and allow it to heat up and undergo sterilization before introducing new batches of chicks to the flock. Taking a proactive approach significantly lowers the likelihood of poultry contracting parasitic infections [32]. Furthermore, it is crucial to prevent overcrowding by maintaining an optimal number of birds. Enhancing parasitic control can be achieved by separating birds according to their age, rather than using the "all in-all out" approach. This is important since older birds might harbor various parasitic infections without displaying obvious clinical symptoms. To reduce the presence of infectious parasitic eggs, a crucial measure is the regular replacement of litter in pens, whether the birds are housed indoors or outdoors, and this should be conducted at least once weekly. Furthermore, it is crucial to maintain a dry floor to discourage parasitic infestations. The most practical and cost-efficient method for preventing and controlling parasitic infections involves regular deworming, and adhering to the appropriate dosage and administration guidelines. This comprehensive approach is vital for sustaining the health and productivity of poultry [25]. The use of insecticides to kill the intermediate hosts is not advisable. It is virtually impossible to eliminate all the potential intermediate hosts with insecticides. And it would be highly detrimental to the environment because it would kill not only the intermediate hosts but numerous beneficial insects and other invertebrates as well.

## CONCLUDING REMARKS

Nematode infestations pose a serious threat to poultry health and production, leading to significant economic and health-related losses. The wide range of nematode species affecting poultry necessitates prompt and accurate diagnostic methods for effective control. While various treatment options, including piperazine, albendazole, and ivermectin, have shown promise, prevention through proper hygiene, environmental management, and regular deworming remains crucial. The production of recombinant antigens for helminth vaccines remains unresolved, making vaccine development an unlikely solution at this time. As a result, breaking the parasite's life cycle through alternative methods, such as the strategic use of deworming agents, seems to be the most effective approach for controlling infections.

## REFERENCES

[1] Al-Quraishi MA, Al-Musawi HS, Al-Haboobi ZA. Pathological study of *Ascaridia galli* in poultry. EurAsian J Biosci 2020; 14(2): 3327-9.

[2] Anderson RC. Nematode parasites of vertebrates Their development and transmission. 2nd ed. Wallingford, Oxon, UK: CAB International 2000; pp. 290-9.
[http://dx.doi.org/10.1079/9780851994215.0000]

[3] Ashour AA. Scanning electron microscopy of *Ascaridia galli* (Schrank, 1788), Freeborn, 1923 and A. columbae (Linstow, 1903). J Egypt Soc Parasitol 1994; 24(2): 349-55.
[PMID: 8077754]

[4] Belete A, Addis M, Ayele M. Review on major gastrointestinal parasites that affect chickens. J Biol Agric Healthc 2016; 6(11): 11-21.

[5] El-Kholy H, Kemppainen BW. Levamisole residues in chicken tissues and eggs. Poult Sci 2005; 84(1): 9-13.
[http://dx.doi.org/10.1093/ps/84.1.9] [PMID: 15685936]

[6] Enigk VK, Dey-Hazra A. Zum verhalten der exogen entwicklungformen von *Amidostomum anseris* (Strongyloidea, Nematoda). Arch Geflugelkd 1969; 33: 259-73.
[http://dx.doi.org/10.1016/S0003-9098(25)01674-1]

[7] Gary DB, Richard DM. Intestinal Parasites in Backyard Chicken Flocks: Cooperative Extension Service, Institute of Food and Agricultural Sciences. University of Florida, Gainesville 2012; 76:

32611.

[8]     Greiner F. In: Altmann RB, Clubb SL, Dorrestein G Avian Me dicine and Surgery Philadelphia:. W.B.Saunders Company 1997; pp. 332-49.

[9]     Shohana NN, Rony SA, Ali MH, *et al. Ascaridia galli* infection in chicken: Pathobiology and immunological orchestra. Immun Inflamm Dis. 2023 Sep;11(9):e1001. [http://dx.doi.org/10.1002/iid3.1001]

[10]    Hall HTB. The Nematode Parasites of Poultry: Diseases and Parasites in Livestock in the Tropics. 2nd ed. UK: London Scientific and Technical, Longan Group 1985; pp. 237-61.

[11]    Helmboldt CF, Eckerlin RP, Penner LR, Wyand DS. The pathology of capillariasis in the blue jay. J Wildl Dis 1971; 7(3): 157-61. [http://dx.doi.org/10.7589/0090-3558-7.3.157] [PMID: 5156481]

[12]    Höglund J, Daş G, Tarbiat B, Geldhof P, Jansson DS, Gauly M. *Ascaridia galli* - An old problem that requires new solutions Int J Parasitol Drugs Drug Resist 2023; 23: 1-9. [http://dx.doi.org/10.1016/j.ijpddr.2023.07.003] [PMID: 37516026] [PMCID: PMC10409999]

[13]    Hurst GA, Turner LW, Tucker FS. Capillariasis in penned wild turkeys. J Wildl Dis 1979; 15(3): 395-7. [http://dx.doi.org/10.7589/0090-3558-15.3.395] [PMID: 501843]

[14]    Jacobs RD, Hogsette JA, Butcher JD. Nematode parasites of poultry (and where to find them) The Institute of Food and Agricultural Sciences (IFAS) series PS18. USA: University of Florida 2003; pp. 1-3.

[15]    Lalchhandama K. On the structure of *Ascaridia galli*, the roundworm of domestic fowl. Sci Vis 2010; 10(1): 20-30.

[16]    Lee EA, Irving AC, Pomproy WE. *Oxyspirura* sp. in the eye of a New Zealand Kaka (Necator meridionalis). N Z J Zool 2006; 28: 227-31. [PMID: 22735854]

[17]    Pinto RM, Menezes RC, Gomes DC. First report of five nematode species in *Phasianus colchicus* Linnaeus (Aves, Galliformes, Phasianidae) in Brazil. Rev Bras Zool 2004; 21(4): 961-70. [http://dx.doi.org/10.1590/S0101-81752004000400034]

[18]    Mathey WJ, Gutter AE. *Capillaria perforans* Kotlan and Orosz 1931 in vulturine guinea fowl. Poult Sci 1979; 58: 1083.

[19]    McDougald LR. Internal Parasites. In Diseases of Poultry. 11th ed., Y. M. Saif, H. G. Barnes, J. R. Glisson, A. M. Fadly, L. R. McDonald, and D. E. Swayne (eds). Iowa State Press, Ames 2003; 1: pp. 931-71.

[20]    Moravec F, Prokopic J, Shlikas AV. The biology of nematodes of the family Capillariidae Neveu-Lemaire, 1936. Folia Parasitol (Praha) 1987; 34(1): 39-56. [PMID: 3583129]

[21]    Nagarajan K, Thyagarajan D, Raman M. *Subulura brumpti* infection - An outbreak in Japanese quails (*Coturnix coturnix japonica*). Vet Res Forum 2012; 3(1): 67-9. [PMID: 25653749]

[22]    Okaeme AN, Agbontale J. Ivermectin in the treatment of helminthiasis in caged raised adult guinea-fowl (*Numida meleagris galeata* Pallas). Rev Élev Méd Vét Pays Trop 1989; 42(2): 227-30. [http://dx.doi.org/10.19182/remvt.8841] [PMID: 2626577]

[23]    Oladosu OJ, Hennies M, Gauly M, Daş G. A copro-antigen ELISA for the detection of ascarid infections in chickens. Vet Parasitol 2022; 311: 109795. [http://dx.doi.org/10.1016/j.vetpar.2022.109795] [PMID: 36108471]

[24]    Panich W, Tejangkura T, Chontananarth T. Feasibility of a DNA biosensor assay based on loop-mediated isothermal amplification combined with a lateral flow dipstick assay for the visual detection

of *Ascaridia galli* eggs in faecal samples. Avian Pathol 2023; 52(3): 209-18.
[http://dx.doi.org/10.1080/03079457.2023.2196251] [PMID: 36971233]

[25]    Permin A, Hansen JW. Diagnostic methods: Epidemiology, diagnosis and control of poultry parasites. FAO animal health manual, no 4. Rome, Italy: Food and Agriculture Organization of the United Nations 1998; pp. 33-118.

[26]    Pinto RM, Tortelly R, Menezes RC, Gomes DC. Trichurid nematodes in ring-necked pheasants from backyard flocks of the State of Rio de Janeiro, Brazil: frequency and pathology. Mem Inst Oswaldo Cruz 2004; 99(7): 721-6.
[http://dx.doi.org/10.1590/S0074-02762004000700010] [PMID: 15654428]

[27]    Puttalakshmamma G, Ananda K, Prathiush P, Mamatha G, Rao S. Prevalence of gastrointestinal parasites of Poultry in and around Banglore. Vet World 2008; 2(2): 201-2.
[http://dx.doi.org/10.5455/vetworld.2008.201-202]

[28]    Ramadan H, Abou Znada N. Morphology and life history of *Ascaridia galli* in the domestic fowl that are raised in Jeddah. Magalat Game'at al-Malik Abdul Aziz Al-U'lum 1992; 4(1): 87-99.
[http://dx.doi.org/10.4197/Sci.4-1.9]

[29]    Ransom BH. Manson's eye worm of chickens: with a general review of nematodes parasitic in the eyes of birds. U.S. Department of Agriculture. Bureau Animal Industry Bulletin Government Printing Office, Washington 1904; 78(60).

[30]    Simon MS. Emeritus Enteric Diseases: ASA Handbook on Poultry Diseases. 2nd ed. American Soybean Association 2005; pp. 133-43.

[31]    Soulsby EJL. Helminthes, arthropods, and protozoa of domestic animals. 7th ed. London: Bailliere, and Tindall 1982; pp. 83-115.

[32]    Soulsby EJL. Helminths, Athropods and Protozoa of Domesticated Animals. Edn 7, Baillière Tindall, London, UK; c1982. 1982; pp. 163-5.

[33]    Tanveer S, Ahad S, Chishti MZ. Morphological characterization of nematodes of the genera *Capillaria, Acuaria, Amidostomum, Streptocara, Heterakis*, and *Ascaridia* isolated from intestine and gizzard of domestic birds from different regions of the temperate Kashmir valley. J Parasit Dis 2015; 39(4): 745-60.
[http://dx.doi.org/10.1007/s12639-013-0401-7] [PMID: 26688646]

[34]    Taylor S, Kenny J, Houston A, Hewitt S. Efficacy, pharmacokinetics and effects on egg-laying and hatchability of two dose rates of in-feed fenbendazole for the treatment of *Capillaria* species infections in chickens. Vet Rec 1993; 133(21): 519-21.
[http://dx.doi.org/10.1136/vr.133.21.519] [PMID: 8310628]

[35]    Gjevre AG, Kaldhusdal M, Eriksen GS. Gizzard erosion and ulceration syndrome in chickens and turkeys: a review of causal or predisposing factors. Avian Pathol. 2013;42(4):297–303.
[http://dx.doi.org/10.1080/03079457.2013.817665]

[36]    Ybañez RHD, Resuelo KJG, Kıntanar APM, Ybañez AP. Detection of gastrointestinal parasites in small-scale poultry layer farms in Leyte, Philippines. Vet World 2018; 11(11): 1587-91.
[http://dx.doi.org/10.14202/vetworld.2018.1587-1591] [PMID: 30587893]

# CHAPTER 12

# Tapeworm (Taeniasis) Infection

**Vivek Agrawal**[1,*], **Nidhi S. Choudhary**[2], **Pradeep Kumar**[3], **Saroj Kumar**[4], **Tanmoy Rana**[5] and **Mukesh Shakya**[1]

[1] *Department of Veterinary Parasitology, College of Veterinary Sciences & A.H., Nanaji Deshmukh Veterinary Science University, Mhow, Indore 453446, Madhya Pradesh, India*

[2] *Department of Medicine, College of Veterinary Sciences & A.H Nanaji Deshmukh Veterinary Science University, Mhow, Indore 453446, Madhya Pradesh, India*

[3] *Department of Veterinary Parasitology, Uttar Pradesh Pandit Deen Dayal Upadhyaya Pashu Chikitsa Vigyan Vishwavidyalaya Evam Go-Anusandhan Sansthan, Mathura 281001, Uttar Pradesh, India*

[4] *Department of Veterinary Parasitology, Faculty of Veterinary and Animal Sciences, Institute of Agricultural Sciences, Banaras Hindu University, Varanasi 221005, Uttar Pradesh, India*

[5] *Department of Veterinary Clinical Complex, West Bengal University of Animal & Fishery Sciences, Kolkata, India*

**Abstract:** The chapter "Tapeworm (Taeniasis) Infection" highlights the critical role of poultry farming, encompassing species such as chickens, turkeys, swans, and quails, in providing essential protein and economic benefits globally. However, tapeworms present a significant threat to poultry health, especially in free-range systems. These parasites have complex life cycles involving intermediate hosts like earthworms and beetles and can infect the intestines of poultry, disrupting nutrient absorption and reducing feed conversion efficiency. Common tapeworm species affecting poultry include *Raillietina, Davainea proglottina, Amoebotaenia cuneata, Choanotaenia infundibulum, Hymenolepis cantaniana*, and *Hymenolepis carioca*. Infected birds experience impaired nutrient absorption, slower growth rates, and increased production costs, alongside heightened susceptibility to other diseases. Effective management requires precise identification of tapeworm species, control of intermediate host populations, and strict biosecurity measures. Understanding the life cycles of these parasites and implementing targeted interventions are crucial for mitigating their impact on poultry health and productivity. Key strategies include reducing intermediate host populations, preventing poultry from ingesting these hosts, maintaining hygiene, managing waste, and using insecticides. A comprehensive understanding of tapeworm life cycles is vital for developing effective treatments and improving the overall health and productivity of poultry flocks.

* **Corresponding author Vivek Agrawal:** Department of Veterinary Parasitology, College of Veterinary Sciences & A.H., Nanaji Deshmukh Veterinary Science University, Mhow, Indore 453446, Madhya Pradesh (India); E-mail: dragrawalin76@gmail.com

**Keywords:** *Amoebotaenia cuneata*, Chicken, *Choanotaenia infundibulum*, Duck, *Davainea proglottina*, Diagnosis, Epidemiology, Geese, *Hymenolepis cantaniana*, *Hymenolepis carioca*, Life cycle, *Raillietina* spp, Turkey.

## INTRODUCTION

In the diverse and vibrant world of poultry, a variety of bird species can be found, from chickens and turkeys to swans and quails. These birds are integral to both backyard settings and commercial production systems globally. Poultry not only provides a rich source of protein through its meat and eggs but also serves as a means of generating income. Additionally, the organic manure produced by poultry is highly fertile, making it valuable in agriculture [1]. Endoparasites, particularly tapeworms, pose a significant threat to poultry production, especially in free-range or backyard systems. The presence of these parasites can lead to substantial economic losses by reducing the efficiency with which chickens convert their feed into energy, delaying their growth and development, and increasing medication and production costs [2].

## TAPEWORMS: LIFE CYCLE AND IMPACT

Tapeworms have a complex life cycle involving various intermediate hosts such as earthworms, snails, slugs, beetles, ants, and houseflies, depending on the species. These parasites infiltrate the intestines of chickens, depleting vital nutrients and disrupting nutrient absorption. This parasitic invasion leads to a decrease in feed conversion efficiency, requiring more feed to produce the same amount of meat or eggs [3]. Infected birds often face delayed growth and development, resulting in lower market value and decreased turnover rates. Additionally, the presence of tapeworms necessitates increased medication and production costs, further burdening poultry farmers. Heavy parasitic infections can also diminish the chickens' resistance to other infections, compounding the health issues within the flock [4].

## COMMON TAPEWORM SPECIES IN POULTRY

Tapeworms are responsible for causing cestodiasis in both domestic and wild birds worldwide, with over 1400 species identified. Some common species that infect the small intestine of chickens include:

- *Raillietina echinobothrida*
- *Raillietina tetragona*
- *Raillietina cesticillus*
- *Davainea proglottina*
- *Choanotaenia infundibulum*

- *Amoebotaenia cuneata*
- *Hymenolepis cantaniana*
- *Hymenolepis carioca*

## ANATOMY AND IDENTIFICATION

Tapeworms are elongated, segmented, and ribbon-like, typically white in appearance. The front part of a tapeworm called the scolex or head, is equipped with four suckers that help it attach to the lining of the small intestine. These suckers are primarily attachment organs and do not consume food. Tapeworms lack a mouth or alimentary canal and absorb nutrients through their body wall, known as the cuticle [3].

The scolex may feature a specialized organ called the rostellum, resembling an anchor, which aids in securing the tapeworm to the intestinal mucosa. This rostellum may have hooks that further assist in anchoring. The neck, located just behind the scolex, is the growth region from which the rest of the tapeworm's body, known as the strobila, develops. The strobila comprises many segments or proglottids, categorized into immature, mature, and gravid based on their proximity to the head and neck [5].

Gravid proglottids contain reproductive organs that have degenerated, leaving behind only a uterus filled with eggs. These eggs consist of an oncosphere, a striated shell, and a delicate membrane. Tapeworms are hermaphroditic, with each proglottid containing both male and female reproductive organs, allowing for both cross-fertilization and self-fertilization [4].

## DIAGNOSIS AND CONTROL

Precise identification of tapeworm species is crucial for developing effective prevention and control strategies, as different species can vary significantly in their pathogenicity. Diagnosticians often rely on examining the scolex, eggs, or individual proglottids of recently shed, live specimens. Differential staining can reveal internal organs of mature proglottids, aiding in species identification [5].

In poultry, tapeworms are more frequently found in warmer seasons when intermediate hosts are abundant. Many species of tapeworms are now considered rare in intensive poultry-rearing regions due to the lack of contact with intermediate hosts. However, beetles and houseflies inhabiting poultry houses can still act as intermediate hosts for some large chicken tapeworms, such as *Raillietina cesticillus* and *Choanotaenia infundibulum* [3].

Effective control measures often involve breaking the life cycle of the tapeworms by altering flock management practices to reduce contact with intermediate hosts. This may include maintaining cleaner environments, reducing the presence of intermediate hosts, and implementing regular deworming programs [2].

Tapeworms are a significant threat to poultry health and productivity. Understanding their life cycle, identifying the specific species, and implementing effective control measures are crucial for mitigating their impact. Through diligent management and preventive strategies, poultry farmers can protect their flocks from these parasitic adversaries, ensuring better health and productivity for their birds [3].

## *Davainea proglottina*

*Davainea proglottina* is a diminutive but highly pathogenic tapeworm commonly found in poultry. Measuring approximately 0.5 to 4 mm in length and composed of 4 to 9 segments, this parasite primarily inhabits the duodenal loop of the small intestine, where it can cause significant health issues in its avian hosts. *Davainea proglottina* can be identified in the duodenal mucosa by the protrusion of gravid proglottids above the villi when the intestine is floated in the water. Key diagnostic features include:

- **Size:** Mature worms reach up to 4 mm in length and have no more than 9 proglottids.
- **Suckers:** Armed with 3–6 rows of hooks.
- **Rostellum:** Armed.
- **Genital Pores:** Regularly alternating and positioned near the anterior margin of the proglottid.
- **Cirrus:** Disproportionately large.
- **Embryonal Hooks:** Distinctive, measuring 10–11 μm long. The eggs lack distinctive membranes.

Various species of slugs and snails act as intermediate hosts for the larval stages of *D. proglottina*. Proglottids containing mature eggs are typically expelled in the feces of infected birds during the afternoon or night. These segments can move and crawl up plants, making them accessible to slugs and snails. Once consumed by the intermediate hosts, the proglottids release eggs that develop into bladder worms, known as cysticercoids, within the body cavity of the slugs and snails. The infectivity of these cysticercoids lasts for over 11 months, and susceptible slugs can harbor over 1500 cysticercoids in their digestive tract. Infected snails or slugs are then ingested by birds, leading to their infection. After being digested, the cysticercoids release young tapeworms that attach themselves to the wall of the gut and develop into adults. The prepatent period, or the time from initial infection to the first egg shedding, lasts around 2 to 3 weeks (Fig. **1**).

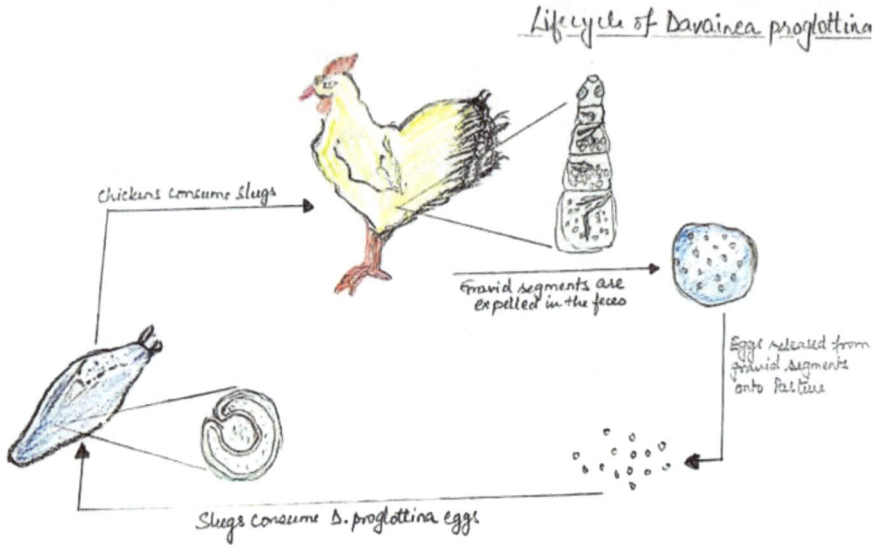

**Fig. (1).** Lifecycle of *Davainea proglottina*.

*Davainea proglottina* poses a significant threat to poultry health due to its compact size and rapid reproductive capabilities. Its presence can cause extensive damage to the intestinal mucosa in the duodenal loop, resulting in poor nutrient absorption and a decline in the overall health and productivity of birds. Infected birds may exhibit symptoms such as emaciation, dull plumage, lethargy, breathing difficulties, thickened mucosal membranes leading to hemorrhage and fetid mucus, leg weakness, paralysis, and in severe cases, death. Controlled experiments have documented a 12% reduction in growth rate due to infection. Infected birds can harbor up to 300 worms, and in some cases, more than 3000 worms have been recovered from a single bird.

Implementing effective control and prevention strategies is essential to minimize the economic losses caused by *D. proglottina* in poultry production systems. Developing a comprehensive understanding of the life cycle and transmission dynamics of *D. proglottina* is crucial to effectively control its spread through targeted interventions. This involves managing populations of intermediate hosts and implementing measures to enhance biosecurity and reduce the likelihood of infection in poultry flocks.

## *Raillietina* Species

*Raillietina* species are significant tapeworms commonly observed in poultry. Among these, *Raillietina tetragona*, *Raillietina echinobothrida*, and *Raillietina cesticillus* are notable for their prevalence and impact on poultry health. These tapeworms inhabit the intestines of chickens and other birds, often leading to various health issues [3].

### *Raillietina tetragona*

*Raillietina tetragona* is a prevalent tapeworm species known for its considerable size, with adults reaching up to 25 cm in length. This tapeworm typically resides in the posterior half of the small intestine of chickens. The scolex is relatively small compared to *Raillietina echinobothrida*, with a rostellum equipped with one or two rows of hooks and oval suckers bearing 8-12 rows of tiny hooks. The genital pores are generally unilateral, and the uterus divides into capsules containing 6-12 eggs. The cirrus sac is small, measuring 75-100 mm, positioned towards the front of the proglottid margin. The eggs range in diameter from 25 to 50 µm [5].

The life cycle of *Raillietina tetragona* involves the development of cysticercoids within ants of the Pheidole and Tetramorium genera. The pre-patent period, the time from the ingestion of cysticercoids to the appearance of eggs in the feces, ranges from 13 days to 3 weeks [4].

Controlled experiments have demonstrated that infections in poultry can lead to weight loss and reduced egg production. Infected chickens show a decrease in glycogen levels in the liver and intestinal mucosa [3].

### *Raillietina echinobothrida*

*Raillietina echinobothrida* is considered the most pathogenic among *Raillietina* species. This tapeworm is similar in size to *Raillietina tetragona*, measuring approximately 25 cm in length, but can be distinguished by its larger strobila, measuring 34 cm in length and 4 mm in width. The scolex has rounded suckers containing 200-250 hooks arranged in 8-15 rows. The genital pores are located in the posterior half of the proglottid, and the cirrus sac is significantly larger, measuring 130-180 mm. The gravid proglottids often loosen from each other in the center, creating a distinctive window-like pattern [5].

The life cycle of *Raillietina echinobothrida* also involves various species of ants as intermediate hosts. Concurrent infections with *Raillietina tetragona* cysticercoids have been observed in ants. After ingestion by chickens, the pre-patent period is around 20 days [4].

*Raillietina echinobothrida* is known for its high pathogenicity, often causing nodular disease in chickens. Experimental infections have shown parasitic granulomas and associated catarrhal hyperplastic enteritis, with lymphocytic, polymorphonuclear, and eosinophilic infiltration [3].

### *Raillietina cesticillus*

*Raillietina cesticillus* is another notable species within the *Raillietina* genus, identifiable by its lack of a neck and a large scolex with a wide, flat rostellum equipped with a double row of 300-500 hammer-shaped hooks. The organism firmly attaches to the mucosa of the duodenum or jejunum. It possesses four unarmed, weak suckers and irregularly arranged genital pores. The proglottid contains 20-30 testes located towards the posterior end. The eggs are fully developed, measuring 75-88 μm in diameter, with two distinctive funnel-shaped filaments between the inner and middle membranes [5].

*Raillietina cesticillus* utilizes over 100 species of beetles from 10 families as natural or experimental intermediate hosts. The minute histerid beetle (*Carcinops pumilio*) serves as the natural intermediate host in broiler houses. A single ground beetle can harbor up to 930 cysticercoids. After ingestion by chickens, the pre-patent period is around 20 days [4].

Early reports indicated that *Raillietina cesticillus* causes emaciation, villous degeneration, and inflammation, reduced blood sugar and hemoglobin levels, and decreased growth rates. However, extensive controlled experiments with broilers and layers on optimal diets did not confirm these effects. Experimental infections showed no significant reduction in weight gain or egg production compared to uninfected controls [3].

The *Raillietina* species in poultry are significant due to their prevalence and impact on poultry health. While *Raillietina tetragona* and *Raillietina echinobothrida* can lead to weight loss and reduced egg production, *Raillietina echinobothrida* is particularly pathogenic, causing nodular disease and enteritis. *Raillietina cesticillus*, despite early reports of pathogenicity, has shown minimal impact on weight gain and egg production in controlled experiments. Understanding the life cycles, physical traits, and pathogenicity of these species is crucial for managing and controlling their impact on poultry health [3 - 5].

## *Amoebotaenia cuneata (Amoebotaenia sphenoides)* in Poultry

*Amoebotaenia cuneata*, also known as *Amoebotaenia sphenoides*, is a small, slim, thread-like tapeworm that resides in the duodenum of domestic fowl. It measures around 4 mm in length and typically has up to 20 proglottids, giving it a triangular appearance [5].

The presence of *Amoebotaenia cuneata* is indicated by whitish projections in the villi of the duodenum. The worm has a wedge-shaped appearance due to its triangular anterior end and pointed scolex. The unarmed suckers are complemented by a rostellum that features a single row of 12 to 14 hooks. The genital pores are usually randomly distributed towards the anterior margin of the proglottid. The proglottid also contains 12 to 15 testes arranged in a single row across its posterior end. The hexacanth embryos are encased in unique granular layers, while the uterus has a sac-like structure with slight lobes [5].

*Amoebotaenia cuneata* utilizes various species of earthworms as intermediate hosts. These earthworms belong to genera such as *Allotophora, Pheritima, Ocnerodrilus,* and *Lumbricus,*. Chickens typically contract the infection during rainy periods when earthworms emerge from the soil. The pre-patent period, which is the time between the ingestion of cysticercoids and the appearance of eggs in the feces, lasts approximately 4 weeks [3].

Earthworms infected with the cysticercoids of *Amoebotaenia cuneata* play a crucial role in the transmission of this parasite. When chickens consume these infected earthworms, the cysticercoids are released during digestion. The juvenile tapeworms then attach to the lining of the duodenum and mature into adult worms. During the pre-patent period, the tapeworms grow and start reproducing within the host, ensuring the continuation of their life cycle [4]. A deep understanding of the life cycle of *Amoebotaenia cuneata* is essential for devising effective control and prevention measures in poultry production systems. Reducing the population of intermediate hosts, such as earthworms, and preventing their ingestion by chickens are crucial steps in managing this parasitic infection effectively. By implementing such measures, poultry producers can significantly reduce the incidence of *Amoebotaenia cuneata* infections, thereby improving the overall health and productivity of their flocks [3].

## *Choanotaenia infundibulum*

*Choanotaenia infundibulum* is a tapeworm commonly found in domestic fowl. Notable for its size and strength, this parasite resides in the small intestine and is distinguished by its remarkably white coloration [5].

Adult *Choanotaenia infundibulum* tapeworms can grow up to about 23 cm in length. These unarmed tapeworms possess a large rostellum adorned with a single row of 16 to 22 hooks. The genital pores are arranged irregularly, and the worm has 25 to 60 testes clustered in the posterior section of each proglottid. The segments exhibit a distinct difference in width, with the posterior end being noticeably wider than the anterior end, resulting in a unique saw-edged appearance. The eggs feature unique elongated filaments [4]. *Choanotaenia infundibulum* has an indirect life cycle, depending on intermediate hosts such as house flies (*Musca domestica*) and beetles from the genera *Geotrupes, Aphodius, Calathus,* and *Tribolium* [3].

**Release of Proglottids**: The life cycle begins when gravid proglottids containing eggs are released in the feces of infected birds [5].

- *Ingestion by Intermediate Hosts:* House flies and beetles consume these proglottids, and the eggs develop into cysticercoids within these intermediate hosts [4].
- *Infection of Chickens:* Chickens become infected by consuming these intermediate hosts. During digestion, the cysticercoids are released and develop into juvenile tapeworms [3].
- *Development into Adults:* The juvenile tapeworms latch onto the lining of the small intestine and mature into fully grown adults. The pre-patent period, the time from infection to the release of initial eggs, typically lasts for approximately 2 to 4 weeks [5].

*Choanotaenia infundibulum* can cause significant health issues in infected poultry. When these parasites attach to the upper half of the small intestine, they can disrupt nutrient absorption, leading to decreased feed conversion and slower growth rates in affected birds [3]. Implementing efficient management and prevention strategies is crucial to minimize the negative impact of this parasite on poultry health and production.

Developing targeted interventions requires a thorough understanding of the life cycle of *Choanotaenia infundibulum*. Effective control measures include:

- *Reducing Intermediate Hosts:* Efforts should be directed towards decreasing the population of intermediate hosts such as house flies and beetles [4].
- *Preventing Ingestion by Chickens:* Ensuring that chickens do not consume these intermediate hosts is vital.
- *Improved Sanitation:* Maintaining cleanliness in poultry environments helps reduce the presence of flies and beetles [3].
- *Proper Waste Management:* Efficient handling of waste can minimize the breeding grounds for intermediate hosts.

• *Use of Insecticides:* Applying insecticides can help control the populations of flies and beetles in poultry houses.

By implementing these measures, poultry producers can effectively manage *Choanotaenia infundibulum* infections, thereby improving the overall health and productivity of their flocks.

## *Hymenolepis cantaniana*

*Hymenolepis cantaniana* is a small tapeworm from the Hymenolepididae family, commonly found in avian hosts. Measuring up to approximately 2 cm in length, this parasite closely resembles the larger *Hymenolepis carioca.*

*Hymenolepis cantaniana* is generally considered an unarmed tapeworm, although some instances have reported the presence of rostellar hooks. The genital pores are unilaterally located on the proglottid, positioned towards the anterior end.

*Hymenolepis cantaniana* has an indirect life cycle involving dung beetles from the Scarabaeidae family as intermediate hosts.

• **Cysticercoid Carriage:** Each beetle can carry over 100 cysticercoids, which develop from a single oncosphere through a budding process.
• **Infection of Birds:** Birds become infected by consuming beetles containing cysticercoids. Once ingested, these cysticercoids are released in the bird's digestive tract, where they mature into adult tapeworms.
• **Egg Release and Continuation:** The adult tapeworms lay eggs, which are excreted in the bird's feces. These eggs are then ingested by dung beetles, perpetuating the cycle.

Despite its small size, *Hymenolepis cantaniana* can adversely affect the health of infected birds. The parasite can interfere with nutrient absorption, leading to decreased growth rates and a general decline in the health of the host, particularly in poultry.

Effective control of *Hymenolepis cantaniana* involves managing the population of dung beetles and preventing their ingestion by poultry. Key strategies include:

• **Reducing Intermediate Hosts:** Efforts should focus on reducing dung beetle populations in poultry environments.
• **Preventing Ingestion by Birds:** Measures should be taken to ensure birds do not consume these beetles.
• **Improved Sanitation:** Maintaining cleanliness and proper waste management can reduce beetle populations.
• **Use of Insecticides:** Applying insecticides can help control beetle populations.

By implementing these control measures, poultry producers can mitigate the risks associated with *Hymenolepis cantaniana*, improving the overall health and productivity of their flocks.

## *Hymenolepis carioca*

*Hymenolepis carioca*, described by Magalhães in 1898, is a remarkably slender tapeworm commonly found in the duodenum of chickens and turkeys. This parasite is characterized by its extremely narrow body, making it appear thread-like rather than worm-like.

Key features of *Hymenolepis carioca* include:

- **Size:** This tapeworm is very slender, approximately 1 mm in diameter, giving it a thread-like appearance due to the numerous proglottids.
- **Suckers:** The tapeworm has unarmed suckers, lacking hooks or other attachment mechanisms.
- **Rosellum:** The presence of rudimentary rostellar sacs is noted.
- **Testes:** It typically has three testes arranged in a straight line.
- **Genital Pores:** The genital pores are unilateral and located anterior to the middle of the proglottid margin.
- **Onchosphere:** The onchosphere is encased in an inner membrane that is elongated into a football shape, with granular deposits at the poles.
- **Embryonal Hooks:** The embryonal hooks measure approximately 10–12 mm.

*Hymenolepis carioca* utilizes a variety of intermediate hosts in its life cycle. These include twenty-six beetle species from nine different families and one termite species, with dung and ground beetles being the most common sources of infection. There have been claims suggesting the involvement of houseflies; however, these are likely incorrect.

Experimental infections with several hundred *Hymenolepis carioca* worms per bird have shown no significant effect on the weight gain of the hosts. This observation suggests that the parasite is relatively nonpathogenic, causing minimal harm to infected poultry.

## TAPEWORMS OF TURKEYS

Tapeworms are easily transmitted between wild and domestic turkeys, making wild turkeys a reservoir for tapeworm infections in domestic flocks. Due to the lack of controlled experiments, the pathogenicity of these tapeworms remains largely unknown. This chapter focuses on two species with established life cycles, providing descriptions and diagnostic characteristics for identification. The morphological features of the scolex and proglottids are illustrated to aid in the differentiation of species, particularly when complete specimens are not available.

## *Raillietina georgiensis* (Reid and Nugara 1961)

*Raillietina georgiensis* is a large tapeworm, measuring 15–38 cm in length and 3.5 mm in width, found in both domestic and wild turkeys. The scolex is armed with a double row of 230 rostellar hooks, each 12–23 mm in length, and 8–10 circles of acetabular hooks, 8–13 mm long (Fig. **2**). The genital pores are unilateral and centrally located in the proglottid. The eggs are contained within uterine capsules, similar to those of *R. tetragona* and *R. echinobothrida*.

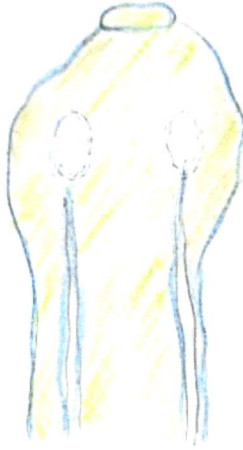

**Fig. (2).** *Raillietina georgiensis* (Tape worm in Turkey).

A small brownish ant, *Pheidole vinelandica*, commonly found in turkey habitats, serves as the intermediate host. Infected ants are ingested by turkeys, leading to the appearance of gravid proglottids in the birds' droppings within three weeks. This species has been introduced to domestic farms through wild turkeys.

Enteritis may occur if the parasites are present in large numbers. Damage to the host is presumed, based on the close relationship to *R. echinobothrida* in chickens.

## *Metroliasthes lucida* (Ransom 1900)

*Metroliasthes lucida* is a long tapeworm, reaching up to 20 cm, primarily found in turkeys and guinea fowl, with rare occurrences in chickens(Fig. **3**). The scolex and suckers are unarmed, measuring 200–250 mm in diameter. The genital pores alternate irregularly; they are located near the middle of the proglottid margin in mature segments but are positioned posteriorly in gravid proglottids. A distinctive feature is the para uterine organ, comprising two sacs visible to the naked eye in gravid proglottids. The eggs are characterized by three membranes and measure 75 × 50 mm.

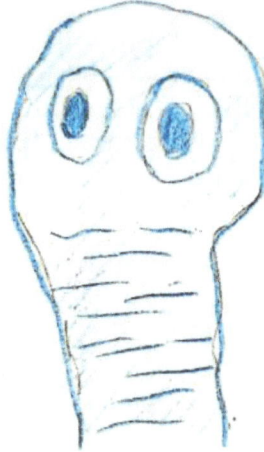

**Fig. (3).** *Metroliasthis lucida* .

The intermediate hosts for *Metroliasthes lucida* include several species of grasshoppers. The development of cysticercoids within these hosts requires 15–42 days, depending on environmental temperatures.

The pathogenicity of *Metroliasthes lucida* remains unknown. These descriptions and details provide critical information for the identification and understanding of turkey tapeworms. Accurate identification and knowledge of life cycles are essential for managing these parasites in poultry populations, minimizing their impact on health and productivity.

## TAPEWORMS OF DUCKS AND GEESE

Ducks and geese are hosts to several species of tapeworms, some of which occasionally infect chickens as well. The life cycles of these parasites typically involve crustaceans or other aquatic invertebrates. This section describes two of the more common species found in these birds. As with many avian tapeworms, there have been no controlled studies on the pathogenicity of these species.

### *Fimbriaria fasciolaris* (Pallas 1781)

*Fimbriaria fasciolaris* is a large tapeworm, measuring between 5 and 43 cm in length and 1 to 5 mm in width. It is notable for its twisted appearance and distinctive flaring anterior neck region, referred to as the pseudoscolex (Fig. **4**).

The strobila is unsegmented, but cross-striations give the appearance of segmentation. The minute scolex, attached to the pseudoscolex, measures 100–130 mm in width. The suckers are unarmed, and the retractile rostellum is equipped with 10–12 hooks, each measuring 17–22 mm. The genital pores are unilateral and closely packed together. The onchospheres measure 35–45 mm in diameter, with hooks approximately 16 mm long [5].

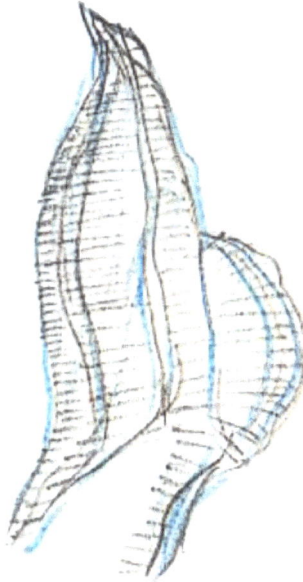

**Fig. (4).** *Fimbriaria fasciolasis .*

The life cycle of *Fimbriaria fasciolaris* involves cysticercoids developing in copepod crustaceans, particularly species of *Diaptomus* and *Cyclops*. These intermediate hosts are ingested by the definitive host through drinking water, facilitating the transmission of the tapeworm [3].

The pathogenicity of *Fimbriaria fasciolaris* remains unknown, as there have been no controlled studies to assess its impact on the health of infected birds [5] These tapeworms illustrate the diversity of parasitic species that can inhabit aquatic and semi-aquatic avian hosts. While the full extent of their impact on bird health is not well understood, identifying and studying these parasites are essential for effective management and control in both wild and domestic bird populations.

## *Hymenolepis megalops*

*Hymenolepis megalops* is a parasitic tapeworm species first described by Nitzsch in 1829, as documented by Creplin. This species is predominantly found in ducks worldwide and measures approximately 3-6 mm in length. It is distinguishable by its large scolex, which ranges from 1-2 mm in width and attaches to either the cloaca or the bursa of Fabricius (Fig. **5**). Notably, the scolex lacks any defensive structures such as suckers and rostellum hooks; the rostellum is characterized by a simple central pit. The eggs of *H. megalops* are unique in that they are not encapsulated.

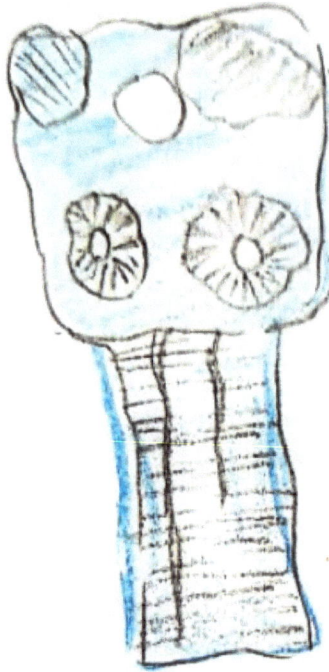

**Fig. (5).** *Hymenolepsis megalops* .

Onchospheres of *H. megalops* undergo metamorphosis into cysticercoids within ostracod crustaceans over a period of 18 days. These crustaceans are subsequently ingested by the definitive host, leading to the infection.

The pathogenicity of *H. megalops* can vary significantly, with reports indicating that it can range from causing severe disease to potentially leading to death, especially when associated with other related species such as *H. coronula* and *H. furcigera*. The impact of this tapeworm on the health of its host depends on several factors, including the presence of co-infecting organisms.

# EPIDEMIOLOGY, CLINICAL PRESENTATION, AND CONTROL

## Epidemiology

Tapeworm infections are prevalent across a broad range of avian species, affecting both domestic and wild birds. Species such as chickens, turkeys, ducks, geese, swans, guinea fowl, pigeons, peafowl, ostriches, pheasants, and quails can all be hosts to these parasites. This wide host range underscores the diversity and adaptability of cestodes in various avian environments [4].

Tapeworms are distributed worldwide, with infections more common in developing countries where poultry are often raised in free-range systems. Regions in Africa, Asia, and Latin America frequently report tapeworm infestations due to inadequate sanitation and close interaction with potential intermediate hosts [3].

The prevalence of tapeworms varies significantly by region. For example, in Ethiopia, infections are more common in lowland areas during warmer seasons, which favor the proliferation of intermediate hosts. In contrast, the higher altitudes with colder temperatures present harsher conditions for these hosts, reducing the rate of transmission [6]. In developed countries, intensive poultry production systems have led to a decline in tapeworm infections. However, even with controlled environments, some cestodes, such as *Choanotaenia infundibulum* and *Raillietina cesticillus*, persist due to the presence of intermediate hosts like flies and beetles. These infections often peak during warmer months when these hosts are most active [3]. The prevalence of tapeworm infections is influenced by climate and seasonal changes, which affect the availability of intermediate hosts. Warmer climates and seasons typically lead to higher infection rates due to the abundance of beetles, flies, and other invertebrates [5].

Altitude plays a crucial role in the survival and transmission of intermediate hosts. Warmer lowlands support the growth of these hosts, while cooler highlands inhibit their survival, thus affecting the transmission of tapeworms [6].

Free-range systems with poor sanitation are more prone to frequent tapeworm infections. Conversely, intensive systems with improved sanitation practices see significantly reduced infection rates (Hofstad *et al.*, 1984). Effective control of tapeworm infections in poultry involves targeting intermediate hosts and improving overall sanitation. Measures include proper waste management, regular cleaning, and disinfection of poultry houses, as well as monitoring and controlling the population of intermediate hosts [4].

## Clinical Presentation and Diagnosis

Tapeworm infections can lead to nutrient depletion, stunted growth, and reduced productivity in poultry. While many infections are mild, severe cases can cause significant symptoms such as emaciation, weight loss, ruffled plumage, slow movement, rapid breathing, diarrhea, and in extreme cases, death. Clinical signs may also include catarrhal enteritis, hemorrhage, intestinal obstruction, and nodular growth [5]. Accurate identification of tapeworms is crucial for understanding their impact and implementing effective control measures. This process involves examining specific attributes of the tapeworm, including the scolex, eggs, and individual proglottids of freshly shed and intact living specimens.

To identify tapeworms, one can examine the scolex, the eggs, or the individual proglottids. Differential staining can reveal the internal organs of fully developed proglottids, but this method is too time-consuming for most diagnostic facilities. Preservation in alcohol or formalin, while necessary prior to staining, often conceals valuable features required for swift identification [4].

To expose the area where the scolex is attached, it is most effective to use scissors to open the gut underwater, allowing the strobila to float freely. Retrieving the scolex is highly valuable since its distinctive features alone can potentially determine the species. To free the scolex, one can either:

• Separate the mucosa using two dissecting needles.
• Create a deep gouge in the mucosa beneath the attachment point with a sharp scalpel.
• Leave the intestine soaked in saltwater for a few hours in the refrigerator [3].

By examining wet-mount preparations of the scolex under a coverglass with a magnification of 3,100 or higher, it is possible to identify the species based on the observed characteristics. Hook features may necessitate assessment using an ocular micrometre at increased magnification [5].

To create semipermanent cleared preparations of scolices, one can use a drop of Hoyer's solution. This solution is formed by sequentially adding the following ingredients to 50mL of distilled water: 30g of gum arabic flakes, 200g of chloral hydrate, and 20g of glycerin [4].

Teasing apart a gravid proglottid under a coverglass can reveal distinctive egg characteristics. By examining wet preparations of mature or gravid proglottids under low magnification, one can identify diagnostic features such as:

- The location, size, and shape of the cirrus pouch.
- The location of the genital pores and the gonads [5].

If further information about the internal organisation of the proglottid is needed for identification purposes, it may be necessary to euthanise, preserve, and apply the dye, remove the dye, remove moisture, and permanently prepare the specimen for examination [4].

## Control

The most effective way to control tapeworm infections is to prevent birds from accessing intermediate hosts. Implementing strict sanitation and management practices, such as regular cleaning of poultry houses, proper disposal of droppings, and thorough cleaning of feeders and drinkers, is essential [3].

Control measures should also focus on eliminating intermediate hosts, such as beetles, flies, snails, and other invertebrates. For instance, controlling houseflies can reduce the prevalence of *Choanotaenia infundibulum*, while beetle control can help manage *Raillietina cesticillus* [7].

In the United States, there are no feed-based treatments specifically for tapeworms in poultry. Historically, butynorate was used to treat various tapeworm species. However, current control efforts focus on prevention by reducing intermediate host populations. Other drugs, such as praziquantel and niclosamide, have been used to treat tapeworm infections, but their effectiveness is limited if intermediate hosts are not controlled [5].

The shift from backyard or free-range systems to confinement rearing in large houses has significantly reduced tapeworm infections in poultry. These controlled environments limit the birds' access to the intermediate hosts required for the parasites' life cycles [3].

Tapeworm infections in poultry, especially in backyard systems with poor management, can lead to severe health issues and economic losses. In Ethiopia, species such as *Davainea proglottina, Raillietina echinobothrida, Raillietina cesticillus, Raillietina tetragona, Amoebotaenia cuneata, Choanotaenia infundibulum, Hymenolepis carioca*, and *Hymenolepis cantaniana* are of particular concern [6].

Effective management strategies include:

- **Minimizing Interaction:** Isolate infected birds and ensure new arrivals are quarantined and dewormed.
- **Sanitation:** Maintain clean housing conditions, regularly replace bedding, and

disinfect poultry houses.

- **Control of Intermediate Hosts:** Implement measures to eliminate intermediate hosts from the environment.
- **Education and Awareness:** Educate farmers about the risks and prevention strategies for tapeworm infections.
- **Strategic Deworming:** Develop a deworming schedule to manage tapeworm infections effectively.

By adopting these practices, poultry farmers can significantly reduce the prevalence of tapeworm infections, leading to healthier flocks and improved productivity.

## CONCLUDING REMARKS

In conclusion, tapeworms, including species like *Raillietina, Davainea proglottina, Choanotaenia infundibulum,* and *Amoebotaenia cuneata*, pose significant threats to poultry health by disrupting nutrient absorption and reducing feed conversion efficiency. These parasites, which rely on intermediate hosts such as earthworms, snails, beetles, and houseflies, can cause various health issues, including growth delays and increased susceptibility to other infections. Effective management strategies include precise identification of tapeworm species, controlling intermediate host populations, maintaining strict sanitation, and regular deworming. Understanding the life cycles and biology of these parasites is crucial for developing targeted interventions. Comprehensive control measures, including proper waste management and environmental hygiene, are essential for reducing economic losses and improving poultry health and productivity. Educating farmers on prevention techniques further supports the welfare and sustainability of poultry production.

## ACKNOWLEDGEMENTS

The authors are grateful to Bentham Science publishers for providing the opportunity to publish this book chapter. The authors also thank their family members for their ongoing support, inspiration, encouragement, and sacrifices, without which this chapter would not have been possible to complete. The authors will always be grateful to the contributors who provided constructive criticism for this work.

## REFERENCES

[1]    Botero H, Reid WM. The effects of the tapeworm *Raillietina cesticillus* upon body weight gains of broilers, poults and on egg production. Poult Sci. 1969 Mar;48(2):536-42.
       [http://dx.doi.org/10.3382/ps.0480536] [PMID: 5389871]

[2]    Permin A, Ranvig H. Genetic resistance to *Ascaridia galli* infections in chickens. Vet Parasitol. 2001

Dec 3;102(1-2):101-11.
[http://dx.doi.org/10.1016/s0304-4017(01)00525-8] [PMID: 11811920]

[3]     Hofstad MS, Barnes HJ, Calnek BW, Reid WM, Yoder HW. Diseases of Poultry. 8$^{th}$ ed., Iowa State University Press 1984.

[4]     Reid WM, Norton RA, Ruska HW. Cestodes and cestodiasis. Diseases of Poultry. Iowa State University Press: In: Hofstad MS, Barnes HJ, Calnek BW, Reid WM, Yoder HW, editors. 1972.

[5]     Soulsby EJL. Helminths, arthropods and protozoa of domesticated animals. 7$^{th}$ ed., Bailliere Tindall 1982.

[6]     Ashenafi H, Eshetu Y. Study on gastrointestinal helminths of local chickens in central Ethiopia. Rev Med Vet 2004; 155(10): 504-7. [http://revmedvet.com/2004/RMV155_504_507.pdf].

[7]     Butboonchoo P, Wongsawad C, Rojanapaibul A, Chai JY. Morphology and molecular phylogeny of *Raillietina* spp. (Cestoda: Cyclophyllidea: Davaineidae) from domestic chickens in Thailand. Korean J Parasitol. 2016 Dec;54(6):777-786.
[http://dx.doi.org/10.3347/kjp.2016.54.6.777]

# CHAPTER 13

# Protozoan Parasitic Infection

**R.L. Rakesh[1], Saroj Kumar[2,\*], Pradeep Kumar[3], Alok Kumar Singh[4], Souti Prasad Sarkhel[5], Anupam Brahma[6] and Vivek Agarwal[7]**

[1] *Department of Veterinary Parasitology, Veterinary College, Hassan 573202, KVAFSU, Bidar, India*

[2] *Department of Veterinary Parasitology, Faculty of Veterinary and Animal Sciences, Institute of Agricultural Sciences,Banaras Hindu University, Varanasi 221005, Uttar Pradesh, India*

[3] *Department of Veterinary Parasitology, Uttar Pradesh Pandit Deen Dayal Upadhyaya Pashu Chikitsa Vigyan Vishwavidyalaya Evam Go-Anusandhan Sansthan, Mathura 281001, Uttar Pradesh, India*

[4] *Department of Veterinary Parasitology, College of Veterinary Science & Animal Husbandry, Kuthuliya, Rewa 486001, Madhya Pradesh, India*

[5] *Faculty of Veterinary and Animal Sciences, Institute of Agricultural Sciences, Banaras Hindu University, Varanasi 221005, Uttar Pradesh, India*

[6] *Faculty of Veterinary and Animal Sciences, Institute of Agricultural Sciences, Banaras Hindu University, Varanasi 221005, Uttar Pradesh, India*

[7] *Department of Veterinary Parasitology, College of Veterinary Sciences & A.H, Nanaji Deshmukh Veterinary Science University, Mhow, Indore 453446, Madhya Pradesh, India*

**Abstract:** Poultry has protozoa that are classified into multiple taxonomic groupings. In poultry, two types of parasites are significant: the coccidia and the mastiogophora (flagellates). Some parasites, which cause coccidiosis, have short, direct life cycles and are therefore preferred, while other parasites that involve intermediate hosts typically do not pose a threat to commercial poultry. A significant exception is blackhead disease (histomoniasis), which has a complex life cycle involving intermediate hosts, but relies on chickens as reservoir hosts and spreads easily among turkeys within a flock. Most coccidia found in poultry belong to the genus *Eimeria*, however, there are also some species of *Isospora* and *Cryptosporidium*. The most well-known are the *Eimeria*, of which seven significant species have been identified in chickens and several more in turkeys. Anywhere chickens are raised, whether in huge commercial operations or tiny backyard flocks, parasites are an issue that can result in severe financial losses. This chapter will provide a quick overview of the main poultry protozoan parasitic species, along with some pathophysiology.

\* **Corresponding author Saroj Kumar:** Department of Veterinary Parasitology, Faculty of Veterinary and Animal Sciences, Institute of Agricultural Sciences,Banaras Hindu University, Varanasi 221005, Uttar Pradesh, India; E-mail: saroj.kumar@bhu.ac.in

Tanmoy Rana (Ed.)

**Keywords:** *Ascaridia galli, Capillaria, Coccidia, Cryptosporidium, Haemoprotozoa, Heterakis gallinarum, Oxyspirura mansoni, Poultry Nematodes, Poultry parasites, Protozoa, Round worms, Subulura brumpti, Syngamus trachea, Tetrameres* sp.

## INTRODUCTION

Protozoan parasites of poultry usually inhabit the lumen of the intestinal tract, present within the cells of many tissues or extracellularly in their blood and other body fluids. Some protozoa are host-specific, while others can infect a wide range of poultry species. Sometimes protozoa, which are relatively non-pathogenic may cause severe clinical disease in birds that are stressed or immune-compromised or have co-morbidities. Protozoan parasites that infect poultry come from various taxonomic groups, with many belonging to the phylum Apicomplexa [1 - 4]. This group includes intracellular protozoa distinguished by the presence of an apical complex during the sporozoite stage. The genera in this group include *Eimeria, Tyzzeria, Wenyonella, Plasmodium, Haemoproteus, Leucocytozoon, Toxoplasma, Sarcocystis,* and *Cryptosporidium*. Flagellates such as *Trypanosoma, Histomonas, Chilomastix, Spironucleus, Cochlosoma,* and amoebas from the genera *Entamoeba* and *Endolimax* also infect poultry. The microsporidian, *Encephalitozoon cuniculi* has recently been found in chickens [2 - 5].

## POULTRY COCCIDIOSIS

Poultry coccidiosis is caused by apicomplexan protozoa from three genera: *Eimeria, Tyzzeria* and *Wenyonella*. It affects virtually all domestic and wild birds, causing enteric disease, which is marked by symptoms such as pallor, diarrhoea (with or without blood), poor feed conversion, weight loss, and occasionally mortality [7 - 10]. Coccidiosis mainly caused by various *Eimeria* spp., is the most significant parasitic disease in the global poultry industry, leading to substantial economic losses due to the costs associated with preventing and controlling both sub-clinical and clinical disease [11 - 13]. Coccidiosis alone represents 30% of total expenditures on pharmacological control for all potential poultry diseases [14 - 18]. The disease typically affects immunologically naïve birds or those that are stressed or overcrowded, leading to severe infections. In general, clinical parasitic disease is less of a concern in backyard poultry compared to commercially raised birds for two reasons: 1) Parasite replication is self-limiting due to a fixed number of asexual cycles, and 2) Hosts develop protective immunity following infection [19 - 22].

## Etiology and Life Cycle

Poultry coccidiosis is a parasitic disease caused by protozoa from the phylum Apicomplexa, specifically the genus *Eimeria*. These are obligate intracellular protozoan parasites that infect and replicate within the intestinal epithelial cells of birds. In domestic chicken (*Gallus gallus domesticus*), although nine species of *Eimeria* have been identified, only seven are widely accepted (Fig. **1**). The species responsible for hemorrhagic disease are *E. brunetti*, *E. necatrix*, and *E. tenella*. *E. acervulina*, *E. maxima*, *E. mitis*, and *E. praecox* are considered mildly pathogenic and are associated with malabsorptive disease [22]. Concurrent infections with two or more species of *Eimeria* are common. However, each species develops in a specific site of the small intestine (upper, middle, lower, rectum, and caeca) and leads to distinct, recognizable diseases that are independent of the other species of *Eimeria* infecting that poultry species.

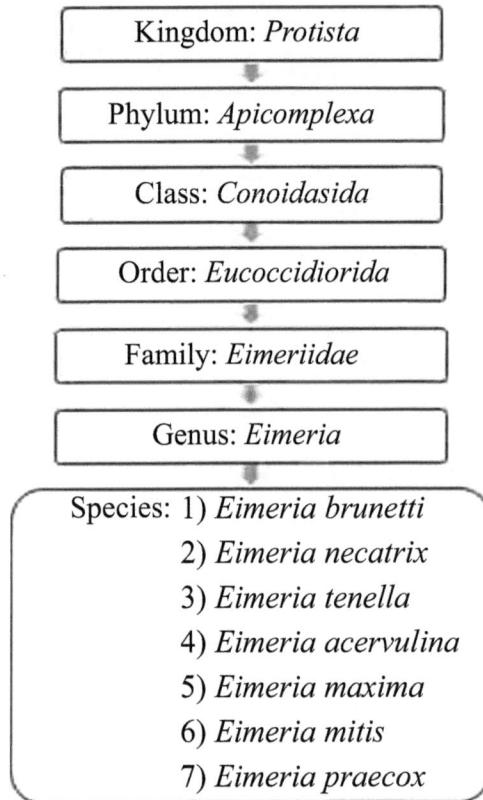

| Kingdom: *Protista* |
| :---: |
| Phylum: *Apicomplexa* |
| Class: *Conoidasida* |
| Order: *Eucoccidiorida* |
| Family: *Eimeriidae* |
| Genus: *Eimeria* |

Species: 1) *Eimeria brunetti*
2) *Eimeria necatrix*
3) *Eimeria tenella*
4) *Eimeria acervulina*
5) *Eimeria maxima*
6) *Eimeria mitis*
7) *Eimeria praecox*

**Fig. (1).** Taxonomy of *Eimeria* spp. in chickens (Adapted from Conway and McKenzie [18]).

Naïve chickens of all ages and breeds are vulnerable to infection. However, immunity develops after mild infections, which helps limit future infections.

Since there is no stimulation of cross-protective immunity among *Eimeria* species, multiple outbreaks of coccidiosis can occur within the same flock, each involving different species. Disease outbreaks are frequently observed in chickens aged 3 to 6 weeks [23-25]. In certain cases, infections can occur as early as 1 week of age. Breeder pullets and layer pullets are at the highest risk since they are kept in litter for 20 weeks or longer. Typically, infections with *E. acervulina, E. maxima, E. mitis, E. praecox,* and *E. tenella* occur between 3 and 6 weeks of age, while *E. necatrix* is observed at 8 to 18 weeks of age. *E. brunetti* can be found both early and late in the life cycle [26 - 28].

The life cycle of the *Eimeria* is complex, but there are no intermediate hosts. *Eimeria* spp., have developmental cycles that include an exogenous phase in the environment. During this phase, the resistant stages known as oocysts, which are excreted by chickens, undergo a differentiation process called sporulation, making them infective. Sporulation is the process that transforms oocysts into an infective form, requiring optimal conditions of temperature (25°–30°C), moisture, and adequate aeration (oxygen). Under ideal circumstances, sporulation for most poultry *Eimeria* spp., takes place within 24 to 72 hours. The degree and speed of sporulation of excreted oocysts are crucial factors that impact the infection pressure within a flock, thereby influencing the epidemiology of these infections [29 - 32]. Infective sporulated oocysts contain four sporocysts, with each sporocyst housing two sporozoites.

When a chicken ingests the oocysts, mechanical abrasion of the oocyst wall in the bird's gizzard (ventriculus) releases the sporozoites, which are then further digested enzymatically as the sporocyst wall breaks down in the upper intestinal lumen. This excystation process is aided by trypsin, bile, and carbon dioxide. Depending on the species, the liberated sporozoites migrate to their preferred sites within the bird's intestine, penetrate the villous epithelial cells in the mucosa, and initiate the endogenous phase of their development. Sporozoites of certain species, such as *E. brunetti* and *E. praecox* develop within the cells at the site of penetration. In contrast, sporozoites of other species, including *E. acervulina, E. maxima, E. necatrix,* and *E. tenella,* are transported to different locations, specifically the crypt epithelium, where they continue their development [33 - 37].

Upon entering the host cell, each sporozoite transforms into a feeding stage called a trophozoite within 12 to 48 hours. The trophozoite begins to enlarge, and the parasite's nucleus undergoes a process of asexual division known as schizogony or merogony. At this stage, the parasite is referred to as a schizont or meront. Within the schizont, smaller parasitic forms develop, known as merozoites. When the schizont matures, it ruptures, releasing the merozoites, most of which invade other epithelial cells to continue their development through the trophozoite and schizogonous stages. Merozoites from the second schizogonous cycle again penetrate the host's epithelial cells, with some or all potentially undergoing a third schizogonous cycle, depending on the species, before differentiating into male (microgametocytes) or female (macrogametocytes) gametocytes. The male gametocyte matures and ruptures, releasing numerous small, motile, biflagellate microgametes. The macrogametocyte grows into a larger macrogamete. When fertilized by a microgamete, the macrogamete forms a zygote, which develops a thickened wall around it, resulting in a young or immature oocyst. Eventually, these mature into unsporulated oocysts, which break out of the host cells in the intestinal mucosa and are excreted in the faeces of the infected chicken [38 - 41] (Fig. **2**).

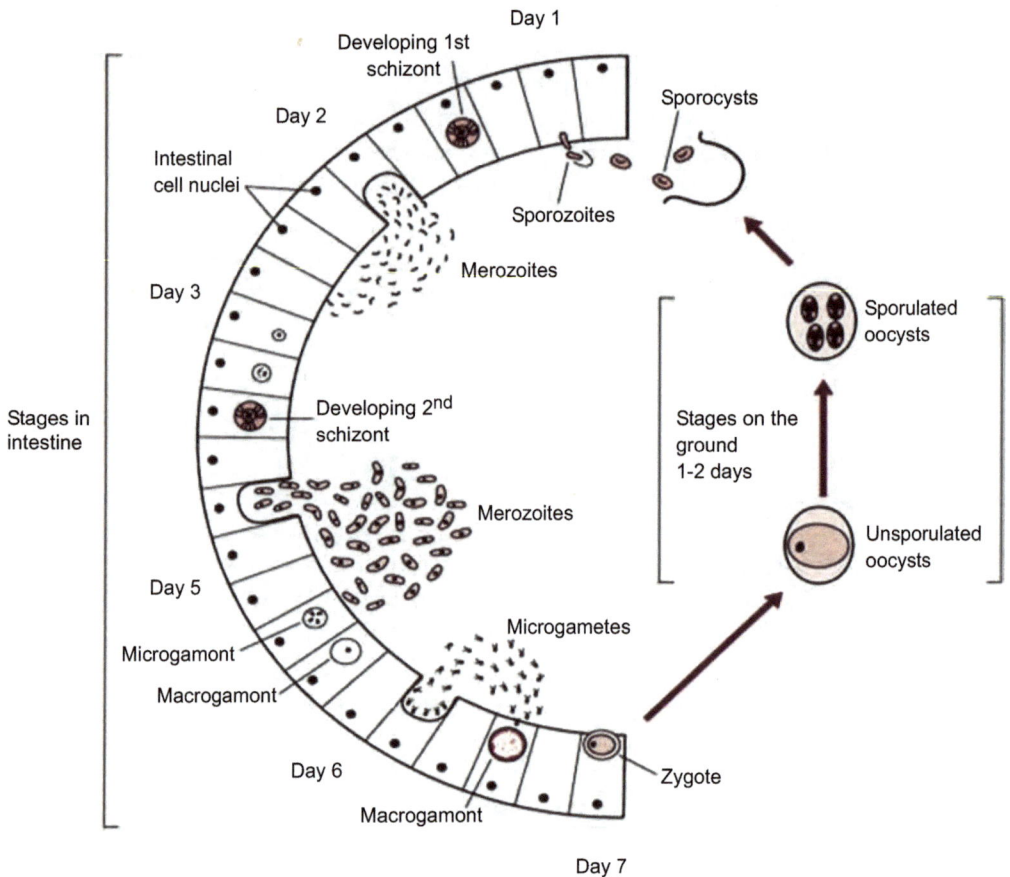

**Fig. (2).**  Typical life cycle of *Eimeria* spp. (Adopted from Pattison *et al.* [43]).

The prepatent period typically ranges from 4 to 6 days after oral infection, depending on the species. While oocysts can be shed for several days once patency is established, the highest output of oocysts usually occurs between 7 to 14 days post-infection. Oocysts are very resistant and remain viable in poultry litter for many months. Most of the chickens are carriers of various strains of the *Eimeria* spp., but not all become infected with the disease. Young chickens (under six months of age) are most susceptible to coccidiosis, where the immune system is immature. Adult chickens can also be infected with the disease and transmit the infection to other members of the flock through their droppings. The strict host specificity of *Eimeria* spp., excludes wild birds as sources of infection, although they can act as mechanical vectors. However, the primary mode of disease transmission is mechanical, often *via* personnel who move between pens, houses, or farms [42].

## Pathogenicity and Clinical Signs

The lesions and clinical signs produced by *Eimeria* infections depend on several factors, including: 1) The number of oocysts ingested; 2) The site of infection; 3) The age and immune status of the bird; and 4) Concurrent infections, among other factors. In some species, such as *E. tenella* and *E. necatrix*, maximum tissue damage may occur when second-generation schizonts rupture to release merozoites. In contrast, other species may have small, scattered schizonts that cause minimal damage, while their gametocytes can provoke a strong reaction, leading to cellular infiltration and thickened, inflamed tissues (*e.g.*, *E. maxima*) [44 - 46]. The lesions associated with the disease are typically found along the intestinal tract and often exhibit distinctive locations and appearances that aid in diagnosis (Table **1**). The most common and pathogenic form of the disease is caecal coccidiosis caused by *E. tenella*, followed by intestinal coccidiosis caused by *E. necatrix*.

Table 1. Predilection sites of different *Eimeria* species and their pathogenicity (Adapted from Permin and Hansen [47], Conway and McKenzie [18]).

| Species | Predilection site of the intestinal tract | Level of pathogenicity | Gross lesions |
|---|---|---|---|
| *Eimeria brunetti* | The lower small intestine, rectum, and caeca | High | Coagulation necrosis, mucoid, and bloody enteritis. |
| *Eimeria necatrix* | Middle intestine and caeca | High | Ballooning of the mid-intestine, small white spots, and petechial hemorrhages on the serosal surface (resembling "salt and pepper"), along with a mucoid, blood-filled exudate. |
| *Eimeria tenella* | Caeca | High | Hemorrhages into the lumen, thickened whitish mucosa, and cores of clotted blood. |

*(Table 1) cont.....*

| Species | Predilection site of the intestinal tract | Level of pathogenicity | Gross lesions |
|---|---|---|---|
| *Eimeria acervulina* | Upper intestine | Medium | In light infections: whitish round lesions on the mucosal surface of the duodenum and upper middle intestine. In heavy infections: coalescing plaques and a thickened intestinal wall. |
| *Eimeria maxima* | Middle intestine | Medium | Thickened intestinal wall, mucoid exudate, and petechial hemorrhages |
| *Eimeria mitis* | Ileum | Low | - |
| *Eimeria praecox* | Upper intestine | Low | - |

Tissue damage and alterations in intestinal tract permeability and function may create conditions favorable for colonization by various harmful enteric bacteria, such as *Clostridium perfringens*, leading to necrotic enteritis [48 - 50] or salmonellosis [51]. Caecal coccidiosis (*E. tenella*) has been shown to exacerbate the severity of *Histomonas meleagridis*, the pathogen responsible for blackhead disease in chickens. Experimental infections involving both organisms were associated with a higher incidence of liver disease compared to infections with *H. meleagridis* alone [52].

Coccidiosis develops quickly, with an incubation period of 5 to 7 days. Clinical signs may appear suddenly or develop gradually depending upon the intensity of infection. Common clinical signs seen in the affected birds include: lack of appetite (reduced feed and water intake), listlessness and weakness, ruffled feathers, severe diarrhoea, often mucoid or bloody diarrhoea, decreased growth rate (in young chickens) or weight loss (in older chickens) with a high percentage of visibly sick birds, anaemia, depigmentation (pale comb or skin), development of culls, decreased egg production and high mortality in the flock. Though, the survivors of severe infections recover in 10-14 days, but may never regain their lost performance.

## Diagnosis

Diagnosis is made through the demonstration of oocysts during the faecal examination and by histopathological examination of mucosal scrapings from the dead birds during necropsy. The oocyst count in faeces shows little correlation with the severity of the clinical disease. Additionally, the detection of a few oocysts in microscopic smears from mucosal scrapings suggests infection but does not confirm a diagnosis of clinical coccidiosis. In practical terms, a diagnosis is justified only when there are significant gross lesions. Therefore, diagnosing coccidiosis should rely on identifying these lesions and confirming microscopic stages during necropsy of representative birds from the flock, rather than relying solely on culled individuals [53].

The severity of lesions is generally related to the number of sporulated oocysts ingested by the bird and is associated with other factors like reduced weight gain, loss of skin pigmentation, and increased feed conversion ratios. The most commonly used method follows the system developed by Johnson and Reid (1970), which is a post-mortem examination scoring system. This system ranks lesions on a scale from 0 to +4 (where 0 indicates no lesions, +1 indicates mild lesions, +2 indicates moderate lesions, +3 indicates severe lesions, and +4 indicates extremely severe lesions) to assess the severity of poultry coccidiosis based on macroscopically visible lesions in the intestines caused by *Eimeria* spp. The complete intestine (between gizzard and rectum) should be dissected under a bright light source and the mucosal surface and serosal surface are carefully observed for lesions, nonetheless, microscopic observations are required to check smears taken from susceptible lesions for *Eimeria* parasites when lesions are not visible clearly [18, 54].

## Treatment and Control

Effective control of poultry coccidiosis typically involves implementing sanitary procedures, maintaining strict biosecurity, using prophylactic in-feed synthetic drugs (anticoccidials) or ionophore antibiotics—referred to as chemoprophylaxis, utilizing disease-resistant chicken breeds, and enhancing flock immunity. The most effective programs for preventing and controlling coccidiosis rely on building flock immunity and enforcing appropriate sanitary and biosecurity measures.

One approach to developing flock immunity is through feed medication with anticoccidial drugs. These anticoccidials can be categorized based on their specific modes of action: (i) Chemicals that impact parasite metabolism, such as amprolium, clopidol, decoquinate, halofuginone, and sulfamethazine, or (ii) Polyether ionophore antibiotics, like lasalocid, monensin, narasin, maduramycin, salinomycin, and semduramicin, which modify ion transport and disrupt the osmotic balance within the parasite's cells. Ionophore antibiotics are now the primary method for controlling coccidiosis [55]. It is concerning that there are reports of the development of resistance against most anticoccidial drugs, including ionophores [55, 56]. To address this resistance issue, poultry producers are implementing shuttle medication programs, which involve using a chemical drug in the starter feed followed by an ionophore in subsequent feeds, as well as rotational programs that utilize different anticoccidials with successive flocks.

These strategies aim to slow the development of resistance to any single medication.

Another approach to achieving controlled immunity is through coccidiosis vaccination using live attenuated or naturally selected strain sporulated oocyst vaccines (Table **2**). Vaccination has become an important control method due to the growing resistance to anticoccidial drugs [56]. It is already predominantly used for coccidiosis control in long-lived birds, such as breeding and egg-laying populations. The routine vaccination of broilers against coccidiosis is on the rise and may eventually replace controlled immunity through feed medication [57].

**Table 2. Commercially available coccidiosis vaccines (Adopted from Shivaramaiah *et al.* [58]).**

| Name | Manufacturer | Type | Composition | Method of administration |
|---|---|---|---|---|
| Advent® | Novus International Inc., St Charles, MO, USA | Live | *E. acervulina, E. maxima, E. tenella* | Oral |
| Coccivac-B® | Merck Sharp and Dohme Ltd, Whitehouse Station, NJ, USA | Live | *E. acervulina, E. maxima, E. mivati, E. tenella* | Oral, spray, intraocular |
| Coccivac-D® | Merck Sharp and Dohme Ltd | Live | *E. acervulina, E. brunetti, E. hagani, E. maxima, E. mivati, E. necatrix, E. praecox, E. tenella* | Oral, spray |
| Coccivac-T® | Merck Sharp and Dohme Ltd | Live | *E. adenoeides, E. dispersa, E. gallopavonis, E. meleagrimitis* | Subcutaneous |
| Eimeriavax 4M® | Bioproperties Pty Ltd, Ringwood, Australia | Live | *E. acervulina, E. maxima, E. necatrix, E. tenella* | Intraocular |
| Inovocox® | Pfizer Inc., New York, NY, USA | Live | *E. acervulina, E. maxima, E. tenella* | *In ovo* |
| Immucox I ® | Ceva, Libourn, France | Live | *E. acervulina, E. maxima, E. necatrix, E. tenella* | Oral, gel spray |
| Immucox II® | Ceva | Live | *E. acervulina, E. maxima, E.necatrix, E. tenella,E. brunetti* | Oral, gel spray |
| Immucox-T® | Ceva | Live | *E. adenoeides, E. meleagrimitis* | Oral, gel spray |
| Hatchpak Cocci III® | Sanofi, Paris, France | Live | *E. acervulina, E. maxima, E. tenella* | Spray |
| Paracox-5® | Merck Sharp and Dohme Ltd | Attenuated | *E. acervulina, E. maxima, E. mitis, E. tenella* | Oral |
| Paracox-8® | Merck Sharp and Dohme Ltd | Attenuated | *E. acervulina, E. brunetti, E. mitis, E. maxima, E. necatrix, E. praecox, E. tenella* | Oral |

(Table 2) cont.....

| Name | Manufacturer | Type | Composition | Method of administration |
|------|--------------|------|-------------|--------------------------|
| Livacox Q® | Biopharm, San Mateo, CA, USA | Attenuated | *E. acervulina, E. maxima, E. necatrix, E. tenella* | Oral, Spray |
| Livacox T® | Biopharm | Attenuated | *E. acervulina, E. maxima, E. tenella* | Oral, Spray |
| Coxabic® | Phibro Animal Health Corp, Teaneck, NJ, USA | Subunit | Purified *E. maxima* antigens from microgametocyte stages | Oral |
| Hipracox | Hipra, Girona, Spain | Attenuated | *E. acervulina, E. maxima, E. mitis, E. praecox, E. tenella* | Oral |

## COCCIDIOSIS IN TURKEYS

Coccidiosis is common in turkeys but often goes unrecognized because the lesions are less distinctive than those found in chickens. Of the seven species of coccidia that infect turkeys, only four are considered pathogenic: *E. adenoides, E. dispersa, E. gallopavonis,* and *E. meleagrimitis. E. innocua, E. meleagridis,* and *.E subrotunda* are classified as non-pathogenic. Oocysts begin to sporulate within 1 to 2 days after being expelled from the host, with a prepatent period of 4 to 6 days. Typical signs of coccidiosis in turkeys include mucoid or watery diarrhoea, blood-stained faeces, anorexia, ruffled feathers, and general signs of illness. While turkeys of all ages are susceptible to primary infections, those older than 6 to 8 weeks tend to be more resistant, likely due to acquired natural immunity. Although older turkeys may experience weight loss and morbidity, they are not as easily affected as younger birds [59, 60].

## COCCIDIOSIS IN DUCKS

While approximately 23 species of coccidia have been documented in both domestic and wild ducks, the validity of some of these descriptions is questionable. The presence of *Eimeria, Tyzzeria,* and *Wenyonella* species has been confirmed. *Tyzzeria perniciosa* is a recognized pathogen that leads to symptoms such as anorexia, distress, weakness, weight loss, and morbidity, and can result in mortality rates of up to 70%. There will be hemorrhages into the lumen leading to ballooning of the entire small intestine with caseous or bloody exudate and cores of clotted blood. *Wenyonella philiplevinei* occasionally leads to petechial hemorrhages accompanied by diffuse congestion in the lower intestinal mucosa [14, 61]. Interestingly, *Eimeria mulardi* develops within the host cell nucleus.

# CRYPTOSPORIDIOSIS

## Introduction

Cryptosporidiosis is caused by small coccidian parasites of the genus *Cryptosporidium*, which inhabit the microvillous region of epithelial cells in the gastrointestinal tracts, and occasionally in the respiratory tracts of vertebrates. While *Cryptosporidium* spp., are common in poultry, their significance is not well understood, apart from occasional outbreaks of respiratory cryptosporidiosis in turkey poults [62].

## Etiology and Life Cycle

Infections from at least nine different avian hosts have been observed in nature. The primary pathogens affecting chickens, turkeys, and quails are *C. baileyi* and *C. meleagridis*, which can cause respiratory and/or intestinal diseases, leading to illness and death [63].

The oocysts of *Cryptosporidium* spp. are excreted in the faeces of infected birds and can be ingested from contaminated environments. Like other true coccidias in the suborder Eimeriorina, their life cycle consists of six key developmental stages: excystation (release of infective sporozoites), schizogony (asexual reproduction within epithelial cells), gametogony (formation of male and female gametes), fertilization (union of gametes), oocyst wall formation (creating a resistant form), and sporogony (development of infective sporozoites within the oocyst wall). However, there are notable differences between this life cycle and that of *Eimeria* spp., which are also the reason behind the infection in birds [64].

The intracellular stages of *Cryptosporidium* spp. are localized to the microvillous region of the host cell. Oocysts sporulate within the host cell, rather than in the environment, and become infective upon being released in the faeces. There are two types of oocysts: thin-walled and thick-walled. Thin-walled oocysts lack environmental resistance and contain sporozoites encased in a single-unit membrane, allowing them to invade neighboring host cells upon release. In contrast, the more common thick-walled oocysts have a multilayered wall and are excreted in the faeces of infected birds. Unlike *Eimeria* spp., which are limited to the gut epithelium, these oocysts can establish infections in the mucosal epithelium of various organs. *C. baileyi* can infect the cloaca, cloacal bursa, upper and lower respiratory tracts, and eyelids (Fig. **3**) [65].

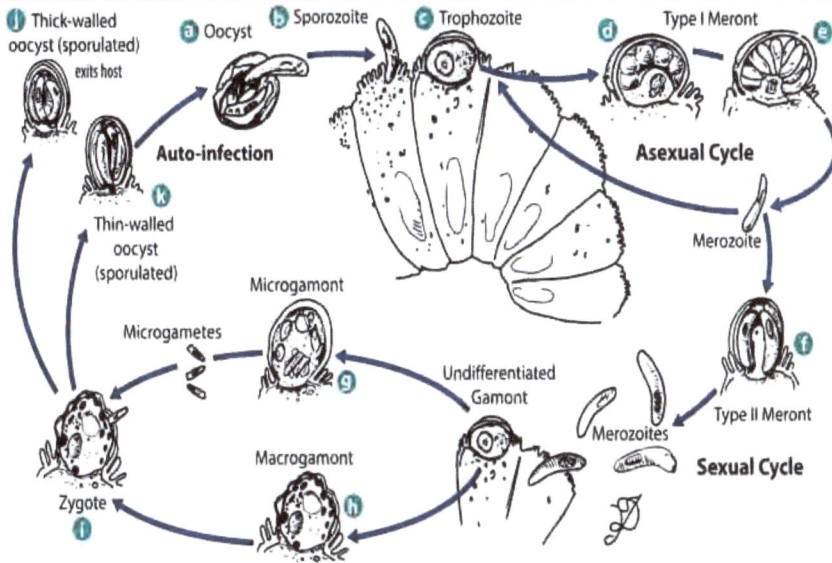

**Fig. (3).** Life cycle of the *Cryptosporidium* spp. (Source accessed from https://www.cdc.gov/dpdx/ cryptosporidiosis/modules/Cryptosporidium_LifeCycle_lg.jpg).

## Pathogenicity and Clinical Signs

Cryptosporidiosis in birds presents as enteritis, respiratory disease, or renal disease. Typically, only one condition is evident during an outbreak, although combinations of the three forms have been noted. Clinical signs of intestinal cryptosporidiosis include diarrhoea (non-bloody) and dehydration. In cases of respiratory infections, affected birds may experience rales, difficulty in breathing, coughing, and sneezing [66].

## Diagnosis

Since cryptosporidiosis in birds can present as enteritis, respiratory disease, or renal disease, there are no distinct clinical signs that specifically indicate the infection. While the examination of paraffin-embedded, hematoxylin and eosin-stained tissue sections has been the preferred diagnostic method, acid-fast staining can quickly identify developmental stages in cytological samples and oocysts in faecal smears [67]. The oocysts are small, measuring approximately 5 μm in diameter, with walls about 0.5 μm thick. They are colorless and lack a micropyle. Oocysts can be detected in faecal samples using Sheather's sugar flotation method. The Ziehl-Neelsen acid-fast staining technique is the most widely used, resulting in red-stained oocysts contrasted against a blue-green background of faecal material.

## Treatment and Control

Currently, there are no known effective treatments or vaccines for avian cryptosporidiosis. Enrofloxacin has shown limited effectiveness, while paromomycin significantly reduced oocyst output by 67-82%. Additionally, paromomycin positively impacted weight gain [68].

The oocysts of *Cryptosporidium* spp., which infect poultry, are highly resistant to most chemical disinfectants that effectively eliminate viral, bacterial, and fungal pathogens. As a result, while proper sanitation can help manage cryptosporidiosis, no proven control programs have been established [69]. Similar to other coccidial infections, cryptosporidiosis primarily affects confined birds or those in large populations in a given area. Implementing management practices that reduce bird density can lower the risk of parasite transmission [70]. Frequent removal of faeces from the area and exposing the affected space to direct sunlight are the most effective strategies for controlling outbreaks.

## HISTOMONOSIS

### Introduction

Histomonosis is caused by the parasite *Histomonas meleagridis*, which primarily affects turkeys. This disease is also known by several other names, including blackhead disease, typhlohepatitis, and infectious enterohepatitis (Clarke *et al.*, 2017). Characteristic lesions develop in the liver and caeca of gallinaceous birds, and untreated cases in turkey flocks can result in mortality rates of up to 80-100 percent. In chickens, the disease is generally less lethal, with lesions typically limited to the caeca [14, 15].

### Etiology and Life Cycle

*Histomonas meleagridis* is a pleomorphic flagellate protozoan that belongs to the phylum Parabasalia, class Tritrichomonadea, order Tritrichomonadida, family Dientamoebidae, and genus *Histomonas* [70]. When found in the lumen or free within the contents of the caeca, *Histomonas meleagridis* appears as an elongated flagellated form. However, once it reaches the tissues, it loses its flagellum and takes on three distinct tissue forms: (1) The invasive stage, which measures 8-17 μm, is amoeboid in shape and appears to form pseudopods at the peripheral areas of lesions; (2) The vegetative stage is longer (12–21 μm), more numerous, and clusters in vacuoles within degenerating tissue; and (3) A third stage, found in older lesions, is eosinophilic, smaller, and may indicate a degenerating form [71].

The life cycle of *Histomonas meleagridis* can be direct, but it typically involves a complex cycle with intermediate hosts and carriers. It reproduces rapidly through binary fission within infected birds. Free trophozoites are highly sensitive and can only survive for a few hours in the external environment. Infection is often transmitted *via* the eggs of *Heterakis gallinarum* (caecal worm). Female nematodes likely ingest the histomonads or become infected during mating, incorporating the protozoan into their eggs before shell formation [71, 72]. Infected birds later shed the eggs in their faeces. Even carrier birds, such as chickens, can harbor caecal worms and release infected heterakid eggs into the environment. This allows trophozoites to remain viable for years within these resilient eggs under suitable conditions. Common earthworms have been found to consume the eggs of the caecal worm, where they hatch and survive as infective larvae, acting as transport hosts. Susceptible birds contract *H. meleagridis* infection by ingesting *Heterakis gallinarum* eggs from the excreta or earthworms from their environment. Recent research indicates that turkeys can also transmit the protozoan directly from one bird to another, even without caecal worms and earthworms, through a process known as cloacal drinking. This involves contaminated fecal material in litter being drawn into the colon *via* rhythmic cloacal contractions or reverses peristaltic movement toward the vent region [73].

After ingestion, when *Heterakis gallinarum* reaches the caeca of the bird, the histomonads exit the worm larva and begin to multiply in the lumen and mucosa. They then migrate into the submucosa and muscularis mucosa, leading to severe necrosis. Within 2–3 days, these tissue forms enter the bloodstream and are transported to the liver *via* the hepatic portal system. In the liver, they cause characteristic focal coagulation necrosis, resulting in crater-like lesions (Fig. **4**).

**Pathogenicity and Clinical Signs**

Turkeys are the most susceptible to histomonosis, while chickens are less affected but can serve as asymptomatic reservoirs for the infection [74]. Clinical signs are primarily observed in poults (young turkeys), with chickens showing fewer symptoms. Early signs in turkeys include droopiness, loss of appetite, weakness, listlessness, closed eyes, dropped and ruffled feathers, and emaciation. Sick birds often huddle together, and their heads may appear cyanotic. Turkeys typically exhibit sulfur-yellow faeces, while chickens may have bloody caecal discharge. In turkeys, *Histomonas meleagridis* causes extensive and severe necrosis of the mucosa and submucosa of the caeca. The caeca becomes enlarged, with thickened walls and contents often mixed with serous and hemorrhagic exudate. In advanced cases, dense caseous plugs form crusts in the caeca, thickening the intestinal wall and narrowing the lumen, resulting in caseous caecal cores. In the liver parenchyma, focal areas of irregularly outlined, depressed coagulation necrosis appear with various sizes (diameter of 0.5–2 cm) and color (yellowish-green to yellowish-brown), presenting as 'target-like' or 'crater-like' lesions. These lesions can sometimes be worsened by other pathogens, such as coccidia and *Escherichia coli*. Concurrent infections with *Salmonella typhimurium* and *E. coli* have also been associated with high mortality rates, even in broiler chickens [75].

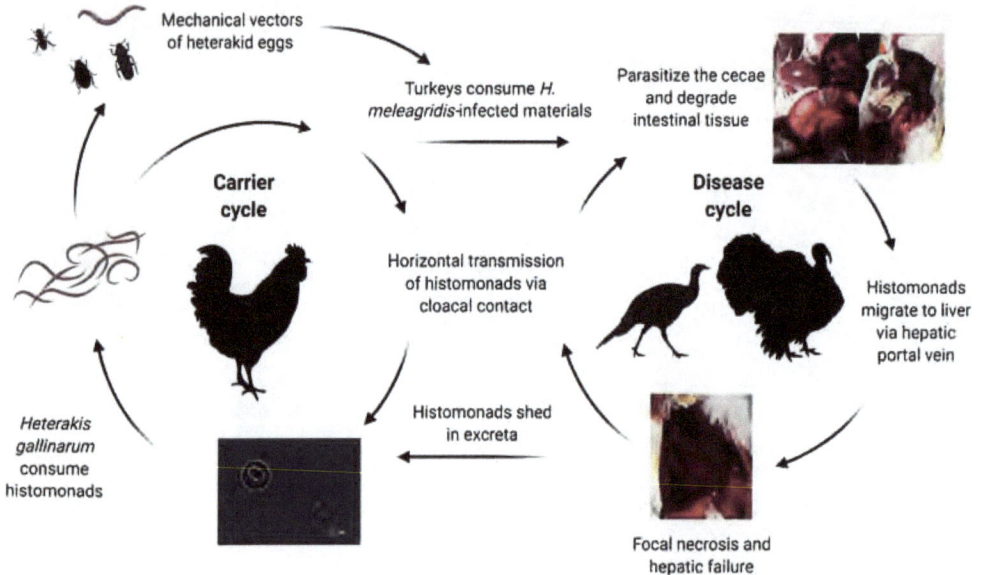

**Fig. (4).** Complex transmission of *Histomonas meleagridis* (Adopted from Beer *et al.* [12]).

## Diagnosis

Experienced veterinarians diagnose histomonosis in turkeys during necropsy in the field by assessing the gross appearance of lesions. Laboratory confirmation may be necessary to exclude concurrent infections with other pathogens affecting the caeca or liver, such as coccidiosis, salmonellosis, aspergillosis, and trichomonosis [1, 7].

## Treatment and Control

Presently, there are no approved treatments or vaccines for histomoniasis. Historically nitroimidazole compounds like dimetridazole, ipronidazole, and ronidazole were used for prevention and treatment from the 1960s through the 1980s and were highly effective [20 - 22]. Response to treatment was also both dose-dependent and time-dependent [11]. However, the extra-label use of this class of drugs in food-producing animals or birds is strictly prohibited in the United States. Paromomycin, an aminoglycoside antibiotic, has been effective as a prophylactic treatment against histomonosis when added to feed. Unfortunately, paromomycin appears to have limited therapeutic effects and is primarily used for prevention. Its use has also raised concerns about the development of antibiotic-resistant bacteria in the birds' gut [17].

In the absence of approved effective drugs or vaccines, the primary strategy for preventing disease is to minimize exposure to *H. meleagridis*. Implementing treatment programs for the caecal worm using benzimidazole drugs like albendazole and fenbendazole, along with effective flock management to limit *Heterakis gallinarum* and transport hosts such as earthworms and other invertebrates, can help reduce the incidence of histomonosis. This is because histomonads cannot survive for extended periods if shed unprotected directly into the environment [12]. Since chickens show much lower mortality rates and often remain carriers, their environments can serve as a source of infection due to the presence of intermediate hosts (*H. gallinarum*) and transport hosts (earthworms). Therefore, it is advisable to avoid keeping turkeys alongside chickens.

## HAEMOPROTOZOAN INFECTIONS OF POULTRY

Poultry kept in free-range systems or on pastures are exposed to various invertebrate hosts that transmit protozoan diseases. These blood protozoan parasites are primarily found in poultry in tropical regions, with the following genera commonly reported: *Plasmodium* spp., *Haemoproteus* spp., *Leucocytozoon* spp., and T*rypanosoma* spp.

## AVIAN MALARIA

### Introduction

Avian malaria is a widespread mosquito-transmitted disease in birds, caused by protozoan parasites belonging to the genus *Plasmodium* (phylum Apicomplexa, class Aconoidasida, order Haemosporidia, family Plasmoiidae). The avian species of *Plasmodium* exhibit morphological and developmental characteristics similar to those of related haemosporidian parasites in the genera *Haemoproteus* and *Leucocytozoon* [5]. In contrast to mammalian *Plasmodium* species, which exclusively infect erythrocytes, the exoerythrocytic stages in avian malaria can cause significant damage to various tissues and organs [10].

### Etiology and Life Cycle

Infections are caused by a complex of over 40 species that vary significantly in terms of host range, geographic distribution, vectors, and pathogenicity. While each Plasmodium species has a restricted host range, they are not strictly host-specific [11]. *P. gallinaceum* is found in jungle fowl and domestic hens; *P. juxta nucleare* infects domestic hens and turkeys; while *P. durae, P. griffithsi, P. hermani, P. kempi,* and *P. lophura* are present in turkeys (Beckstead, 2020). Many asymptomatic carrier birds exist, typically harboring parasitemias of less than 0.1% of erythrocytes. Additionally, non-pathogenic strains can be present in the same avian species that are susceptible to pathogenic strains [14].

*Plasmodium* species that infect birds have a complex life cycle, featuring sexual stages and sporogony in invertebrate hosts and asexual stages in vertebrate hosts. The invertebrate hosts for birds include mosquitoes from the *Aedes, Culex, Mansonia,* and *Armigeres* genera.

The life cycle begins when infective sporozoites in the mosquito's saliva are injected into a susceptible host during feeding [18]. This is followed by a schizogony stage in the reticuloendothelial cells of the liver, spleen, and bone marrow (pre-erythrocytic schizogony). A second schizogony stage may occur if merozoites produced in the first stage invade additional reticuloendothelial cells. Later, merozoites are released to invade erythrocytes, where they develop into schizonts and undergo multiple stages of schizogony, breaking out and destroying the erythrocytes at each stage. At some point, the merozoites trigger gametogony in other erythrocytes, resulting in the formation of sexual stages *viz.,* microgametocytes (male) and macrogametocytes (female) (Vogelnest, 1990). An exchange of parasites between the blood and reticuloendothelial tissues may occur, leading to secondary exoerythrocytic schizonts (phanerozoites), particularly in the spleen, kidney, and liver endothelial cells. When the mosquito feeds on infected birds, it ingests these gametocytes. Inside the mosquito, gamete formation takes place, followed by the development of oocysts and sporogony, which results in the production of sporozoites in the mosquito's salivary glands.

Infection can also be transmitted directly from bird to bird through blood transfer, without the need for an intermediate host, due to the transfer of schizonts found in the erythrocytes [25].

**Pathogenicity and Clinical Signs**

Avian malaria primarily affects the blood and reticuloendothelial system, with the progression of the disease and clinical symptoms closely linked to increases in parasite numbers in the peripheral circulation [11]. Clinical disease is more common in newly introduced, naïve birds rather than as relapses in chronically infected birds [26]. Depending on the strain, the pathological effects of avian malaria in infected birds can range from no noticeable symptoms to severe anaemia and death. Clinical signs are associated with endothelial damage caused by schizogony in various organs and the erythrocytic damage from released stages, meaning symptoms can appear before an erythrocytic parasite is detected. *P. durae*, *P. gallinaceum*, and *P. juxtanucleare* are the most pathogenic for domestic fowl and can result in up to 90% mortality [19].

Infected birds usually display symptoms such as anaemia, loss of appetite, lethargy, and ruffled feathers. Domestic chickens infected with *P. gallinaceum* and *P. juxtanucleare* show signs of lethargy, pale combs, green droppings, diarrhoea, and may experience partial or complete paralysis. Young turkeys infected with *P. durae* often show few clinical symptoms until right before death, when they may exhibit severe convulsions [26]. Adult turkeys typically show igns of lethargy and loss of appetite, and they frequently develop right pulmonary hypertension due to hypoxic pulmonary arterial hypertension [44]. Additionally, these birds may experience swollen legs and gangrene of the wattles. Infected birds can also exhibit neurological signs and paralysis before death, which is caused by blockage of cerebral capillaries by developing exoerythrocytic schizonts [11, 18].

## Diagnosis

Diagnosing *Plasmodium* spp., infection usually requires a microscopic examination of Giemsa-stained thin blood smears. This process allows for the observation of multinucleated schizonts within erythrocytes. Furthermore, gametocytes within the erythrocytes can be identified by their distinct dark golden-brown malarial pigment granules. These gametocytes may appear either round, displacing the erythrocyte's nucleus, or elongated, without displacing it. Individual *Plasmodium* species are typically classified based on the size and shape of intraerythrocytic gametocytes and schizonts, the number of merozoites produced by mature schizonts, alterations in the morphology of host erythrocytes, and other biological characteristics such as host range, susceptibility to different mosquito species, and the morphology and location of exoerythrocytic schizonts [24]. Comprehensive keys and descriptions of avian *Plasmodium* spp., have been provided by [72].

The intraerythrocytic gametocytes of *Plasmodium* spp., are often confused with those of *Haemoproteus* spp., because of their similar refractile pigment granules. However, *Plasmodium* gametocytes usually occupy less than 50 percent of the host cell's cytoplasm, and in certain species, they can displace the erythrocyte nucleus [10]. Two key features that aid in identifying Plasmodium are the presence of schizogony in peripheral blood and the detection of gametocytes or schizonts in blood cells other than erythrocytes.

During the necropsy of birds that died from avian malaria, various lesions can be observed, including significant hepatomegaly, splenomegaly, spleenic infarcts, subcutaneous hemorrhages, pigmented liver, lung, and spleen, as well as pericardial effusion and pulmonary oedema [71].

## Treatment and Control

Currently, there is no approved drug therapy for avian malaria [10, 14]. However, chloroquine phosphate, primaquine phosphate, pyrimethamine-sulfadoxine combinations, and mefloquine have shown effectiveness in treating various *Plasmodium* spp., infecting birds [65]. In turkeys, infections with *P. durae* were successfully treated using a combination of sulfachloropyrazine and sulfamonomethoxine, while treatment with halofuginone showed partial effectiveness [35]. To control avian malaria, efforts should concentrate on either eradicating the mosquitoes or isolating the flock from the intermediate hosts through appropriate housing.

## *HAEMOPROTEUS* INFECTIONS

### Introduction

*Haemosproteus* spp., are the most frequently encountered genus of avian hemoprotozoan parasites from the phylum Apicomplexa, transmitted by biting flies from the Ceratopogonidae and Hippoboscidae families. In contrast to their close relatives in the genus *Plasmodium*, they reproduce asexually through schizogony within tissues rather than in circulating erythrocytes [10].

### Etiology and Life Cycle

Approximately 140 species of *Haemosproteus* have been reported in birds, with the majority found in wild waterfowl, raptors, and passerines [45]. Species identified in domestic poultry include *H. meleagridis* in domestic and wild turkeys [13, 56], *H. columbae* and *H. saccharovi* in pigeons and doves, and *H. nettionis* in waterfowl [20].

Infections are characterized by schizogony occurring in visceral endothelial cells, the formation of gametocytes within circulating erythrocytes, and the presence of pigment granules in the infected erythrocytes. In the insect hosts, the zygotes formed develop into ookinetes and oocysts, with sporozoites eventually infecting the salivary glands [28]. Atkinson [6] reported that in domestic turkeys experimentally infected with *H. meleagridis*, at least two generations of pre-erythrocytic schizogony take place within the skeletal and cardiac muscles. The first-generation schizonts mature within 5 to 8 days post-infection, while second-generation megaloschizonts, which can reach lengths of up to 500 μm, develop between 8 and 17 days. These megaloschizonts then rupture to release spherical merozoites that mature into erythrocytic gametocytes [56]. Mature gametocytes that completely encircle the nucleus of the host erythrocyte develop within 7 to 10 days after the invasion of red blood cells [15]. In *H. columbae*, the parasites invade the capillary endothelial cells of the lungs, where they undergo pre-erythrocytic development to form thin-walled, oval or branching schizonts that extend along the pulmonary capillaries.

## Pathogenicity and Clinical Signs

*H. meleagridis* in turkeys causes symptoms like severe lameness, loss of appetite, diarrhoea, depression, and emaciation (Atkinson, 1985). Enlarged livers and anaemia are occasionally observed as well. Wild turkeys exhibit pathology linked to megaloschizonts in their skeletal and cardiac muscles [14]. Additionally, pigeons infected with *H. saccharovi* show enlarged gizzards.

## Diagnosis

The gold standard for diagnosing *Haemoproteus* infections is the identification of erythrocytic gametocytes containing distinct dark golden-brown refractile pigment granules in peripheral blood films, along with the absence of erythrocytic schizonts, which are characteristic of *Plasmodium* spp. (Atkinson, 2008). This is because schizogony in *Haemoproteus* spp., occurs only in tissues such as the liver, lungs, and spleen [12]. A mature gametocyte generally occupies more than 50 percent of the erythrocyte's cytoplasm, partially encircling the host cell nucleus in a distinctive "halter shape" while causing minimal displacement of the nucleus. It is rare to find more than one mature gametocyte in a single cell. Macrogametocytes appear blue when stained with Romanowsky stains and contain pigment granules dispersed throughout their cytoplasm. In contrast, smaller microgametocytes stain pale blue to pink, with pigment granules clustered into spherical aggregates [17]. PCR assays and restriction enzyme tests have been created to distinguish among *Haemoproteus* spp., *Plasmodium* spp., and *Leucocytozoon* spp [11].

## Treatment and Control

Atebrine, plasmochin, chloroquine sulfate, primaquine, mefloquine, and the antitheilerial drug buparvaquone have been shown to be effective in treating infections caused by various *Haemoproteus* spp [10].

In captive settings, *Haemoproteus* infections can be managed by housing birds in screened facilities that are shielded from biting midges and by applying insecticidal dusts to the birds to reduce or eliminate hippoboscid flies.

## LEUCOCYTOZOONOSIS

### Introduction

Leucocytozoonosis is a vector-borne disease of birds caused by apicomplexan protozoan parasites belonging to the genus *Leucocytozoon,* transmitted by biting flies belonging to the Simuliidae and Ceratopogonidae families. While many *Leucocytozoon* spp., exist, only a few are known to cause illness in their hosts. Waterfowl, pigeons, galliforms, raptors, and ostriches are the birds found to be particularly susceptible to this disease [18].

### Etiology and Life Cycle

All *Leucocytozoon* spp., are specific to their avian host orders and, in some cases, to particular host families. For instance, *L. simondi* (also known as *L. anseris* and *L. anatis*) infects members of the Anatidae family, which includes ducks, geese, and swans. In certain cases, they can even be specific to individual host species, such as *L. caulleryi*, which only infects chickens, and *L. smithi*, which exclusively infects turkeys [26].

The lifecycle involves sporogony occurring in insects such as blackflies (vectors for *L. simondi, L. smithi,* and others) or biting midges (vectors for *L. caulleryi*), following their ingestion of blood-containing gametocytes from infected birds. In the insect's midgut, gametocytes mature into macrogametocytes (female), which exhibit red-staining nuclei and dark blue-staining cytoplasm, and microgametocytes (male), characterized by pale pink-staining, diffuse nuclei, and very pale blue-staining cytoplasm when stained with Romanowsky stain [11]. Fertilization of the macro gametocytes results in the formation of zygotes, which elongate into ookinetes that invade the intestinal cells and develop into oocysts. The sporozoites produced within the oocysts then migrate to the salivary glands. This entire process can be completed in 3 to 4 days [15].

Sporozoites enter the bloodstream of the bird host when it is bitten by an infected fly. Once released, the sporozoites migrate and undergo schizogony in endothelial cells, hepatocytes, and the cells of the heart, kidney, spleen, and brain, leading to cellular destruction. Merozoites are subsequently released and can either initiate another schizogonic cycle or enter erythrocytes or erythroblasts to develop into gametocytes. Within the host erythrocyte, the gametocyte is positioned next to the host cell nucleus and takes on a compact, round shape [33]. In *L. caulleryi*, the nucleus of the host cell is reported to disappear after infection, which distinguishes it from other species that have round gametocytes (Forrester and Greiner, 2008). These gametocytes within erythrocytes produce anti-erythrocytic factors that lead to intravascular haemolysis and anaemia [28]. Megaloschizonts, which can grow up to 400 μm in size, form when syncytia are phagocytized by macrophages or reticuloendothelial cells in various organs throughout the body. The megaloschizonts then release merozoites into the bloodstream, which can develop into gametocytes in lymphocytes and other leukocytes. In leukocytes, particularly lymphocytes and monocytes, elongated (sail-like) gametocytes are likely to develop exclusively [29]. Aberrant infections occur when reticuloendothelial cells deposit merozoites in parenchymatous organs, leading to the formation of megaloschizonts without the development of gametocytes in circulating erythrocytes.

## Pathogenicity and Clinical Signs

Strains of varying pathogenicity have been identified for *L. caulleryi* in chickens and *L. simondi* in waterfowl [15, 37]. In cases of *L. caulleryi* infection, clinical signs in chickens usually appear two weeks after infection. Mortality rates can be as high as 100%, depending on the strain involved. Affected chickens may appear lethargic and anaemic, with pale combs and wattles, as well as a decline in egg production. Hemorrhages may be noted in the liver, lungs, and kidneys, with extensive hemorrhaging occurring in the kidneys upon the release of merozoites. Post-mortem examinations commonly reveal hemorrhages in the peritoneal cavity, splenomegaly, and hepatomegaly [12].

Infections with *L. simondi* are found to be highly pathogenic in young ducks and geese, typically manifesting as per-acute to acute infections in these birds. Clinical signs of *L. simondi* infection include loss of appetite, weakness, lethargy, labored breathing, and, in some cases, death within 24 hours. Nervous signs may occasionally be observed before death. These symptoms result from the parasite's effects, which include anaemia, leukocytosis, splenomegaly, and degeneration and hypertrophy of the heart and liver (Beckstead, 2020).

Infections caused by *L. smithi* are more severe in poults than in adult turkeys. Affected birds exhibit signs of anaemia, loss of appetite, and lethargy. In the later stages of infection, they may experience muscular incoordination, fall over, and ultimately succumb to the disease.

## Diagnosis

*Leucocytozoon* spp., can be easily identified from blood films because the large gametocytes grossly distort the infected host cells (usually immature erythrocytes) that they parasitize making cell identification difficult. Similar to *Haemoproteus* spp., only the gametocyte stages of *Leucocytozoon* spp. are present in the peripheral blood of birds [56].

The large, round-to-elongated gametocytes cause the host cell to enlarge, creating the appearance of two nuclei: the host cell nucleus pushed to the edge and the parasite nucleus, which appears as a pale-pink structure within the parasite. The affected cell typically has tapered ends with remnants of the cell membrane extending away from the cell. The macrogametocyte stains dark blue, featuring a condensed nucleus and occasional cytoplasmic vacuoles. In contrast, the microgametocyte stains light blue with a diffuse, pale-pink nucleus. Unlike *Haemoproteus* spp., the gametocytes of *Leucocytozoon* spp. do not contain refractile pigment granules [19].

**Treatment and Control**

There are no approved drugs for treating leucocytozoonosis. Coccidiostatic drugs such as sulphaquinoxaline and pyrimethamine have been used in attempts to prevent and treat this parasite, but there have been no reports of success (Rae, 1995). Controlling leucocytozoonosis involves avoiding the insect host and removing breeding sites, such as running water, from the susceptible bird's environment.

**TRICHOMONOSIS**

Trichomonosis in birds is caused by the flagellated protozoan *Trichomonas gallinae* (phylum Parabasalia, class Trichomonadea, order Trichomonadida, family Trichomonadidae), and affects their upper digestive tracts. This protozoan is very motile and pear-shaped, typically featuring four free flagella that emerge from a basal granule at its anterior end. A slender axostyle usually extends well beyond the rear end of the organism. An undulating membrane begins at the anterior end and extends towards, but does not reach the posterior end, with the enclosed flagellum not trailing free at the rear end [28].

In pigeons, this infection results in a condition known as canker. Chickens, turkeys, and various wild birds can also be infected, showing differing levels of pathogenicity (Levine, 1985). *Trichomonas gallinae* reproduces by longitudinal binary fission, and cysts, sexual stages, or vectors have not been observed. Squabs typically become infected when they first consume 'pigeon milk' from the crops of adult pigeons, and they usually remain carriers for life. In chicken and turkey flocks, trichomonosis spreads through direct contact or by ingesting contaminated food or water [5].

Virulent strains can lead to mortality rates of up to 50% before sufficient protective immunity is established. Pigeons are often involved in transmitting trichomonosis to turkeys and chickens. Depending on the species, infections may be localized in the mouth, oropharynx, oesophagus, crop, and trachea, or may spread to pulmonary and hepatic tissues. Pathogenic strains cause inflammation and white plaques on the gastrointestinal mucosa, or necrosis with the accumulation of cheesy material that can obstruct the trachea and oesophagus. Overcrowding and poor hygiene can worsen infections in individual birds and increase disease incidence within a flock. Advanced cases with significant necrotic masses are difficult to treat and usually have a poor prognosis.

## SPIRONUCLEOSIS (HEXAMITOSIS)

*Hexamita meleagridis,* a bilaterally symmetrical pear-shaped binucleate flagellate, is now categorized under the order Diplomonadida, family Hexamitidae, and genus *Spironucleus* [45]. However, the illness caused by this protozoan, known as spironucleosis, is still more frequently called hexamitiasis or hexamitosis [67, 69].

Flagellates of the genus *Spironucleus* alternate between a motile trophozoite and a nonmotile cyst, which is shed into the environment during their life cycle. The cysts of the parasite are probably the infectious forms, with transmission occurring *via* the faecal-oral route. *Spironucleus meleagridis* is responsible for infectious catarrhal enteritis in turkey poults. This organism has also been found in quails, chukar partridges, pheasants, and peafowls, which may act as sources of infection for turkeys that are raised on pasture. It possesses eight distinct flagella: four at the front, two anterolateral, and two at the back, with the four anterior flagella being recurved along the body [10].

Clinically, the infected poults become nervous and exhibit foamy, watery diarrhoea. At first, feed intake will be normal, but as the disease advances, affected birds may become lethargic and huddle together, experiencing rapid weight loss. In the final stages, they may have convulsions, go into a coma, and finally die. Adult birds usually carry the organism in their large intestine, releasing it into the environment, which can then infect the small intestines of younger birds or those with compromised immune systems, resulting in clinical symptoms. Generally, resistance to the infection tends to improve with age [14].

The diagnosis can be established through the observation of foamy, watery diarrhoea and the microscopic identification of flagellated *S. meleagridis* in wet smears of very fresh faeces or cloacal scrapings. These parasites can be readily differentiated from other flagellates due to their smaller size and quick, darting movements [19]. There is currently no effective treatment or vaccine for this parasite. To minimize transmission, it is advised to remove carrier birds, keep older stock separate from poults, and prevent other avian species from entering the area where the poult flock is located.

Other parasitic protozoa present in the intestinal tract of poultry include

*Tetratrichomonas gallinarum*, *Chilomastix gallinarum*, *Cochlosoma anatis*, and *Giardia* spp. These parasites are known to cause occasional infections in birds and are typically diagnosed through microscopic examination of the organism isolated from the infection site.

Tissue cyst-forming coccidian infections in poultry are primarily caused by *Toxoplasma gondii* and *Sarcocystis* spp. While these infections are found globally in wild birds, they are relatively rare in domestic poultry [28]. These parasites result in symptoms including muscle cysts, decreased growth rates, poor egg production, and, in severe cases, death. Infections can be diagnosed using histological methods, serological tests, and PCR techniques.

## CONCLUDING REMARKS

Protozoan parasites of poultry are broadly divided into two groups: intestinal protozoan parasites and haemoprotozoan parasites. These protozoan parasites typically inhabit the lumen of the gastrointestinal (GI) tract, reside within the cells of various tissues, or exist intracellularly in blood cells and extracellularly in blood and other body fluids. Some protozoan species of poultry are host and site-specific, while others can infect a wide range of poultry species. Sometimes protozoa which are relatively non-pathogenic, may cause severe clinical disease in birds that are stressed or immune-compromised or have co-morbidities. The major groups of protozoan parasites of poultry belong to the phylum Apicomplexa and genus *Eimeria*, *Tyzzeria*, *Wenyonella*, *Plasmodium*, *Haemoproteus*, *Leucocytozoon*, *Toxoplasma*, *Sarcocystis*, and *Cryptosporidium*. Most of these are intracellular protozoan parasites that are highly host-, cell-, and site-specific, causing some of the most important diseases in poultry. Several flagellate protozoan parasites such as *Trypanosoma*, *Histomonas*, *Chilomastix*, *Spironucleus*, *Cochlosoma*, and amoebas of the genera *Entamoeba* and *Endolimax* also infect the poultry. Young birds are more susceptible to these infections due to their immature immune systems; however, adults can also contract the disease, become carriers, and spread it to other susceptible flocks. The diagnosis of poultry protozoan parasites primarily relies on the microscopic examination of faecal samples or blood smears from suspected birds to identify parasitic stages. Additionally, a necropsy may be performed to observe the gross appearance of typical lesions. In recent years, several studies have been conducted to develop advanced diagnostics for parasitic diseases. These include molecular technique-based approaches, immunoassays, and proteomics for accurate and prompt diagnosis of the parasites. For the control and prevention of protozoan parasites, several chemotherapeutic drugs are available on the market. Although several vaccines are available for controlling coccidiosis, most other protozoan infections lack approved vaccines or effective treatments.

# REFERENCES

[1]   Aarthi S, Dhinakar Raj G, Raman M, Gomathinayagam S, Kumanan K. Molecular prevalence and preponderance of *Eimeria* spp. among chickens in Tamil Nadu, India. Parasitol Res 2010; 107(4): 1013-7.
[http://dx.doi.org/10.1007/s00436-010-1971-2] [PMID: 20607286]

[2]   Abbas RZ, Iqbal Z, Blake D, Khan MN, Saleemi MK. Anticoccidial drug resistance in fowl coccidia: the state of play revisited. Worlds Poult Sci J 2011; 67(2): 337-50.
[http://dx.doi.org/10.1017/S004393391100033X]

[3]   Al-Sheikhly F, Al-Saieg A. Role of Coccidia in the occurrence of necrotic enteritis of chickens. Avian Dis 1980; 24(2): 324-33.
[http://dx.doi.org/10.2307/1589700] [PMID: 6254485]

[4]   Arakawa A, Baba E, Fukata T. *Eimeria* tenella infection enhances *Salmonella typhimurium* infection in chickens. Poult Sci 1981; 60(10): 2203-9.
[http://dx.doi.org/10.3382/ps.0602203] [PMID: 7329903]

[5]   Atkinson CT, Forrester DJ. Myopathy associated with megaloschizonts of *Haemoproteus meleagridis* in a wild turkey from Florida. J Wildl Dis 1987; 23(3): 495-8.
[http://dx.doi.org/10.7589/0090-3558-23.3.495] [PMID: 3114504]

[6]   Parsa FR, Bayley S, Bell F, *et al.* Epidemiology of protozoan and helminthic parasites in wild passerine birds of Britain and Ireland. Parasitology. 2023 Mar;150(3):297-310.
[http://dx.doi.org/10.1017/S0031182022001779]

[7]   Atkinson CT. Epidemiology and Pathogenicity of *Haemoproteus meleagridis* Levine 1961 from Florida Turkeys. PhD Dissertation 1985.

[8]   Atkinson CT. Haemoproteus. In: Atkinson CT, Thomas NJ, Hunter DB, Eds. Parasitic Diseases of Wild Birds. State Avenue, Iowa, USA: Blackwell Publishing 2008; pp. 13-34. b
[http://dx.doi.org/10.1002/9780813804620.ch2]

[9]   Augustine PC, Barta JR, Innes L, Müller N. Chasing coccidia – new tools enter the race. Trends Parasitol 2001; 17(11): 509-11.
[http://dx.doi.org/10.1016/S1471-4922(01)02121-3] [PMID: 11872382]

[10]  Baba E, Furata T, Arakawa A. Establishment and persistence of *Salmonella typhimurium* infection stimulated by *Eimeria tenella* in chickens. Res Vet Sci 1982; 33(1): 95-8.
[http://dx.doi.org/10.1016/S0034-5288(18)32366-X] [PMID: 6753076]

[11]  Beckstead R. Miscellaneous and sporadic protozoal infections. In: DE Swayne Ed, 14ᵗʰ ed Diseases of poultry Diseases of Poultry. In: DE Swayne (Ed.), 14ᵗʰ ed. Wiley Blackwell Press, Hoboken, NJ, USA. 2020; pp. 1231-42.

[12]  Beer LC, Petrone-Garcia VM, Graham BD, Hargis BM, Tellez-Isaias G, Vuong CN. Histomonosis in poultry: A comprehensive review. Front Vet Sci 2022; 9: 880738.
[http://dx.doi.org/10.3389/fvets.2022.880738] [PMID: 35601402]

[13]  Campbell TW. Hematology. In: Ritchie BW, Harrison GJ, Harrison LR, Eds. Avian medicine: Principles and application. Lake worth, Florida: Wingers Publishing, Inc. 1994; pp. 176-98.

[14]  Cervantes HM, McDougald LR, Jenkins MC. Coccidiosis. Diseases of poultry. In: DE Swayne (Ed.), 14ᵗʰ ed. Wiley Blackwell Press, Hoboken, NJ, USA. 2020; pp. 1193-216.

[15]  Chapman HD, Barta JR, Blake D, *et al.* A selective review of advances in coccidiosis research. Adv Parasitol 2013; 83: 93-171.
[http://dx.doi.org/10.1016/B978-0-12-407705-8.00002-1] [PMID: 23876872]

[16]  Chapman HD. Biochemical, genetic and applied aspects of drug resistance in *Eimeria* parasites of the fowl. Avian Pathol 1997; 26(2): 221-44.
[http://dx.doi.org/10.1080/03079459708419208] [PMID: 18483904]

[17] Clarke LL, Beckstead RB, Hayes JR, Rissi DR. Pathologic and molecular characterization of histomoniasis in peafowl ( *Pavo cristatus* ). J Vet Diagn Invest 2017; 29(2): 237-41.
[http://dx.doi.org/10.1177/1040638716687002] [PMID: 28065124]

[18] Conway DP, McKenzie ME. Poultry Coccidiosis: Diagnostic and Testing Procedures. 3rd ed. State Avenue, Iowa, USA: Blackwell Publishing 2007; p. 164.
[http://dx.doi.org/10.1002/9780470344620]

[19] Current WL, Upton SJ, Haynes TB. The life cycle of *Cryptosporidium baileyi* n. sp. (Apicomplexa, Cryptosporidiidae) infecting chickens. J Protozool 1986; 33(2): 289-96.
[http://dx.doi.org/10.1111/j.1550-7408.1986.tb05608.x] [PMID: 3735157]

[20] Current WL. Techniques and laboratory maintenance of *Cryptosporidium*. In: Dubey JP, Speer CA, Fayer R, Eds. Cryptosporidiosis of man and animals. Boca Raton, FL: CRC Press 1990; pp. 31-50.

[21] Eide A, Fallis AM. Experimental studies of the life cycle of *Leucocytozoon simondi* in ducks in Norway. J Protozool 1972; 19(3): 414-6.
[http://dx.doi.org/10.1111/j.1550-7408.1972.tb03494.x] [PMID: 4627525]

[22] Forrester DJ, Greiner EC. Leucocytozoonosis. In: Atkinson CT, Thomas NJ, Hunter DB, Eds. Parasitic diseases of wild birds. State Avenue, Iowa, USA: Blackwell Publishing 2008; pp. 54-107.
[http://dx.doi.org/10.1002/9780813804620.ch4]

[23] Ganapathy K, Salamat MH, Lee CC, Johara MY. Concurrent occurrence of salmonellosis, colibacillosis and histomoniasis in a broiler flock fed with antibiotic-free commercial feed. Avian Pathol 2000; 29(6): 639-42.
[http://dx.doi.org/10.1080/03079450020016000] [PMID: 19184862]

[24] Garnham PCC. Malaria parasites and other haemosporidia. Oxford: Blackwell Scientific Publications 1966.

[25] Geng T, Ye C, Lei Z, *et al.* Prevalence of *Eimeria* parasites in the Hubei and Henan provinces of China. Parasitol Res 2021; 120(2): 655-63.
[http://dx.doi.org/10.1007/s00436-020-07010-w] [PMID: 33409626]

[26] Gerhold R. Parasitic diseases. In: Greenacre CB, Morishita TY, Eds. Backyard poultry medicine and surgery: A guide for veterinary practitioners. 2nd ed. Hoboken, NJ, USA: Wiley Blackwell Press 2021; pp. 206-17.
[http://dx.doi.org/10.1002/9781119511816.ch11]

[27] Gibbs BJ. The occurrence of the protozoan parasite *Histomonas meleagridis* in the adults and eggs of the cecal worm *Heterakis gallinae*. J Protozool 1962; 9(3): 288-93.
[http://dx.doi.org/10.1111/j.1550-7408.1962.tb02622.x] [PMID: 13898352]

[28] Goodwin MA, Latimer KS, Brown J, *et al.* Respiratory cryptosporidiosis in chickens. Poult Sci 1988; 67(12): 1684-93.
[http://dx.doi.org/10.3382/ps.0671684] [PMID: 3241775]

[29] Greiner EC, Forrester DJ. *Haemoproteus meleagridis* Levine 1961: redescription and developmental morphology of the gametocytes in turkeys. J Parasitol 1980; 66(4): 652-8.
[http://dx.doi.org/10.2307/3280524] [PMID: 6775070]

[30] Greiner EC, Ritchie BW. Parasites. In: Ritchie BW, Harrison GJ, Harrison LR, Eds. Avian medicine: Principles and application. Lake Worth, Florida: Wingers Publishing, Inc. 1994; pp. 1007-29.

[31] Griffiths HJ. A handbook of veterinary parasitology: Domestic animals of North America. Minneapolis, Minnesota, USA: University of Minnesota Press 1978; pp. 23-5.

[32] Hess M, McDougald LR. Histomoniasis (Histomonosis, Blackhead Disease). DE Swayne (Ed.), 14th ed. Wiley Blackwell Press, Hoboken, NJ, USA. Diseases of poultry 2020; 1223-30.

[33] Hess M, Liebhart D, Bilic I, Ganas P. *Histomonas meleagridis*—New insights into an old pathogen. Vet Parasitol 2015; 208(1-2): 67-76.

[http://dx.doi.org/10.1016/j.vetpar.2014.12.018] [PMID: 25576442]

[34]　Hoerr FJ, Ranck FM Jr, Hastings TF. Respiratory cryptosporidiosis in turkeys. J Am Vet Med Assoc 1978; 173(12): 1591-3.
[http://dx.doi.org/10.2460/javma.1978.173.12.1591] [PMID: 748302]

[35]　Hu J, Fuller L, McDougald LR. Infection of turkeys with *Histomonas meleagridis* by the cloacal drop method. Avian Dis 2004; 48(4): 746-50.
[http://dx.doi.org/10.1637/7152] [PMID: 15666855]

[36]　Huchzermeyer FW. Avian pulmonary hypertension syndrome. IV. Increased right ventricular mass in turkeys experimentally infected with *Plasmodium durae.*. Onderstepoort J Vet Res 1988; 55(2): 107-8.
[PMID: 2969087]

[37]　Huchzermeyer FW. Pathogenicity and chemotherapy of *Plasmodium durae* in experimentally infected domestic turkeys. Onderstepoort J Vet Res 1993; 60(2): 103-10.
[PMID: 8332320]

[38]　Huff CG, Coulston F. The development of *Plasmodium gallinaceum* from sporozoite to erythrocytic trophozoite. J Infect Dis 1944; 75(3): 231-49.
[http://dx.doi.org/10.1093/infdis/75.3.231]

[39]　Jeffers T. Tyzzer to tomorrow: control of avian coccidiosis into the next millenium. In: Shirley MW, Tomley FM, Freeman BM, Eds. Proceedings of 7th International Coccidiosis Conference. 16.

[40]　Johnson J, Reid WM. Anticoccidial drugs: Lesion scoring techniques in battery and floor-pen experiments with chickens. Exp Parasitol 1970; 28(1): 30-6.
[http://dx.doi.org/10.1016/0014-4894(70)90063-9] [PMID: 5459870]

[41]　Kreier JP, Ed. Parasitic Protozoa. New York: Academic Press 1978; 2: pp. 2-138.

[42]　Lal K, Bromley E, Oakes R, *et al.* Proteomic comparison of four *Eimeria tenella* life-cycle stages: Unsporulated oocyst, sporulated oocyst, sporozoite and second-generation merozoite. Proteomics 2009; 9(19): 4566-76.
[http://dx.doi.org/10.1002/pmic.200900305] [PMID: 19795439]

[43]　Pattison M, McMullin P, Bradbury JM, Alexander D. Parasitic diseases: Coccidiosis. Poultry Diseases. Elsevier Limited, Elsevier's Health Sciences Rights Department, 1600 John F. Kennedy Boulevard, Philadelphia. 2007; pp. 444-56.

[44]　Levine ND, Campbell GR. A check-list of the species of the genus *Haemoproteus* (Apicomplexa, Plasmodiidae). J Protozool 1971; 18(3): 475-84.
[http://dx.doi.org/10.1111/j.1550-7408.1971.tb03358.x] [PMID: 5002336]

[45]　Levine ND. The Taxonomy of *Sarcocystis* (Protozoa, Apicomplexa) Species. J Parasitol 1986; 72(3): 372-82.
[http://dx.doi.org/10.2307/3281676] [PMID: 3091802]

[46]　Levine ND. Veterinary Protozoology. Ames, IA: Iowa State University Press 1985.

[47]　Permin Aand Hansen JW. FAO Animal Health Manual No. 4, Epidemiology, diagnosis and control of poultry parasites. Food and Agriculture Organization of The United Nations. Viale delle Terme di Caracalla,Rome, Italy 1998; p. 160.

[48]　Lindsay DS, Blagburn BL. Cryptosporidium. In: Atkinson CT, Thomas NJ, Hunter DB, Eds. Parasitic diseases of wild birds. State Avenue, Iowa, USA: Blackwell Publishing 2008; pp. 195-203.
[http://dx.doi.org/10.1002/9780813804620.ch10]

[49]　Lollis L, Gerhold R, McDougald L, Beckstead R. Molecular characterization of *Histomonas meleagridis* and other parabasalids in the United States using the 5.8S, ITS-1, and ITS-2 rRNA regions. J Parasitol 2011; 97(4): 610-5.
[http://dx.doi.org/10.1645/GE-2648.1] [PMID: 21506848]

[50]　McDougald LR, Hu J. Blackhead disease (*Histomonas meleagridis*) aggravated in broiler chickens by

concurrent infection with cecal coccidiosis (*Eimeria tenella*). Avian Dis 2001; 45(2): 307-12.
[http://dx.doi.org/10.2307/1592969] [PMID: 11417809]

[51]    McDougald LR. Blackhead disease (histomoniasis) in poultry: a critical review. Avian Dis 2005; 49(4): 462-76.
[http://dx.doi.org/10.1637/7420-081005R.1] [PMID: 16404985]

[52]    McDougald LR. Cryptosporidiosis. Diseases of poultry. DE Swayne (Ed.), 14$^{th}$ ed. Wiley Blackwell Press, Hoboken, NJ, USA 2020; 14: pp. 1217-22.

[53]    Kumar S, Garg R, Ram H, Maurya PS, Banerjee PS. Gastrointestinal parasitic infections in chickens of upper gangetic plains of India with special reference to poultry coccidiosis. J Parasit Dis. 2015 Mar;39(1):22-6
[http://dx.doi.org/10.1007/s12639-013-0273-x]

[54]    Morgan UM, Monis PT, Xiao L, *et al.* Molecular and phylogenetic characterisation of Cryptosporidium from birds. Int J Parasitol 2001; 31(3): 289-96.
[http://dx.doi.org/10.1016/S0020-7519(00)00164-8] [PMID: 11226456]

[55]    Morii T, Nakamura K, Lee YC, Iijima T, Hoji K. Observations on the Taiwanese strain of *Leucocytozoon caulleryi* (Haemosporina) in chickens. J Protozool 1986; 33(2): 231-4.
[http://dx.doi.org/10.1111/j.1550-7408.1986.tb05597.x] [PMID: 3090239]

[56]    Quiroz-Castañeda RE. Avian coccidiosis, new strategies of treatment. Farm animals diseases, recent omic trends and new strategies of treatment. London, UK: IntechOpen 2018; pp. 119-33.
[http://dx.doi.org/10.5772/intechopen.74008]

[57]    Rae M. Hemoprotozoa of Caged and Aviary Birds. Seminars in avian and exotic pet medicine. 1995; 4: pp. (3)131-7.
[http://dx.doi.org/10.1016/S1055-937X(05)80037-4]

[58]    Shivaramaiah C, Barta JR, Hernandez-Velasco X, Téllez G, Hargis BM. Coccidiosis: recent advancements in the immunobiology of *Eimeria* species, preventive measures, and the importance of vaccination as a control tool against these Apicomplexan parasites. Vet Med (Auckl) 2014; 5(5): 23-34.
[PMID: 32670843]

[59]    Ranck FM Jr, Hoerr FJ. *Cryptosporidia* in the respiratory tract of turkeys. Avian Dis 1987; 31(2): 389-91.
[http://dx.doi.org/10.2307/1590893] [PMID: 3619834]

[60]    Venkateswara Rao P, Raman M, Gomathinayagam S. Sporulation dynamics of poultry *Eimeria* oocysts in Chennai. J Parasit Dis 2015; 39(4): 689-92.
[http://dx.doi.org/10.1007/s12639-013-0403-5] [PMID: 26688635]

[61]    Reid AJ, Blake DP, Ansari HR, *et al.* Genomic analysis of the causative agents of coccidiosis in domestic chickens. Genome Res 2014; 24(10): 1676-85.
[http://dx.doi.org/10.1101/gr.168955.113] [PMID: 25015382]

[62]    Ruff MD. Important parasites in poultry production systems. Vet Parasitol 1999; 84(3-4): 337-47.
[http://dx.doi.org/10.1016/S0304-4017(99)00076-X] [PMID: 10456422]

[63]    Soulsby EJL. Helminths, arthropods, and protozoa of domesticated animals. 7$^{th}$ ed. Bailliere Tindall. Greycoat Place, London: Bailliere Tindall 1982; p. 809.

[64]    Sréter T, Széll Z, Varga I. Anticryptosporidial prophylactic efficacy of enrofloxacin and paromomycin in chickens. J Parasitol 2002; 88(1): 209-11.
[http://dx.doi.org/10.1645/0022-3395(2002)088[0209:APEOEA]2.0.CO;2] [PMID: 12053972]

[65]    Sullivan TW, Grace OD, Aksoy A. Influence of level, timing and duration of ronidazole water medication on histomoniasis in turkeys. Poult Sci 1977; 56(2): 571-6.
[http://dx.doi.org/10.3382/ps.0560571] [PMID: 564505]

[66]    Swarbrick O. Hexamitiasis and an emaciation syndrome in pheasant poults: clinical aspects and differential diagnosis. Vet Rec 1990; 126(11): 265-7.
[PMID: 2327046]

[67]    Tewari AK, Maharana BR. Control of poultry coccidiosis: changing trends. J Parasit Dis 2011; 35(1): 10-7.
[http://dx.doi.org/10.1007/s12639-011-0034-7] [PMID: 22654309]

[68]    Tudor DC. Pigeon Health and Disease. Iowa: Iowa State University Press 1991.

[69]    Uzal FA, Sentíes-Cué CG, Rimoldi G, Shivaprasad HL. Non- *Clostridium perfringens* infectious agents producing necrotic enteritis-like lesions in poultry. Avian Pathol 2016; 45(3): 326-33.
[http://dx.doi.org/10.1080/03079457.2016.1159282] [PMID: 27009483]

[70]    Valkiunas GA. Avian malaria parasites and other haemosporidia. Boca Raton, New York: CRC Press 2005.

[71]    Van der Heyden N. Haemoparasites. In: Rosskopf W, Woerpel R, Eds. Diseases of cage and aviary birds. 3rd ed., Baltimore: Williams and Wilkins 1996.

[72]    van Riper C, Atkinson CT, Seed TM. Plasmodia of birds. In: Kreier JP, Ed. Parasitic Protozoa. New York: Academic Press 1994; 7: pp. 73-140.
[http://dx.doi.org/10.1016/B978-0-12-426017-7.50007-4]

[73]    Vogelnest L. Avian malaria (*Plasmodium* spp.) in blue faced parrot finches (*Erythruratrichroa*) at taronga zoo. Proceedings of the Association of Avian Veterinarians. 21-4.

[74]    Williams RB. Intercurrent coccidiosis and necrotic enteritis of chickens: rational, integrated disease management by maintenance of gut integrity. Avian Pathol 2005; 34(3): 159-80.
[http://dx.doi.org/10.1080/03079450500112195] [PMID: 16191699]

[75]    Wood AM, Smith HV. Spironucleosis (Hexamitiasis, Hexamitosis) in the ring-necked pheasant (*Phasianus colchicus*): detection of cysts and description of *Spironucleus meleagridis* in stained smears. Avian Dis 2005; 49(1): 138-43.
[http://dx.doi.org/10.1637/7250-080204R] [PMID: 15839427]

# CHAPTER 14

# Ectoparasites: Tick Infestation

**V. Gnani Charitha[1,\*], V. C. Rayulu[2] and H. Srinivas Naik[3]**

*[1] Department of Veterinary Parasitology, College of Veterinary Science, Sri Venkateswara Veterinary University, Proddatur 516360, Andhra Pradesh, India*

*[2] YSR Administrative building, Sri Venkateswara Veterinary University, Tirupati 517502, Andhra Pradesh, India*

*[3] Department of Veterinary Pathology, College of Veterinary Science, Sri Venkateswara Veterinary University, Proddatur 516360, Andhra Pradesh, India*

**Abstract:** Most of the domesticated birds are susceptible to a wide range of ectoparasites like flies, fleas, lice, ticks, and mites. Ectoparasites besides causing direct injuries with skin-associated lesions, irritation, and anemia act as vectors with a significant impact on the transmission of a variety of pathogens. Among ectoparasites, ticks are notorious vectors and second in line next to mosquitoes and they belong to the suborder Ixodida within the order Parasitiformes. This suborder comprises three families: hard ticks (Ixodidae), soft ticks (Argasidae), and the monotypic family Nuttalliellidae; while the family Argasidae encompasses 198 species of "soft ticks" (without scutum). Argas persicus popularly known as 'fowl tick' parasitizes domestic poultry, including chickens, ducks, and geese, and is found throughout the dry climatic zones of the world. Heavy tick infestation may lead to anemia and eventually death. Additionally, they play a role in transmitting various parasitic, bacterial, and viral diseases including leucocytozoonosis, aegyptianellosis, pasteurellosis, avian encephalomyelitis, fowl spirochaetosis, and fowl cholera.

**Keywords:** *Argas persicus*, Fowl spirochaetosis, Fowl tick, Hard ticks, Soft ticks, Tick paralysis, Tick toxicosis, Ticks.

## INTRODUCTION

Among the blood-sucking arthropods, ticks are of major public health concern as being vectors for numerous pathogens [1]. The first documented case of cattle fever (caused by *Babesia bigemina*) transmitted through the vector *Rhipicephalus microplus*, marked the beginning of a new era in the discovery of the role of ticks in transmitting some of the life-threatening diseases. Ticks are second in line next to mosquitoes in the transmission of a variety of pathogenic organism *viz.*,

---
*\* **Corresponding author V. Gnani Charitha:** Department of Veterinary Parasitology, College of Veterinary Science, Sri Venkateswara Veterinary University, Proddatur 516360, Andhra Pradesh, India; E-mail: dr.charithagnani@gmail.com

bacteria, viruses, rickettsia, and protozoa to humans, animals, and birds. In addition to their vector potentiality, ticks are important as pests causing tick paralysis, toxicosis, irritation, bite allergies, immune responses, and economic losses due to blood loss. Additionally, they can cause serious illnesses in the host by injecting proteins (Lipocalins) along with their saliva. Meanwhile, the major economic detriment to the poultry industry is ancillary effects by ectoparasite infestations with ticks, lice, and mites [1]. Heavy tick infestation may lead to anemia and eventually death. Additionally, they are known to transmit diseases such as leucocytozoonosis, Aegyptianellosis, avian encephalomyelitis, fowl cholera, and paralysis in different domestic birds [2].

*In toto*, ticks are obligate blood-sucking arthropods and nearly 850 species are known worldwide. The suborder Ixodida comprises three families: Ixodidae, Argasidae, and the monotypic family Nuttalliellidae. The family Ixodidae comprises "hard ticks," which have a protective scutum on their dorsal side. This family contains 14 genera, with *Ixodes* being the largest tick genus, estimated to include around 200 species followed by *Haemophysalis* (155 species); *Amblyomma* (102 species); *Rhipicephalus* (75 species); *Dermacentor* (30 species); *Hyalomma* (30 species) and *Boophilus* (5 species). However, the family *Argasidae* encompasses 198 species of "soft ticks" (without scutum) distributed among five genera of significance. Of these, the genus: *Ornithodorus* comprises 101 species followed by *Argas* (61 species); *Antricola* (10 species); *Otobius* (2 species), and the monospecific genus *Nothoaspis*. *Argas persicus*, first recorded by Lorenz Oken in 1818 in Mianeh, Persia initially named the parasite *Rhynochoprion persicum* which predominantly parasitizes domestic fowl such as chickens, ducks, and geese.

## GENERAL MORPHOLOGY OF TICKS

Typically body comprises the *capitulum* (Gnathosoma) and *idiosoma*. Gnathosoma has a basic capitulum on which the rostrum is lodged. The rostrum comprises four segmented paired palps, two segmented paired chelicera, and a hypostome with recurved teeth (Fig. **1**). The chelicerae cut through host tissues thus facilitating the attachment. The body without mouthparts *viz.,* idiosoma is further divided into two regions: the anterior part, which contains the legs and the genital pore, is termed the podosoma, while the posterior section is called the opisthosoma. In hard ticks belonging to the family Ixodidae, mouth parts are visible dorsally and are typically characterized by the presence of a chitinous shield or plate called 'Scutum'. However, in the family Argasidae scutum is absent hence the name soft ticks and capitulum/mouthparts are not visible dorsally due to hood-like expansion. In the soft ticks, the body is leathery and mamillated [3].

Dorsal View                                                    Ventral view

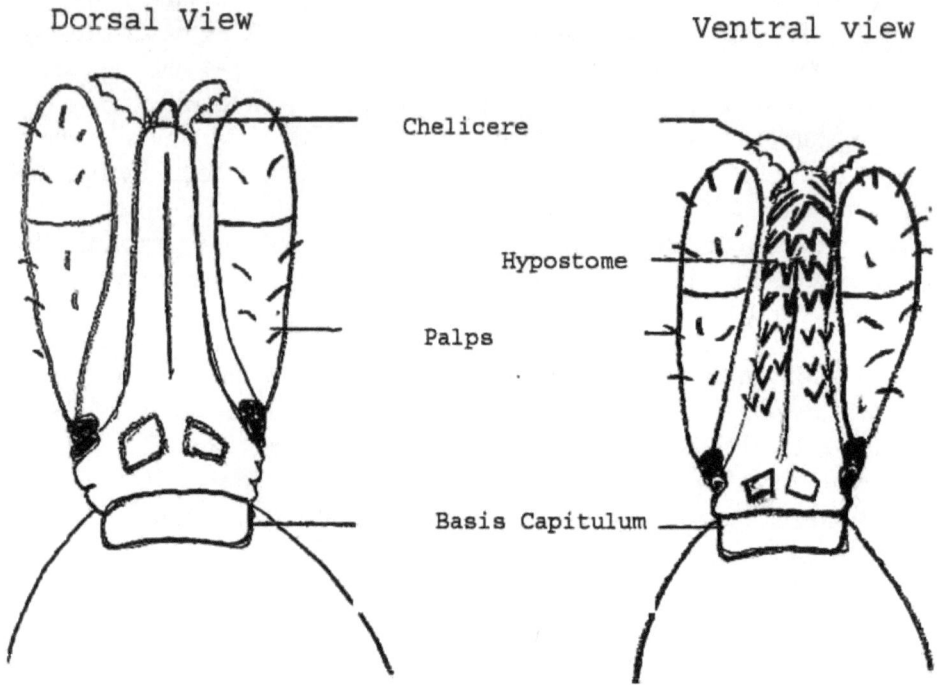

**Fig. (1).** Line diagram of gnathosoma or capitulum of ticks with dorsal and ventral views (image source: Dr. V. Gnani Charitha).

The legs are articulated with the body and consist of six segments: the coxa, trochanter, femur, patella (genu), tibia, and tarsus. Variations in the structure and arrangement of the first coxa help to distinguish several genera. Further, studying the first coxa contributes to the knowledge of tick biology, ecology, and taxonomy, which is essential for controlling tick-borne diseases and understanding their role in ecosystems. Tick larvae are easily identified by the presence of only three pairs of legs, while nymphs and adults possessing four pairs of legs. A pair of claws and a pad-like pulvillus are present on each tarsus of most hard tick species and it is absent in argasid nymphs and adults. The differences between hard ticks and soft ticks are represented in Table **1**.

The internal organs of a tick are bathed in a colorless fluid known as hemolymph. A simple heart located mid-dorsally, filters and circulates this vital body fluid. Ticks respire through paired spiracles that connect internally to the ramified tracheal system. The digestive system facilitates the complete expansion of the midgut when filled with blood. Mouthparts are internally connected to a pair of salivary glands that resemble a bund of grapes. Tick saliva contains a complex mixture of biologically active compounds that serve various functions during the feeding process. The Malpighian tubules in ticks, a pair of long, coiled structures that empty into the rectal sac play a crucial role in excretion and osmoregulation. The activity of the coxal glands can vary in response to changes in hydration levels and environmental conditions of soft ticks and removes excess watery waste taken up during blood meals. The nervous system comprises a mass of fused nerves and syn ganglions that supply to the legs, rostrum, cuticular sensilla, and internal organs. Another prominent system is the reproductive system and ticks are unisexual with male ticks having testes, vas deferentia, seminal vesicles, and ejaculatory duct. The female reproductive system in ticks is adapted to ensure successful reproduction and survival of the next generation, with features that allow for efficient egg production and fertilization with key components *viz.,* the ovary, paired oviducts, uterus, vagina, and the seminal receptacle [4].

**Table 1. Ticks and its host.**

| Family Argasidae<br>Soft Ticks | Family Ixodidae<br>Hard Ticks |
|---|---|
| Mouthparts not visible dorsally covered by hood-like body expansions | M.P visible dorsally |
| Body leathery, mammillated | Smooth |
| Scutum absent | Present, Male entire dorsum, female $1/3^{rd}$ of the dorsum |
| Festoons absent | Present |
| Eyes: Ventrolaterally placed 2 pairs. | Dorso-lateral in position, One pair |
| Spiracles: b/w $3^{rd}$ and $4^{th}$ coxae | Posterior to $4^{th}$ coxae |
| Plates/grooves: Absent | Present |
| Pulvilli: Absent | Present |
| Sexual dimorphism: Not marked | Marked |
| Feeding behaviour: Intermittent feeders | Takes a single blood meal over a period |
| Nymphal instars: Many | Only one |
| Reproduction: 200-300 eggs after each blood meal (Several batches) | The mated fully engorged female lays 10,000-20,000 eggs (Only one batch per tick) |
| Host-seeking behavior: Nidiculous | Non nidiculous, Sit-and-wait strategy |
| Life span: Long-lived Resistant to long periods of starvation | Not so long-lived, dies of starvation |

## Genus *Argas*

Soft ticks in the genus *Argas* are parasites associated mostly with birds. About 61 species have been described under this genus. Argas persicus is primarily found in the Old World, including parts of Europe, Asia, and Africa, but it can also be found in the Americas due to poultry trade. All life stages (larvae, nymphs, and adults) feed on the blood of their hosts. Populations of the tick can reach enormous numbers in poultry barns, leading to significant health issues and high mortality rates in affected birds. Most species are nocturnal and are parasites of birds, bats, reptiles, and occasionally mammals. Species are distributed worldwide and more adapted to dry and arid habitats. Significant species include the fowl tick (*Argas persicus*) and the pigeon tick (*Arags reflexus*). In the New World, the fowl tick exists as a complex of three species, which are often difficult to distinguish from one another. In the New World, the fowl tick exists as a complex of three species-*Argas radiatus*, *A. sanchezi,* and *A. miniatus*. These ticks share many morphological and behavioral characteristics, making it challenging to identify them accurately without careful examination [5].

### *Agras persicus*

It is popularly known as 'Persian Fowl Tick' or 'Chicken Tick' or 'Adobe tick' or 'Blue tick'. The morphology of *Argas persicus* is well adapted to its parasitic lifestyle, allowing it to feed effectively on its avian hosts while providing some camouflage and protection against environmental threats. Understanding these morphological features is crucial for identifying and managing infestations in poultry. The adult tick is oval in shape which allows it to hide in crevices and between the feathers of birds. Females are approximately 8-10 mm in length and males are 5 mm.

When unfed, the tick appears yellow to reddish-brown, but after engorgement, it changes to a slatey-blue color, which is why it is often referred to as the "blue tick." The body is covered with a leathery cuticle that is relatively flexible. The dorsal surface has a wrinkled appearance with numerous small, rounded projections called mammillae. These features help the tick cling to its host. The ventral surface also has a leathery texture, which aids in attachment to the host during feeding. Like all other soft ticks, it has no scutum and four segments of the palps are equal in length. Mouth parts are not visible dorsally due to hood-like projection (Fig. **2**).

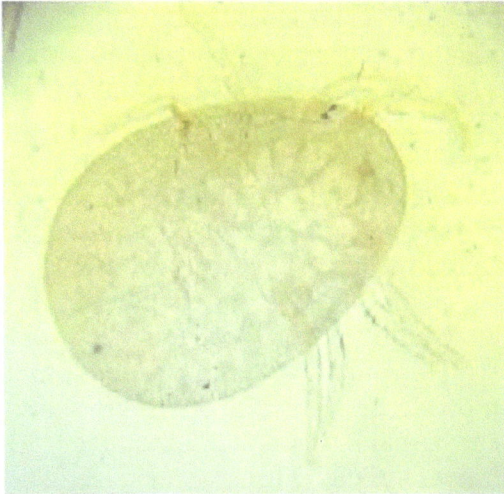

**Fig. (2).** *Argas persicus* processed an image showing ventrally placed mouth parts, oval-shaped body, and a mamillated body surface. (Image Source: Dr. V. Gnani Charitha).

## *Behaviour, Feeding and Life Cycle of Argas persicus*

Most argasid ticks are *nidicolous* or *exhibit host-seeking behavior*. They are typically found away from the host, hiding in bird nests, rock ledges, cracks, building cervices, and on the base of railings or cages (Fig. **3**). They can also live in fissures in walls or trees and can survive long periods of starvation (even up to several years) without feeding on the host.

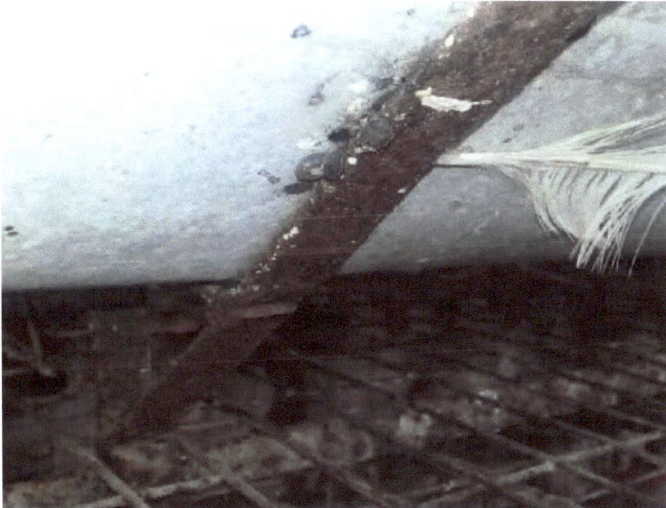

**Fig. (3).** Soft ticks (*Argas persicus*) found off the host, hiding in crates of the poultry house (Image Source: Dr. V. Gnani Charitha).

Diapause in the fowl tick is a crucial survival strategy that allows the tick to delay development or reproduction during unfavorable conditions, particularly when hosts are absent. This dormancy can occur at various life stages, including eggs, larvae, nymphs, or adults, and is triggered by environmental cues such as temperature changes, humidity levels, or the absence of a host. During this phase, physiological processes slow down, enabling the tick to conserve energy and survive for extended periods without feeding. This behavior, combined with their ability to hide in sheltered environments (nidicolous behavior) groups them as endophilic. These behavioral patterns contribute to the resilience of *Argas persicus* and complicate control measures in poultry farming. They are confined to dark environments with low humidity ensuring close proximity to food sources. Further, a combination of sensory cues like odors such as carbon dioxide emitted by the host, radiant heat, visual stimuli, and vibrations trigger the ticks to locate and identify a suitable host for feeding [6].

Ticks undergo incomplete metamorphosis/hemi-metabolism. The entire cycle can last several months to years. The multi-host life cycle of *A. persicus* is complex and involves movement between hosts in different stages. The life cycle includes the egg, larva, nymph (with multiple instars), and adult. Studies indicate that more than two nymphal instars (typically around 6 to 7) have been documented in their development. The reproductive strategy of multiple gonotrophic cycles allows the female tick to copulate only once but facilitates it to lay several batches of eggs (4 to 6) in clutches of 50 to 100 per batch/blood meal. Six-legged larvae hatch out from eggs in a span of one to four weeks and seek out a suitable host in the vicinity. They feed on the host for a few hours to days and leave the host for molting. The first nymphal instar seeks the host (either the same or a different host) and exhibits nocturnal behavior. Nymphal and adult argasid ticks have relatively short feeding duration (30 to 70 min), which allows them to minimize the risk of detection by their hosts. Usually, the life cycle is completed in 30 days under favorable conditions. The ideal temperature and humidity required for the development of *A.persicus* are 22-38°C and 70% to 80%, respectively [7].

### *Significance of Fowl Tick*

Ticks transmit an array of pathogens *viz.,* bacteria, viruses, rickettsia, and protozoans in poultry. Direct injuries associated with their attachment lead to skin abnormalities such as pain, dermatoses, inflammatory reactions, and swelling. The detrimental effects of *Argas persicus* on poultry through blood loss and mortality can have a severe economic impact on poultry farmers, leading to financial losses from reduced production, increased veterinary costs, and the need for pest control measures. It is determined that a single *A. persicus* tick can consume approximately 18.57 mg of blood in one day due to their relatively longer feeding time (> 4 days) before molting to a nymphal stage [6]. In addition, the physical stress of the infested bird with persistent bites; pressure to compensate for the blood loss by boosting erythropoiesis, and the time spent on removing the parasites by self-grooming end up in reduced feed consumption, poor appetite, and depression [5].

*Argas persicus* serves as a natural reservoir for *Borrelia anserina*, a spirochete that can cause avian spirochetosis in birds. Other associated bacteria include those of the genus *Salmonella, Aerobacter, Escherichia, Proteus, Staphylococcus, Flavobacterium, Bacillus, Pseudomonas,* and *Streptococcus* [4]. Avian spirochetosis is a highly fatal disease of turkeys and the affected birds develop signs of high fever, severe greenish diarrhea, and dehydration. Infected birds may show a lack of interest in feeding, leading to weight loss, depression, and pale cyanotic combs. Neurological signs may occur in some cases, such as incoordination or difficulty walking, and paralysis of the legs and wings, although this is less common. In severe cases, particularly among young or immunocompromised birds, the disease can lead to high mortality rates. Before death, the birds tend to become recumbent or stretched out. Birds that survive the above phase will develop a long-lasting immunity.

Although *A. persicus* is not the primary vector for Infectious Bursal Disease (IBD), its role as a blood-feeding ectoparasite may contribute to the epidemiology of the disease. Especially fowl tick larvae can potentially harbor the virus for a period and may transmit it to other birds during subsequent feedings [3]. Moreover, there is a higher risk for co-infections, as the stress from tick feeding can further weaken the immune system of birds already compromised by IBD.

Adding to the complications, the saliva of feeding ticks contains neurotoxins that can interfere with nerve function, leading to paralysis. The signs typically depend on the duration of tick feeding and the number of ticks involved. Common symptoms include weakness, lethargy, and ataxia. As paralysis progresses, birds may experience difficulty standing or moving. In severe instances, it can lead to difficulty breathing due to paralysis of respiratory muscles. Death then follows. Heavy infection in ducks leads to range paralysis.

The public health significance of fowl ticks extends beyond their direct impact on poultry. They play a potential role in disease transmission where the accidental bites lead to localized reactions such as itching, inflammation, and discomfort. In some cases, secondary infections may incidentally be transmitted to humans *viz.,* West Nile Virus [2].

## Control and Management

In summary, *A. persicus* infestation causes serious health problems in chickens. In addition to viral and bacterial diseases caused by fowl ticks, anemia could be the most direct health risk associated with tick infestation. The effective control and management of *A. persicus* require a multifaceted approach that includes monitoring, environmental management, biological control, chemical treatments, and education. By implementing these strategies, poultry producers can reduce tick infestations, improve the health of their flocks, and minimize economic losses associated with fowl ticks. Regular evaluation and adaptation of control measures are essential for sustained success.

The following are key strategies for managing fowl tick infestations:

## Monitoring and Surveillance

Conduct frequent checks for ticks on birds and in their environment. Inspect nesting areas, cracks, and crevices in poultry houses where ticks are likely to hide. Maintain records of tick sightings and infestations to track patterns and identify problem areas.

## Environmental Management

Keep poultry housing clean and free from debris where ticks can thrive. Regularly remove organic matter, such as feathers and waste, to reduce tick habitats. Reduce tick habitats around poultry facilities by clearing brush, tall grass, and other vegetation where ticks may reside. Replace or regularly clean nesting materials to minimize populations in the areas.

## Biological Control

Introduce natural predators of ticks, such as certain birds (*e.g*: guineafowl) that may help reduce tick populations in the environment.

## Chemical Control

Apply acaricides as sprays or dips on infested birds, being mindful of withdrawal periods before slaughter or egg production to comply with food safety regulations. Apply residual acaricides in the poultry house, particularly in areas where ticks are likely to hide.

## *Integrated Pest Management (IPM)*

Implement an IPM approach that combines monitoring, sanitation, biological controls, and targeted use of acaricides to effectively manage tick populations. Regularly assess the effectiveness of control measures and make adjustments as needed to ensure continued success. Educate poultry producers about the life cycle of fowl ticks, signs of infestation, and effective control measures to empower them to manage tick populations proactively. Raise awareness among workers and the public about the importance of tick management in poultry farming and the potential health risks associated with infestations.

Last but the most crucial is professional advice from veterinarians to develop tailored control programs based on specific conditions and challenges in poultry operations.

## CONCLUDING REMARKS

In summary, ectoparasites infestation causes serious health problems in chickens. In addition to viral and bacterial diseases caused by fowl ticks, anemia could be the most direct health risk associated with tick infestation.

## REFERENCES

[1]    Estrada-Peña A, Venzal JM, González-Acuña D, Guglielmone AA. *Argas (Persicargas) keiransi* n. sp. (Acari: Argasidae), a parasite of the Chimango, *Milvago* c. chimango (Aves: Falconiformes) in Chile. J Med Entomol 2003; 40(6): 766-9.
       [http://dx.doi.org/10.1603/0022-2585-40.6.766] [PMID: 14765651]

[2]    Lisbôa RS, Teixeira RC, Rangel CP, Santos HA, Massard CL, Fonseca AH. Avian spirochetosis in chickens following experimental transmission of Borrelia anserina by *Argas (Persicargas) miniatus*. Avian Dis 2009; 53(2): 166-8.
       [http://dx.doi.org/10.1637/8377-061508-Reg.1] [PMID: 19630219]

[3]    Hobbenaghi R, Tavassoli M, Allymehr M, Nasiry S, Pashaie B. Pathological study of experimentally induced tick bitten (*Argas persicus*) in poultry skin. Iran J Vet Sci Technol 2016; 7(2): 1-8.

[4]    Khan MN, Khan LA, Mahmood S, Qudoos A. *Argas persicus* infestation: prevalence and economic significance in poultry. Pak J Agric Sci 2001; 38: 32-4.

[5]    Kilpinen O, Roepstorff A, Permin A, Nørgaard-Nielsen G, Lawson LG, Simonsen HB. Influence of *Dermanyssus gallinae* and *Ascaridia galli* infections on behaviour and health of laying hens ( *Gallus gallus domesticus* ). Br Poult Sci 2005; 46(1): 26-34.
       [http://dx.doi.org/10.1080/00071660400023839] [PMID: 15835249]

[6]    CDC- Centers for Disease Control and Prevention. Laboratory Identification of Parasitic Diseases of Public Health Concern 2016.

[7]    Rosenstein M. Paralysis in chickens caused by larvae of the poultry tick, *Argas persicus*. Avian Diseases. STOR. American Association of Avian Pathologists, Inc. 1976; 20: pp. (2)407-9.
       [http://dx.doi.org/10.2307/1589281]

# CHAPTER 15

# Ectoparasites: Fleas Infestation

**Pradeep Kumar[1,\*], Amit Kumar Jaiswal[1], Alok Kumar Singh[2], Kale Chandrakant Dinkar[1], Rupam Sachan[1] and Gaurav Kumar Verma[3]**

[1] *Department of Veterinary Parasitology, Uttar Pradesh Pandit Deen Dayal Upadhyaya Pashu Chikitsa Vigyan Vishwavidyalaya Evam Go-Anusandhan Sansthan, Mathura 281001, Uttar Pradesh, India*

[2] *Department of Veterinary Parasitology, College of Veterinary Science & Animal Husbandry, Kuthuliya, Rewa 486001, Madhya Pradesh, India*

[3] *COVSc & AH, Uttar Pradesh Pandit Deen Dayal Upadhyaya pashu Chikitsa Vigyan Vishwavidyalaya Evam Go Anusandhan Sansthan (DUVASU), Mathura 281001, Uttar Pradesh, India*

**Abstract:** The most overlooked ectoparasites in the Siphonaptera order are poultry fleas. An estimated USD 2.8 billion is lost economically each year in America alone as a result of flea infestations in various animal species. These are ectoparasites with hopping legs that have been laterally flattened. The main reason fleas bother their hosts is because they itch, which prompts the host to attempt to get rid of the pest by biting, pecking, or scratching. At the location of each bite, a slightly elevated, swollen, and itchy nodule with a single puncture point in the center, resembling a mosquito bite, forms on the epidermis. This can result in flea allergic dermatitis, an eczematous, itchy skin condition that affects numerous host species, including poultry. The bites might itch and become inflamed for a few weeks after they occur, and they frequently occur in groups or rows of two bites. In severe circumstances, they might also result in anemia. The fully mature flea has a thin and flat body that enables it to fit through the feathers of its host. It is usually brown in color and grows to a length of 3 millimeters (1/8 inch). The wings are absent and their posterior legs are mainly adapted for jumping. Their claws keep them immobile, while their mouthparts are intended for piercing flesh and drawing blood. The present chapter discusses the different fleas of poultry life cycle and control measures.

**Keywords:** *Ceratophyllus, Echidnophaga,* Ectoparasite, Flea, Poultry, Siphonaptera.

\* **Corresponding author Pradeep Kumar:** Department of Veterinary Parasitology, Uttar Pradesh Pandit Deen Dayal Upadhyaya Pashu Chikitsa Vigyan Vishwavidyalaya Evam Go-Anusandhan Sansthan, Mathura 281001, Uttar Pradesh, India; E-mail: drpkdiwakar@gmail.com

## INTRODUCTION

The flea is a special pest of poultry, as well as other birds and mammals. In case of poultry, these fleas are seen in groups around the comb, eyes, wattles, and other exposed areas. On the basis of external morphologically, they have their heads embedded in the host's body and cannot be removed by any object. In the poultry industry, chickens are known as naturally resilient and generally free from diseases [1 - 4]. Once the birds are attacked by fleas, they become inactive, which decreases production in poultry farms. Fleas are categorized as the class Insecta, order Siphonaptera, which is derived from the Greek word Siphon apteron, which means the sucking wingless insects. There are so many species present on earth, most of them are present in mammals and few are found in poultry [5 - 7]. These are temporary parasites that are wingless, laterally compressed bodies and have three pairs of legs. They have three pairs of legs; the third pair is designed for jumping on and off of its host. Resilin, a rubber-like elastic protein found on the body, aids in the flea's ability to leap from one location to another. A flea can jump up to 18 cm vertically and 33 cm horizontally [8 - 10].

## MORPHOLOGY

The flea's head and thorax area have numerous protruding spines known as combs or ctenidia. Genal combs, which are also known as genal ctenidium, are found on the head region, whereas pronotal combs, which are also known as pronotal ctenidium, are found on the posterior boundary of the first thoracic segment. These unique features both facilitate quick passage through the host's hairs and prevent detachment from the host hairs. Additionally, fleas have a large number of robust setae that shield them from the impacts of host grooming [12 - 14]. The sexes, male and female, are found apart, and when feeding, the maxillary laciniae pierce and cut the host's skin. The elongated epipharynx enters the blood vessel. The laciniae release saliva, yet this saliva does not enter the blood vessel. Only adults have sucking mouth parts. Mouthparts form short proboscis and are modified for piercing and sucking the body fluids of their hosts. The abdomen has ten segments [15, 16]. The ninth abdominal segment of both sexes has a dorsal sensory plate on its tergum, which is called sensillum or pygidium covered with sensory setae like that of a pin cushion. The function of this body part is still unknown. In males, the tergum of the ninth segment is modified to form the claspers that hold the female during copulation. The chitinous penis, which is also known as aedeagus, projects between the claspers and the sternum of the ninth segment.

## LIFE CYCLE

Once the female has finished her blood meal, she lays her eggs on the host's body. The female flea generally lays about 3 to 18 eggs at a time and usually, between two and six months, up to twenty eggs can be laid at a time; however, occasionally, hundreds of eggs can be laid; most of which fall to the ground a few hours after drying. The eggs are oval about 5 mm long, white and glistening, and rounded at the ends [18 - 20]. The egg hatches in a few days, but it could take up to three weeks depending on the environmental conditions. Both temperature and humidity affect the hatching phenomenon. The larvae may hatch in 2-16 days after laying of the eggs. The young larvae are active, without legs, yellowish-white, elongate, slender, maggot-like, and hiding from light [21 - 24]. Larvae consist of three thoracic and ten abdominal segments, each of which bears a few long hairs. The last abdominal segment bear two hooked processes called the anal struts, which are used for holding on the substrate or for locomotion. The head is more strongly chitinised than the rest of the body. It bears two short antennae; each of which consists of two segments.

Mouth parts of larvae are masticatory types with a pair of mandibles, a pair of first maxillae, and a labium formed by the second pair of maxillae. The larvae eat little food like organic matter, dry blood, and parts of faces [25]. The fully developed larvae need moderate moisture. About seven to ten days or sometimes more in unfavorable conditions, the larvae grow and molt two times and become opaque white. Now it converts into mature maggots and the size becomes about 6 mm long. After a few days, it becomes quiescent and spins a whitish cocoon of about 4 mm x 2 mm inside which it pupates [26]. The cocoon is loosely spun and the free pupa can be seen inside it very easily. The pupal stage runs for a variable period from ten days to about one year as per condition which is present externally. In favorable conditions, the whole life cycle takes place in about 20 days. Once an adult flea develops, it may survive for a very long time without food. They use scents to find the right host, and light, shadow, and temperature cues help them find it. They are able to harbor both the bubonic plague and the tapeworm cysticercoids stage of the disease [27].

There are several genera of flea that infect poultry as well as mammals which are as follows: *Echidnophaga gallinacea* (Fig. **1**); *Ceratophyllus gallinae* (Fig. **2**); *Ceratophyllus garei* (Fig. **3**); *Ceratophyllus niger* (western chicken flea) found in poultry. *Ctenocephalides felis* (cat flea); *Ctenocephalides canis* (dog flea); *Hoplopsyllus anomalus*; *Pulex simulans*; *Xenopsylla cheopis* (rat flea); *Diamanus montanus*; *Nosopsyllus fasciatus* and *Tunga penetrans* are found in mammals. The simple connection between the nesting habitat and many Ceratophyllidae groups is exemplified by the adults' frequent movement between hosts and nests and their sporadic, fleeting relationships with the hosts. However, several Pulicidae species show continuous adult relationships with their hosts. Still, there might be a great deal of variation even within these broad categories. Only a small number of genera continue to be related as adults. These are the "stickfast," or burrowing fleas, the females of which are embedded in skin nodules. These fleas only have a surface-communicating area on their backs, which permits the eggs or larvae to drop to the ground and grow normally [28].

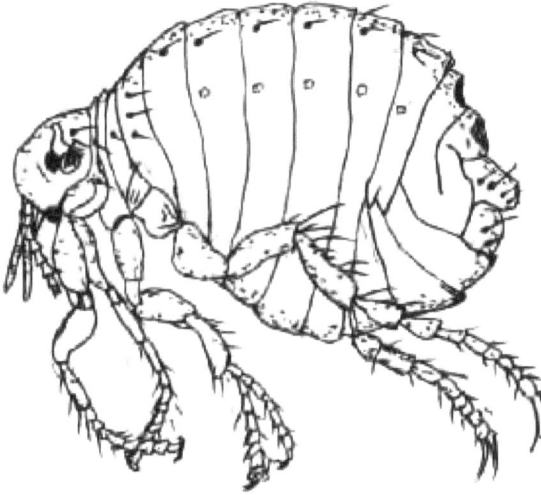

**Fig. (1).** *Echidnophaga gallinacea.*

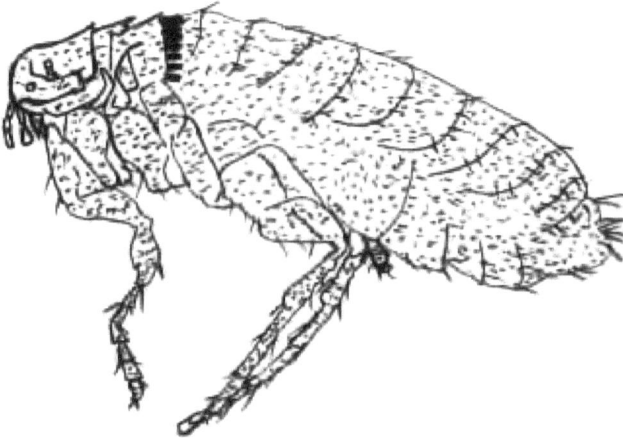

**Fig. (2).** *Ceratophyllus gallinae.*

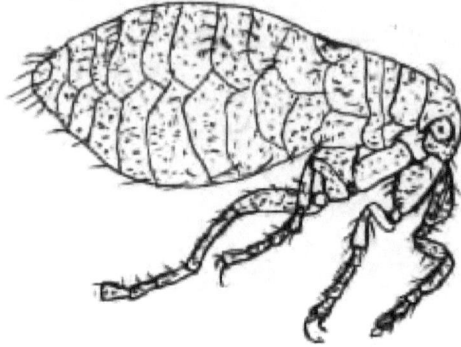

**Fig. (3).** *Ceratophyllus* species.

There are about 239 genera and around 16 families of fleas available on earth; the only families having species of substantial veterinary interest are the Ceratophyllidae and Pulicidae families. The Ceratophyllidae family is thought to have more than 500 species, of which 80 are thought to be avian parasites and the remainder species to be other parasites [29 - 31]. In case of poultry industry, mainly three fleas namely *Echidnophaga gallinacea*; *Ceratophyllus gallinae,* and *Ceratophyllus garei* are found . Being ectoparasites, these fleas live on the skin of their hosts, which are primarily birds. It is important to keep in mind that different *Ceratophyllus* species may favor different hosts, and there may be geographical variations in their distribution. Numerous species in the *Ceratophyllus* genus are specialized to specific hosts and environmental factors. Even though several *Ceratophyllus* fleas have been studied in great detail, there can still be unidentified species. Since fleas have a complex biology and ecology, they can have a significant impact on the health of the animals they inhabit. *Ceratophyllus* is the name of a genus of fleas that belong to the Ceratophyllidae family [32].

Flea infestations can be problematic because some fleas can transmit diseases to humans in addition to the afflicted animals. The Holarctic region is home to the majority of the family's species. Despite the fact that the taxonomic classification of these groups is predicated on a variety of morphological characteristics that, while seemingly unimportant at first glance, truly represent the fundamental distinctions among the groups. The majority of characteristics used for classification at the family or generic level include the morphology of the head and thorax, the arrangement of the combs, the modifications made to the female and male reproductive organs, the general chaetotaxy (bristle arrangement), and other characteristics [33].

A significant proportion of flea species rely on birds as their primary hosts. They can be found in many different kinds of birds, such as songbirds and ducks. These parasites can pose serious problems for birds that breed as well as the young that they raise. All fleas are parasitic and voracious blood eaters. With special mouthparts, they pierce the skin of their hosts to feed on their blood. This eating behavior could be the cause of the hosts' discomfort and health issues. It is well known that fleas, particularly those belonging to the *Echidnophaga* genus, can transmit illness [34]. They can transfer diseases like viruses or parasites from one host to another by way of their eating habits. Fleas have historically played a role in the spread of diseases like the bubonic plague.

## PATHOGENIC EFFECTS OF FLEAS

Among the flea species that feed on both humans and animals are the sticktight flea (*Echidnophaga gallinacea*) and the jigger, or chigoe, flea (*Tunga penetrans*). Parasites that can infest chickens include the European chicken flea (*Ceratophyllus gallinae*) and the American western chicken flea (*Ceratophyllus niger*). Sometimes fleas that feed mostly on birds will attack people, especially if their usual host is absent. Flea infestations can cause unbearable itching and serious skin irritation. Although many animals gain partial immunity following numerous or repetitive assaults, exposure to certain substances can occasionally cause sensitization and allergy development in individuals, notably in humans.

In general, the fleas cause great irritation to their host, sometimes more than other ectoparasites like lice and ticks. The majority of poultry with their infestation are those that are unhealthy or afflicted with a persistent illness that makes their lives difficult. The infested animals become restless, lose their condition, and spoil their coats by biting and scratching [35]. The flea bite site develops a region of ischaemia with surrounding wheal. In hypersensitive birds, this lesion may become flea dermatitis and last for several days.

The females of fleas generally *Echidnophaga gallinacea* mainly attach with comb, wattles, and around the eyes of birds. Generally, young birds are quickly killed by these dangerous fleas while in heavy infestation, adult fleas also die. Adult flea penetrates the skin and causes swelling and may ulcerate where the flea lays its eggs [36].

## TREATMENT AND CONTROL OF FLEAS

The best way to control fleas is to keep all areas used by farm animals occupied and, to the greatest extent feasible, clear of dust, litter, and waste. An all-encompassing strategy is needed to control fleas in birds. Treatment of the bird's host and environment should occur simultaneously. Insecticides should be applied to the birds and their surroundings per the veterinary officers' recommendations. To keep fleas under control, birds should be kept out of the contaminated area for a period of three weeks. Certain fatty or oily materials can be used to treat poultry fleas; these substances prevent mites from breathing, thereby killing them. Petroleum jelly and paraffin are two products that smallholder farmers can easily obtain. Dead fleas take several days to die off. A small number of farmers successfully apply tick grease to a chicken's head, while others employ a few drops of insecticides. Treatment of fleas can be done in two parts; first by the removal of fleas with the help of small forceps followed by the application of a topical antibiotic solution or ointment to prevent secondary bacterial infection; and second by the removal of fleas' eggs and larvae from the bedding of chicken environment by complete replacement of all bedding materials [37]. Nowadays, some tested drugs are available in the market like Fipronil, Permethrin, Malathion, *etc.* which may be used with the advice and supervision of a registered veterinary doctor.

## CONCLUDING REMARKS

Poultry is a major source of egg production and contributes a rich supply of protein to diets worldwide. In addition to directly causing morbidity by sucking blood and irritating the birds, some ectoparasites of poultry, such as fleas, ticks, lice, and mites, are significant contributors to the spread of certain pathogens that cause significant financial losses to the poultry industry. This has a negative impact on the poultry industry's ability to produce poultry economically. The general impact of ectoparasites on the production of farmers and the poultry industry should be made known to the community, and extension personnel should receive training on better feeding, housing, and illness prevention as well as increased productivity of the poultry industry [38 - 42]. The use of insecticides not meant for poultry is prohibited. Certain insecticides meant for yards and sheds are not meant for use on birds, and birds should not even be inside the shed while the pesticides are being applied. Insecticides may be absorbed and show up in the meat or eggs, rendering them unfit for human consumption even if the birds do not appear to be affected by them. This may be due to the birds' care or as a result of them residing in a shed or yard that has been treated. If insecticide exposure is brief, the effects will eventually wear off, returning eggs and meat to safe levels after a "withholding period."

## REFERENCES

[1]    Aksin N. Chewing lice (insecta: Phthiraptera) on mallards (*Anas platyrhynchus*) inTurkey. J Anim Vet Adv 2011; 10(13): 1656-9.
       [http://dx.doi.org/10.3923/javaa.2011.1656.1659]

[2]    American Ornithologists' Union. Check-list of North American Birds. 6th ed., Washington, D.C., USA: Am.Ornithol. Union 1983.

[3]    Baird SJE, Ribas A, Macholán M, Albrecht T, Piálek J, Goüy de Bellocq J. Where are the wormy mice? A reexamination of hybrid parasitism in the European house mouse hybrid zone. Evolution

2012; 66(9): 2757-72.
[http://dx.doi.org/10.1111/j.1558-5646.2012.01633.x] [PMID: 22946801]

[4]     Bandelt HJ, Forster P, Röhl A. Median-joining networks for inferring intraspecific phylogenies. Mol Biol Evol 1999; 16(1): 37-48.
[http://dx.doi.org/10.1093/oxfordjournals.molbev.a026036] [PMID: 10331250]

[5]     Charleston MA, Robertson DL. Preferential host switching by primate lentiviruses can account for phylogenetic similarity with the primate phylogeny. Syst Biol 2002; 51(3): 528-35.
[http://dx.doi.org/10.1080/10635150290069940] [PMID: 12079649]

[6]     Charlesworth B. Effective population size and patterns of molecular evolution and variation. Nat Rev Genet 2009; 10(3): 195-205.
[http://dx.doi.org/10.1038/nrg2526]

[7]     Clayton DH, Bush SE, Johnson KP. Ecology of congruence: past meets present. Syst Biol 2004; 53(1): 165-73.
[http://dx.doi.org/10.1080/10635150490265102] [PMID: 14965911]

[8]     Clayton DH, Bush SE, Johnson KP. Coevolution of Life on Hosts: Integrating Ecology and History. Chicago, USA: University of Chicago Press 2016.

[9]     Clayton DH, Drown DM. Critical evaluation of five methods for quantifying chewing lice (Insecta: Phthiraptera). J Parasitol 2001; 87(6): 1291-300.
[http://dx.doi.org/10.1645/0022-3395(2001)087[1291:CEOFMF]2.0.CO;2] [PMID: 11780812]

[10]    Clayton DH, Walther BA. Influence of host ecology and morphology on the diversity of Neotropical bird lice. Oikos 2001; 94(3): 455-67.
[http://dx.doi.org/10.1034/j.1600-0706.2001.940308.x]

[11]    Detwiler JT, Criscione CD. An infectious topic in reticulate evolution: introgression and hybridization in animal parasites. Genes (Basel) 2010; 1(1): 102-23.
[http://dx.doi.org/10.3390/genes1010102] [PMID: 24710013]

[12]    DiBlasi E, Johnson KP, Stringham SA, *et al.* Phoretic dispersal influences parasite population genetic structure. Mol Ecol 2018; 27(12): 2770-9.
[http://dx.doi.org/10.1111/mec.14719] [PMID: 29752753]

[13]    Eichler WD. Arthropoda. Insecta. Phthiraptera 1. Mallophaga. Bronn's Klassen and Ordnungen des Tierreichs, Leipzig. 1963; 5: p. 290.

[14]    Escalante GC, Sweet AD, McCracken KG, Gustafsson DR, Wilson RE, Johnson KP. Patterns of cryptic host specificity in duck lice based on molecular data. Med Vet Entomol 2016; 30(2): 200-8.
[http://dx.doi.org/10.1111/mve.12157] [PMID: 26753998]

[15]    Excoffier L, Lischer HL. Arlequin suite ver 3.5: a new series of programs to perform population genetics analyses under Linux and Windows. Mol Ecol Resour 2010; 10(3): 564-7.
[http://dx.doi.org/10.1111/j.1755-0998.2010.02847.x] [PMID: 21565059]

[16]    Folmer O, Black M, Hoeh W, Lutz R, Vrijenhoek R. DNA primers for amplification of mitochondrial cytochrome c oxidase subunit I from diverse metazoan invertebrates. Mol Mar Biol Biotechnol 1994; 3(5): 294-9.
[PMID: 7881515]

[17]    Fritz RS, Nichols-Orians CM, Brunsfeld SJ. Interspecific hybridization of plants and resistance to herbivores: hypotheses, genetics, and variable responses in a diverse herbivore community. Oecologia 1994; 97(1): 106-17.
[http://dx.doi.org/10.1007/BF00317914] [PMID: 28313595]

[18]    Galloway TD, Lamb RJ. Abundance of chewing lice (Phthiraptera: Amblycera and Ischnocera) increases with the body size of their host woodpeckers and sapsuckers (Aves: Piciformes: Picidae). Can Entomol 2017; 149(4): 473-81.
[http://dx.doi.org/10.4039/tce.2017.18]

[19]    Gao JF, Hou MR, Cui YC, Wang LK, Wang CR. The complete mitochondrial genome sequence of *Drepanidotaenia lanceolata* (Cyclophyllidea: Hymenolepididae). Mitochondrial DNA A DNA Mapp Seq Anal 2017; 28(3): 317-8.
[http://dx.doi.org/10.3109/19401736.2015.1122762] [PMID: 26714065]

[20]    Gardner W, Mulvey EP, Shaw EC. Regression analyses of counts and rates: Poisson, overdispersed Poisson, and negative binomial models. Psychol Bull 1995; 118(3): 392-404.
[http://dx.doi.org/10.1037/0033-2909.118.3.392] [PMID: 7501743]

[21]    Gillespie GD. Hybridization, introgression and morphometric differentiation between mallard (*Anas platyrhynchos*) and grey duck (*Anas superciliosa*) in Otago, New Zealand. Auk 1985; 102(3): 459-69.
[http://dx.doi.org/10.1093/auk/102.3.459]

[22]    Green J, Wallis G, Williams M. Determining the extent of grey duck x mallard hybridisation in New Zealand. Wellington, New Zealand: Department of Conservation 2003.

[23]    Grossi AA, Sharanowski BJ, Galloway TD. *Anatoecus* species (Phthiraptera: Philopteridae) from Anseriformes in North America and taxonomic status of *Anatoecus dentatus and Anatoecus icterodes*. Can Entomol 2014; 146(6): 598-608.
[http://dx.doi.org/10.4039/tce.2014.12]

[24]    Guay P-J, Williams M, Robinson RW. Lingering genetic evidence of North American mallards (Anas platyrhynchos) introduced to New Zealand. N Z J Ecol 2015; 39: 103-9.

[25]    Hafner MS, Sudman PD, Villablanca FX, Spradling TA, Demastes JW, Nadler SA. Disparate rates of molecular evolution in cospeciating hosts and parasites. Science 1994; 265(5175): 1087-90.
[http://dx.doi.org/10.1126/science.8066445] [PMID: 8066445]

[26]    Heather BD, Robertson HA, Onley DJ. The field guide to the birds of New Zealand. Auckland, New Zealand: Viking 2000; pp. 78-9.

[27]    Hoi H, Darolova A, König C, Kristofík J. The relation between colony size, breeding density and ectoparasite loads of adult European bee-eaters ( *Merops apiaster* ). Ecoscience 1998; 5(2): 156-63.
[http://dx.doi.org/10.1080/11956860.1998.11682455]

[28]    Huelsenbeck JP, Ronquist F. MRBAYES: Bayesian inference of phylogenetic trees. Bioinformatics 2001; 17(8): 754-5.
[http://dx.doi.org/10.1093/bioinformatics/17.8.754] [PMID: 11524383]

[29]    Jaiswal AK, Kumar P, Shanker D. A diagnostic manual for parasites of veterinary importance. International Books & Periodicals Supply Services. 2021; 1.

[30]    Jaiswal AK, Sudan V, Kumar P. Endoparasitic infections in Indian peacocks (*Pavo cristatus*) of Veterinary College Campus, Mathura. J Parasit Dis 2013; 37(1): 26-8.

[31]    Johnson KP, Cruickshank RH, Adams RJ, Smith VS, Page RDM, Clayton DH. Dramatically elevated rate of mitochondrial substitution in lice (Insecta: Phthiraptera). Mol Phylogenet Evol 2003; 26(2): 231-42.
[http://dx.doi.org/10.1016/S1055-7903(02)00342-1] [PMID: 12565034]

[32]    Johnson KP, McKinney F, Sorenson MD. Phylogenetic constraint on male parental care in the dabbling ducks. Proc Biol Sci 1999; 266(1421): 759-63.
[http://dx.doi.org/10.1098/rspb.1999.0702]

[33]    Johnson KP, Shreve SM, Smith VS. Repeated adaptive divergence of microhabitat specialization in avian feather lice. BMC Biol 2012; 10(1): 52.
[http://dx.doi.org/10.1186/1741-7007-10-52] [PMID: 22717002]

[34]    Kabatangb MA, Katule AM. Rural Poultry Production Systems in Tanzania. In: Sonaiya EB, Ed. Conference Proceedings. Jlelfo, Nigeria. 1999; pp. 171-6.

[35]    Kear J. The adaptive radiation of parental care in waterfowl. In: Crook JH, Ed. Social Behavior in Birds and Mammals. London: Academic Press 1970; pp. 357-92.

[36]   Kearse M, Moir R, Wilson A, *et al.* Geneious Basic: An integrated and extendable desktop software platform for the organization and analysis of sequence data. Bioinformatics 2012; 28(12): 1647-9. [http://dx.doi.org/10.1093/bioinformatics/bts199] [PMID: 22543367]

[37]   Kirby RE, Sargeant GA, Shutler D. Haldane's rule and American black duck × mallard hybridization. Can J Zool 2004; 82(11): 1827-31. [http://dx.doi.org/10.1139/z04-169]

[38]   Knox GA. The Natural History of Canterbury. Canterbury Branch of the Royal Society of New Zealand. Wellington, New Zealand: A. H. & A. W. Reed 1969.

[39]   Krasnov BR, Mouillot D, Shenbrot GI, Khokhlova IS, Poulin R. Geographical variation in host specificity of fleas (Siphonaptera) parasitic on small mammals: the influence of phylogeny and local environmental conditions. Ecography 2004; 27(6): 787-97. [http://dx.doi.org/10.1111/j.0906-7590.2004.04015.x]

[40]   Light J, Hafner MS. Phylogenetics and host associations of *Fahrenholzia* sucking lice (Phthiraptera: Anoplura). Syst Entomol 2007; 32(2): 359-70. [http://dx.doi.org/10.1111/j.1365-3113.2006.00367.x]

[41]   Lipovsky LJ. A washing method of ectoparasite recovery with particular reference to chiggers (Acarina: Trombiculidae). J Kans Entomol Soc 1951; 24: 151-6.

[42]   Long JS. Regression models for categorical and limited dependent variables. Thousand Oaks, California, USA: Sage Publications 1997.

# CHAPTER 16

# Ectoparasites: Mites Infestation

**Jayalakshmi Jaliparthi[1,*]** and **Poojasree Alli[2]**

[1] *Department of Veterinary Parasitology, SKPP AHP, S.V.V.U, Ramachandrapuram, Andhra Pradesh, India*

[2] *Department of Veterinary Parasitology, C.V.Sc, P.V.N.R.T.V.U, Rajendranagar, Hyderabad, Telangana, India*

**Abstract:** External parasites, particularly mites belonging to families such as Dermanyssidae, Macronyssidae, and Trombiculidae, pose a significant threat to poultry production worldwide. These pests, including the poultry red mite (PRM), northern fowl mite, tropical fowl mite, and turkey chigger, not only compromise the health and welfare of poultry but also lead to substantial economic losses in the industry. Understanding the biology, behavior, and effective control measures of these parasites is crucial for sustaining the productivity and profitability of poultry operations. The life cycle of poultry mites comprises five stages: larva, egg, protonymph, deutonymph, and adult, each presenting unique challenges for management. Repeated mite bites can cause hens to lose more than 3% of their blood resulting in sub-acute anemia. Additionally, *Dermanyssus gallinae*, besides causing direct injury, serves as a vector for various bacterial and viral diseases affecting birds. Chemical control strategies for mites involve the use of pesticides and essential oils, with careful consideration given to minimizing non-target effects and preventing resistance. Biological control methods utilizing entomo-pathogens like fungi and nematodes, as well as natural enemies such as *Androlaelaps casalis*, show promise but require further research for practical implementation in poultry houses.

**Keywords:** External parasites, Mites, Poultry, Production.

## INTRODUCTION

External parasites pose a significant threat to poultry production worldwide, especially mites from families such as *Dermanyssidae, Macronyssidae*, and *Trombiculidae* are among the most impacting economically. Mites are commonly spread to chickens from wild birds, as all types of birds can suffer from mites [1]. These parasites, including the poultry red mite, northern fowl mite, tropical fowl mite, and turkey chigger, not only affect the health and welfare of poultry but also

* **Corresponding author Jayalakshmi Jaliparthi:** Department of Veterinary Parasitology, SKPP AHP, S.V.V.U, Ramachandrapuram, Andhra Pradesh, India; E-mail: raghava.plr@gmail.com

**Tanmoy Rana (Ed.)**

inflict substantial financial losses on the industry. Understanding the biology, behavior, and control measures of these pests is crucial for maintaining the productivity and profitability of poultry operations (Table **1**).

**Table 1. Name of the parasites and their host.**

| Name | Common name | Hosts |
|------|-------------|-------|
| *Dermanyssus gallinae* | Poultry Red Mite, Roost mite. | Chickens, pigeons, turkeys, ducks and other birds. |
| *Ornithonyssus sylviarum* | The northern fowl mite (NFM). | Fowl, turkey, and other birds. |
| *Ornithonyssus bursa* | Tropical fowl mite. | Chicken, sparrows, pigeons, turkey, and other birds. |
| *Cnemidocoptes gallinae* | Depluming itch mite. | Chickens, pigeons, parrots and pheasants. |
| *Cnemidocoptes mutans* | Scaly leg mite. | Chickens, turkeys, pheasants, and other birds. |
| *Cnemidocoptes pilae* | Scaly face mite. | Budgerigars, and other psittacine species. |
| *Trombicula alfreddugesi* | Common chigger, and Harvest mite. | Animals, birds, and humans. |
| *Neoschongastia americana,* | Turkey chiggers. | Majorly turkey and other birds. |
| *Laminosioptes cysticola* | Fowl cyst mite. | Chickens, turkeys, and pigeons. |

## *Dermanyssus gallinae*

Kingdom: Animalia

Phylum: Arthropoda

Subphylum: Chelicerata

Class: Arachnida

Order: Acarina

Sub Order: Mesostigmata

Family: Dermanyssidae

Genus: *Dermanyssus*

**Synonyms:** Poultry Red Mite, Roost mite.

**Hosts:** Chickens, pigeons, turkeys, ducks, and other domestic and wild birds. Sometimes on humans.

**Morphology:** Adult *D. gallinae*, an obligatory hematophagous ectoparasite measuring 0.75–1 mm in length, often have greyish-white bodies that turn reddish-brown when they are engorged. They have segmented and flattened bodies, with eight well-organized legs. Their dorsal shield is truncated at the back margin and taper towards the back. The setae on the dorsal shield are smaller than those on the skin around the dorsal plate. The anus is on the posterior half of the anal plate. In both sexes, the anal plate has three pairs of setae [2]. Modified piercing-sucking mouthpart aids in the penetration of the host skin and makes blood intake easier.

**Predilection site:** Due to its nocturnal behaviour, *D. gallinae* is present on the host at night only and can be located anywhere on the skin. The mites hide throughout the day in a variety of inconspicuous places, including cardboard boxes, crevices, cracks, beneath cribs and roosts, and walls and floors. Using thigmokinesis, they usually group with larval stages in the middle, females outside, and males on top [3].

**Life Cycle:** The five life stages of this species are larva, egg, protonymph, deutonymph, and adult. During the 14 mins-1 hour mating process, which takes place off the host, the male transfers sperm in a specific sack. Females are reproductive for three weeks, and males can mate up to four times in four days [4].

Following mating, females lay 4-8 eggs per day while fasting for three days in between batches. After the third, fourth, and fifth blood meal, the majority of eggs are generated. The ideal temperature range for egg laying is between 20 and 25 °C with 70% humidity. Eggs remain viable but do not hatch at 5 °C; at 45 °C, they rapidly become dehydrated.

After 13-51 hours, eggs become larvae, which molt into protonymphs after a 24 hour fast. Before developing into deutonymphs, protonymphs consume blood; they then require another blood meal to mature into adults. The life cycle can last anywhere from 5.5 to 17 days, depending on the temperature, and the sex ratio is equal.

**Pathogenesis and Clinical Signs:** Every night, a hen that has been bitten by a mite multiple times may lose more than 3% of her blood volume leading to sub-acute anemia. Hens may potentially die from acute anemia in extreme circumstances of large infestations. In addition to causing direct injury, *Dermanyssus gallinae* acts as a vector for a number of bacterial and viral diseases that affect birds. These include *Salmonella gallinarum* and *S. enteritidis*, *Pasteurella multocida*, *Escherichia coli*, *Borrelia anserine*, *Equine encephalomyelitis viruses*, *Newcastle disease virus*, and *avian influenza A virus*.

Poultry mites serve as reservoirs for these diseases and increase the vector potential. The mite's capacity to resist fasts and live between flocks amplifies its contribution to the persistence of pathogenic pathogens on chicken farms.

Due to pain and skin irritation from repeated bites, poultry red mite infestations in production houses cause severe stress in birds. Infested households have increased noise levels, violent pecking of feathers, cannibalistic behaviour, increased intake of food and water, and an overall decline in bird health as a result of this stress. Affected chickens exhibit increased self-grooming, an indication of anxiousness.

**Diagnosis:** The mites can be seen with the unaided eye when they are engorged.

**Control**: Pesticides and essential oils are used in chemical control strategies for poultry red mites (PRM). In order to limit side effects on non-target species and prevent resistance, choosing the appropriate acaricide is essential. Although essential oils with demonstrated efficacy, such as neem oil, are restricted since they are not registered as biocide.

Utilizing entomo-pathogens like fungi and nematodes as well as natural enemies like *Androlaelaps casalis* constitutes biological control. Their actual usage in chicken homes is still being researched, though. The potential of semiochemicals and growth regulators in controlling PRM is investigated.

The use of lighting and temperature control is physical control. *D. gallinae* can be successfully controlled by heating poultry houses to 55°C in between flocks, however, there are obstacles due to cost and potential structural damage. The mites' feeding cycle is disturbed by brief, sporadic cycles of light and shade.

For physical control, inert materials such as silica, kaolin, and diatomaceous earth (DE) are utilized. By adsorbing lipids, DE, when applied as a fine-particle powder, dehydrates mites. However, at high humidity levels, their effectiveness can be restricted.

## *Ornithonyssus*

Kingdom: Animalia

Phylum: Arthropoda

Subphylum: Chelicerata

Class: Arachnida

Order: Acarina

Sub Order: Mesostigmata

Family: Dermanyssidae

Genus: *Ornithonyssus*

### *Ornithonyssus sylviarum*

**Synonyms:** The northern fowl mite (NFM).

**Hosts:** Fowl, turkey, and other birds in temperate regions.

**Morphology:** Adult mites are oval-shaped and extend to a length of 1 mm. Its dorsal plate, which is broad for two-thirds of its length and tapers to resemble a tongue in the remaining portion, sets it apart from other mites. Dorsal plate setae resemble those of *D. gallinae*. The anus is on the anterior part of the anal plate.

Symptomatic mite infestations are common in birds, with feathers seeming "dirty" from the build-up of eggs, cast skins, mite feces, and mites themselves.

**Predilection Site:** The mite is most commonly found around the vent, tail, and breast of the bird.

**Life Cycle:** The northern fowl mite life cycle was studied in detail by investigators such as Denmark [1]. Hexapod larvae are first produced from eggs, and they spend approximately a day in a rather immobile state without feeding. A non-feeding deutonymph stage comes next, which is followed by an active and blood-feeding protonymph stage. The mites become aggressive, blood-feeding adults after they molt. The full life cycle takes from 5 to 12 days. It is interesting to note that these mites may survive for 1-3 weeks without a host, with protonymphs faring better than adults. Lower humidity levels and higher temperatures have a detrimental effect on the survival of both phases.

**Pathogenesis and Clinical Lesions:** Feathers become darkened due to the defecation of significant numbers of mites. Scabbing may develop in the vent region, with reduced feed intake, decrease in body weight, decreased egg production, anaemia, and pale combs.

**Diagnosis:** Based on clinical signs and history.

Microscopical examination of mites.

**Control**: Farmers often combat northern fowl mites by spraying pesticides on birds. However, because these mites are becoming more resistant, it is becoming more difficult to successfully spray. Alternative techniques of control are becoming more and more necessary as the shift to larger cages and organic production raises concerns about the use of pesticides.

Numerous tactics are being investigated, including plant oils, entomopathogenic fungi, and natural items like garlic. There is hope for vaccine development and selective breeding for mite-resistant chickens. Traditional methods like beak trimming and grooming have drawbacks [4].

Allowing chickens to dustbathe with diatomaceous earth, which helps prevent mites, is an interesting idea. Another choice is to use low-toxicity herbicides in slow-release dust bags. Old but potent pesticide sulfur is also taken into consideration.

In integrated pest management, the economic threshold is critical because it aims to treat pests before costs surpass damage. Reducing mite counts below this critical point is essential for profitable chicken production. To put it briefly, managing mites is a challenging task that farmers are investigating through a combination of conventional and novel approaches [5].

## *Ornithonyssus bursa*

**Synonyms:** Tropical fowl mite

**Hosts:** Chicken, sparrows, pigeons, turkeys, and other birds. Zoonotic in the areas of high bird populations.

**Morphology:** Characteristic morphology; the dorsal plate is wide up to one-third of the body and suddenly tapped to form a tongue-like blunt posterior end. Anus is present at the anterior half of the anal plate (Figs. **1-4**).

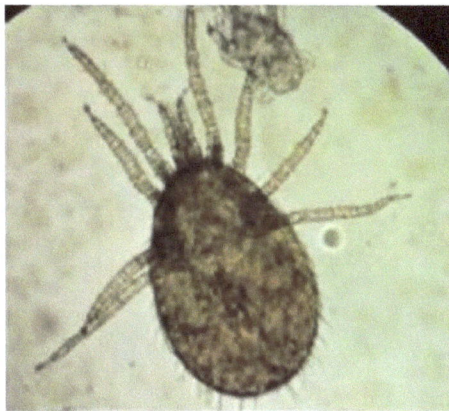

**Fig. (1).** *Ornithonyssus bursa* ventral view.

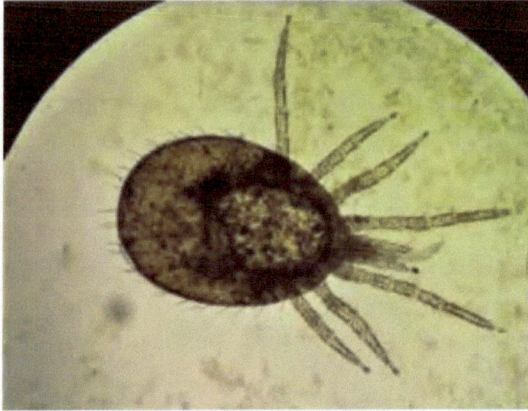

**Fig. (2).** *Ornithonyssus bursa* dorsal view.

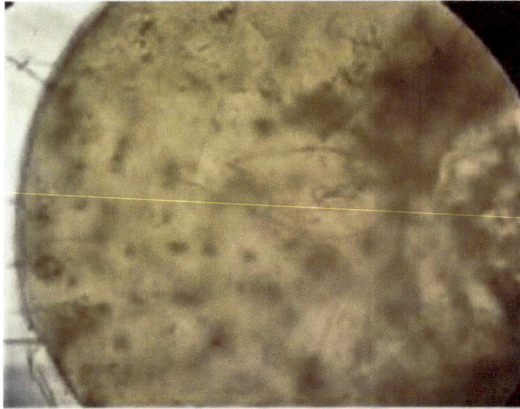

**Fig. (3).** *O.bursa* anal plate.

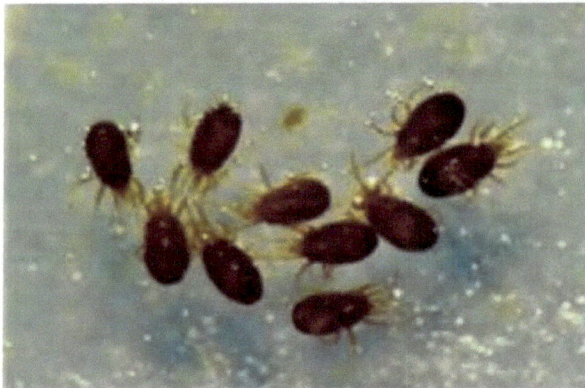

**Fig. (4).** Cluster of *O.bursa*.

## Predilection Site

Mites are found in the down feathers around the vent area, eyes, and beak of birds. They are also found in nesting materials and nest debris, roosting areas, and cracks and crevices.

**Life Cycle:** Mites deposit their eggs on the host or in the nest. Eggs hatch to non-feeding larvae within three days which molt in about 17 hours to protonymph. The protonymph is expected to molt within one or two days, while the duration of the deutonymphal stage remains uncertain. In case of the northern fowl mite, this stage typically lasts about a day. Unlike the northern fowl mite, where only the protonymph and adult stages feed on blood, both nymphs and adults of the tropical fowl mite indulge in the feeding of blood meals [5].

**Pathogenesis and Clinical signs:** Pruritis, reduction in egg production, prolonged itching, hyperkeratosis, and structural damage of feather integrity. Along with the painful bite, these mites also act as vectors in the transmission of viral, rickettsial, and protozoan infections among the birds.

## Diagnosis

• Based on clinical signs and history.
• Microscopical examination of mites.

## Control

Preventing fowl mite infestations is paramount for effective control. Measures such as excluding mite-carrying vectors like wild birds and rodents from poultry houses and ensuring proper cleanliness play a crucial role. Regular monitoring of rodent activity and implementing bait stations can help manage populations [6].

To keep wild birds and rodents out, sealing entry points such as end doors, electrical conduits, fan housings, and damaged siding is essential. Regular monitoring of bird activity is necessary to detect mite issues early on.

In breeder bird flocks, roosters often harbor more northern fowl mites than hens, facilitating their spread. Although no vaccine exists for mites, detecting infestations early can mitigate their impact. Prevention is challenging due to various potential vectors, but isolating infected farms and implementing strict protocols during egg deliveries and pullet movements can significantly reduce the risk of spreading infestations.

## *Cnemidocoptes*

Classification: Class: Arachnida

Sub Order: Sarcoptiformes

Family: Epidermoptidae

Subfamily: Knemidokoptinae

Genus: *Cnemidocoptes*

**Morphology:** The mites have a globose body with interrupted striae that create scales but no spines. From the bases of the pedipalps to the level of the legs, two longitudinal chitinized bars extend; at this point, a transverse bar unites them. The pedicels and legs are stumpy and short. Males have suckers on all the legs but, they are absent in females.

**Life Cycle:** The three-week life cycle of knemidocoptes species mites takes place on their avian hosts. The females are ovo-viviparous. Larvae have three pairs of legs while adults have four pairs of legs. Larvae molt to nymphs (two nymphal stages) and then to adults.

**Transmission:** Transmission is through direct contact with infected birds. From mother to nestling.

## *Cnemidocoptes gallinae*

**Synonyms:** Depluming mite, depluming itch mite

**Hosts:** Chickens, pigeons, parrots, and pheasants.

**Predilection Site:**  Common sites are the feathers on the head, neck, back, abdomen, and upper legs. Mites are smaller than *Cnemidocoptes mutans*. **Pathogenesis and Lesions:** Itching, inflammation, vesicle formation, serous exudation, and crust formation are among the lesions. Feathers break off readily. When the illness becomes worse, leg deformity, lameness, and finger loss are possible.

**Diagnosis:** Based on clinical signs and mites in the lesions

Microscopic examination of skin scraping

**Treatment:** Fipronil can be applied directly to the affected areas.

Ivermectin or moxidectin @ 0.2 mg/kg.

## *Cnemidocoptes mutans*

**Synonyms:** Scaly leg mite

**Hosts:** Chickens, turkeys, pheasants, and other birds.

**Predilection Site:** Primarily affects the unfeathered skin underneath the scales of legs, occasionally, the comb and wattles.

**Pathogenesis and Lesions:** Common burrowing mites cause scaly leg mange in birds that are associated with lameness and arthritis. They produce rough nodules with a powdery appearance on the legs. They cause intense irritation, resulting in affected birds pulling out their body feathers with weight loss and reduced egg production.

**Diagnosis:** Based on clinical signs and mites in the lesions

Microscopic examination of skin scraping

**Treatment:** Fipronil can be applied directly to the affected areas.

Ivermectin or moxidectin @ 0.2 mg/kg.

## *Cnemidocoptes pilae*

**Synonyms:** Scaly face mite

**Hosts:** Predominantly affects budgerigars, although it is rare in other psittacine species.

**Predilection Site:** Commonly located on the face of the birds and rarely on legs and vents.

**Pathogenesis and Lesions:** In budgerigars, characteristic symptoms include white, porous, proliferative encrustations around the corners of the mouth, cere, beak, and occasionally the periorbital area, legs, or vent. Passerine birds, such as canaries and European goldfinches, may develop crusts on their legs and digits, known as "tassel foot."

**Diagnosis:** Recovering mites from facial scrapings, although the clinical appearance is typically distinctive.

**Treatment:** Ivermectin (0.2 mg/kg, orally or intramuscularly) or Moxidectin (0.2 mg/kg, orally or topically). This treatment is usually repeated after 2 weeks to ensure effectiveness in eliminating the mite infestation.

## *Trombicula alfreddugesi*

Kingdom: Animalia

Phylum: Arthropoda

Subphylum: Chelicerata

Class: Arachnida

Order: Trombidiformes

Family: Trombiculidae

Genus: *Trombicula*

Species: *T. alfreddugesi*

**Synonyms:** Common chigger, harvest mite.

**Hosts:** Animals, birds, and humans.

**Morphology:** Adult chiggers are typically small, measuring between 1 to 2 millimeters in size. They are usually reddish in color and covered with numerous feathered hairs both on their dorsal and ventral sides, which gives them a velvety appearance [7, 8]. Each chigger possesses four pairs of legs, each ending in paired claws. The body of the chigger is distinctly constricted between the third and fourth pairs of legs, resulting in an outline resembling the shape of a figure eight. Palps and mouthparts extend in front of the body and are easily visible.

**Life Cycle:** The life cycle of chiggers involves five developmental stages: egg, deutovum, larva, nymphochrysalis, and adult. Eggs laid singly in soil hatch to deutovum which is a larva enclosed in an egg shell within 4-7 days. Deutovum emerges as a six-legged larva, which is the only parasitic stage, and feeds on the host before dropping to the ground to become inactive. Nymphs and adults feed on other arthropods. Adults are ready to deposit eggs within a week, and egg-laying continues for several weeks [9].

**Predilection Site:** Larvae of these chiggers may be found singly or in clusters on the ventral portion of birds.

**Pathogenesis and Lesions:** Birds heavily parasitized by these chiggers may show signs of droopiness, and refusal to eat, and can potentially die from starvation and exhaustion.

**Diagnosis:** Based on symptoms and lesions.

Microscopic identification of mites.

**Treatment:** Controlling chigger infestations on the range can be aided by practices such as keeping the grass cut short and using acaricides for dusting.

## *Neoschongastia americana*

**Synonyms:** Turkey chiggers.

**Hosts:** Majorly turkey and other birds.

**Morphology**. This is similar to other chigger mites. Turkey chiggers are relatively small, typically measuring between 1 to 2 millimeters in size. The life cycle is similar to other chigger mites.

**Pathogenesis and Lesions:** These chiggers feed in groups, with as many as 100 mites per lesion over a period of 8 to 15 days. Turkeys may develop 25 to 30 lesions each, with even a single lesion measuring 3 mm in diameter causing significant downgrading at market time [10].

**Treatment and Control:** The use of acaricidal sprays or dusts is common for combating turkey chigger infestations. Furthermore, a preventive strategy gaining popularity in turkey farming regions involves transitioning from free-range to confined rearing or providing sheltered sheds to protect turkeys from chigger infestations. These practices are implemented to reduce the adverse effects of chigger infestations on turkeys and maintain their quality for market purposes.

## *Laminosioptes cysticola*

**Synonyms:** Fowl cyst mite

**Hosts:** Chickens, turkeys, and pigeons

**Pathogenesis and Lesions:** White to yellowish caseocalcareous nodules, typically measuring around 1 to 3 millimeters in diameter, in the subcutaneous tissue, muscles, lungs, and abdominal viscera of infected birds.

**Diagnosis:** Careful examination of the skin and subcutaneous tissue under a dissecting microscope often reveals the presence of these mites.

**Treatment and Control:** The most effective control method for fowl cyst mites has been to destroy the infected bird. However, ivermectin may also prove to be effective in controlling infestations of these parasites.

## *Cytodites nudus*

Family: Cytoditidae Oudemans, 1908

Genus: *Cytodites nudus*

**Synonyms:** "air sac mite"

**Hosts:** Chickens, turkeys, and pheasants.

**Morphology**: These mites are oval-shaped, creamy-colored, measure between 0.4 to 0.5 mm in diameter, and have legs with suckers but no hairs. They are transmitted *via* contaminated respiratory mucus.

**Pathogenesis and Lesions:** The birds experiencing the condition showed symptoms such as difficulty breathing, gasping for air, coughing, and lethargy [11]. Those severely affected appeared to be in a weakened nutritional state. The observed lesions comprised reddened lung areas with concentrated yellowish pus in the bronchial tubes. Additionally, the air sacs displayed a cloudy appearance and were moderately thickened [8].

**Diagnosis:** Examination of sections of the lungs undera microscope often reveals the presence of mites.

## CONCLUDING REMARKS

External parasites, especially mites, present a severe challenge to poultry production, causing both direct harm to bird health and indirect economic losses. The complex life cycle of these mites requires a comprehensive management strategy that includes chemical, biological, and environmental control measures. While pesticides and essential oils are currently used for chemical control, minimizing non-target impacts and resistance development is critical. Promising biological control methods, such as entomo-pathogens and natural enemies, offer potential long-term solutions, but further research is needed to fully integrate these methods into practical use. A well-rounded approach to mite management is essential for maintaining the health, welfare, and productivity of poultry operations globally.

# REFERENCES

[1]  Denmark HA, Cromroy HL. Tropical Fowl Mite, *Ornithonyssus bursa* (Berlese) (Arachnida: Acari: Macronyssidae). IFAS Extension 2003; 297: 1-3.

[2]  Kavitha S, Yamini SH, Nagarajan B, Latha BR, *et al.* Depluming itch in a parrot. Intas Polivet 2013; 14(2): 312-4.

[3]  Kunz SE, Price MA, Graham OH. Biology and economic importance of the chigger neoschongastia americana on Turkeys1. J Econ Entomol 1969; 62(4): 872-5.
[http://dx.doi.org/10.1093/jee/62.4.872]

[4]  McOrist S. *Cytodites nudus* infestation of chickens. Avian Pathol 1983; 12(1): 151-5.
[http://dx.doi.org/10.1080/03079458308436158] [PMID: 18766772]

[5]  Online Merck veterinary manual, Veterinary / Poultry / Ectoparasites / Mites of poultry 1983.

[6]  Lesley C. The complete guide to chicken mites: Identification. Treatment And More 2024.

[7]  Venu R, Rao PV, Surya UNS. Severe infestation of *Ornithonyssus bursa* in a commercial poultry layer farm and its successful management. J Entomol Zool Stud 2020; 8(6): 1490-2.
[http://dx.doi.org/10.22271/j.ento.2020.v8.i6t.8035]

[8]  Nevin FR. Anatomy of *Cnemidocoptes Mutans* (R. and L.), the scaly-leg mite of poultry. Ann Entomol Soc Am 1935; 28(3): 338-67.
[http://dx.doi.org/10.1093/aesa/28.3.338]

[9]  Service M. Scrub typhus mites (Trombiculidae). Medical Entomology for Students. Cambridge University Press 2008; pp. 246-53.
[http://dx.doi.org/10.1017/CBO9780511811012.023]

[10]  Soulsby EJL. Helminths, athropods and protozoa of domesticated animals. London, UK: Edn 7, Baillière Tindall 1982.

[11]  Sreedevi C, Ramesh P, Mala Kondaiah P, Lakshmi Rani N, Abhishek M. Occurrence of *Knemidokoptes mutans* and *Laminosioptes cysticola* in backyard poultry in India. J Parasit Dis 2016; 40(4): 1627-30.
[http://dx.doi.org/10.1007/s12639-015-0673-1] [PMID: 27876998]

# CHAPTER 17

# Ectoparasites: Lice Infestation

## V. Gnani Charitha[1,*] and C. Sreedevi[2]

[1] *Department of Veterinary Parasitology, College of Veterinary Science, Sri Venkateswara Veterinary University, Proddatur 516360, Andhra Pradesh, India*

[2] *Department of Veterinary Parasitology, NTR College of Veterinary Science, Sri Venkateswara Veterinary University, Gannavaram 521102, Andhra Pradesh, India*

**Abstract:** Avian lice, which belong to the order Phthiraptera, are permanent ectoparasites infesting a wide range of domesticated birds. The chewing lice/bird lice (Amblycera & Ischenocera) are wingless, flat-bodied insects characterized by biting and chewing mouthparts. They primarily feed on the skin, feathers, hair, or scales of their host animals, but sometimes they feed on blood, particularly in the Amblycera species. Lice undergo incomplete metamorphosis with the egg stage followed by three nymph instars, and the entire life cycle can take as little as 2 to 3 weeks, allowing populations to grow quickly if left untreated. Lice are primarily transmitted through close contact between hosts, such as grooming or shared bedding. Bird lice are highly host-specific and inhabit highly specialized host sites. *Menacanthus stramineus,* the chicken body louse, is considered as the most economically significant parasite of poultry farming. Less frequent infestations occur with the shaft louse (*Menopon gallinae*), the wing louse (*Lipeurus caponis*), the head louse (*Cuclotogaster heterographus*), the fluff louse (*Goniocotes gallinae*), the large chicken louse (*Goniodes gigas*), and the brown chicken louse (*Goniodes dissimilis*). Lousiness in infected birds often exhibits poor growth, weight loss, and reduced feed efficiency as their energy is diverted toward coping with the irritation and stress from lice. Bite wounds cause significant skin irritation, leading to scabs, sores, and inflammation that are further complicated by secondary infections. Chewing lice, particularly *Trinoton anserinum* act as an intermediate host for the filarial heartworm *Sarconema eurycerca* that parasitized waterfowls/ swans. Further, louse-borne diseases like fowl cholera and fowl spirochetes prevailed in flocks with heavy lice infestations. This overall view highlights the need for proper control of lice infection with the majority being still relied on chemical pesticides.

**Keywords:** Amblycera, Bird lice, Chewing lice, Control, Disease transmission, Hemimetabolous, Ischenocera.

---

* **Corresponding author V. Gnani Charitha:** Department of Veterinary Parasitology, College of Veterinary Science, Sri Venkateswara Veterinary University, Proddatur 516360, Andhra Pradesh, India;
E-mail: dr.charithagnani@gmail.com

## INTRODUCTION

Domestic and wild birds are susceptible to various ectoparasites such as flies, fleas, lice, bugs, ticks, and mites. Based on the duration of existence on the host, external parasites are classified as either temporary or permanent. Temporary ectoparasites (flies, bugs, and ticks) only engage with their host during feeding or breeding periods. Conversely, permanent parasites (lice and mites) remain on their host throughout their lifecycle. Lice belong to the Phylum Arthropoda, Class Insecta, and Order Phthiraptera. Bird lice are a group of permanent ectoparasites that have remained under-focused for many years. To date, around 5,000 described species of lice have been documented parasitizing both mammals and birds. Of these more than 70% inhabited bird hosts, reflecting the close evolutionary relationship between birds and their lice [1]. In earlier classifications, lice were divided into two separate orders: Anoplura (In Greek: 'anoplos'-unarmed; 'ura'-tail) and Mallophaga (Greek: "Mallos" - lock of wool; Phagus-eating). This distinction has been revised, and all lice are now grouped under the single-order Phthiraptera with four suborders 1. Anoplura (sucking lice); 2. Amblycera; 3. Ischnocera, and 4. Rhynchophthirina (the latter three are popularly grouped as chewing lice or biting lice) [2]. Sucking lice (Suborder: Anoplura), exclusively inhabit mammals, feeding on their blood. These small, wingless insects possess retractable mouthparts adapted for piercing and sucking. Furthermore, the Rhynchophthirina includes lice that parasitize elephants and warthogs. Avian lice, which constitute the primary focus of the present study, fall under two suborders: Amblycera and Ischnocera.

Ectoparasites present a significant health risk and constitute major obstacles in poultry production worldwide. They prompt significant negative impacts on a bird's health, welfare, and productivity. Additionally, biting lice generally takes a toll on skin health, inducing intense itching, pruritus, and abrasions or wounds. Localized alopecia with hair or feather loss, especially around the vent, breast, and neck of the birds, is quite visible. Amblyceran lice target the quills of feathers, causing extensive feather damage, while the Ischenoceran members chew the feathers, causing partial damage. Moreover, they serve as mechanical or biological vectors, transmitting numerous pathogens [3]. However, they often receive less attention compared to endoparasites and infectious diseases. The substantial economic impact of these parasites warrants a comprehensive study that encompasses accurate disease information.

## CLASSIFICATION

Recent molecular phylogenetic analyses reveal that both sucking lice (Anoplura) and chewing lice (Mallophaga) are thought to have evolved from a common, free-living ancestor within the Psocoptera (booklice and bark lice). However, few authors now acknowledge the order Psocodea, encompassing both parasitic lice and book/bark lice. Over time, as lice became more specialized for life on specific hosts, two distinct groups emerged (Anoplura and Mallophaga). This distinction has been again revised, and all lice are now grouped under the single order Phthiraptera with four suborders 1. Anoplura (sucking lice); 2. Amblycera; 3. Ischnocera, and 4. Rhynchophthirina (the latter three are popularly grouped as chewing lice or biting lice) (Fig. **1**). Price *et al.* [4] identified thousand-odd species of chewing lice that primarily parasitize the birds (87.6%). *Amblycera Suborder* has six families (Boopidae; Gyropidae; Laemobothriidae; Menoponidae; Ricinidae and Trimenoponidae) [5].

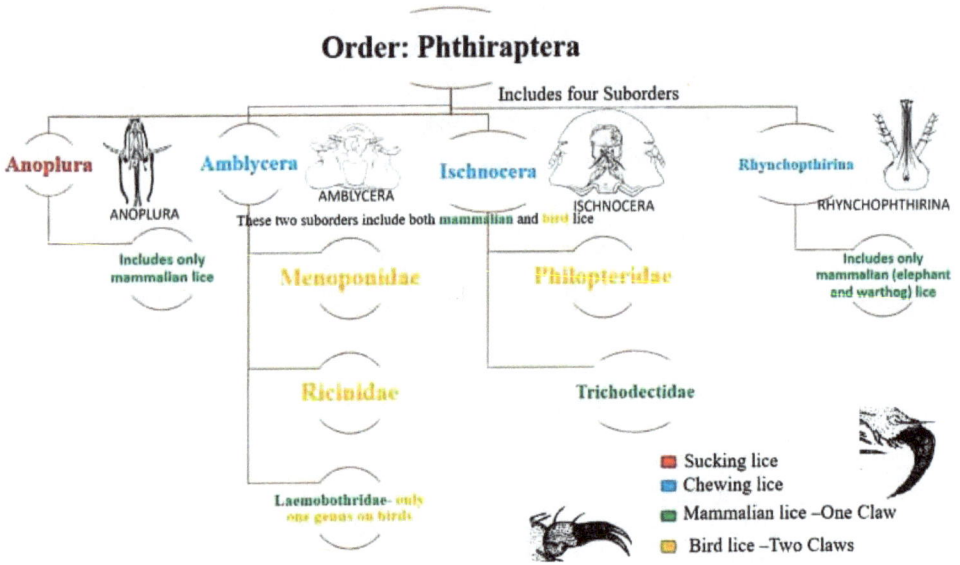

**Fig. (1).** Classification of bird lice under the order: Phthiraptera (Sourcefor Head and mouthparts Anoplura from, Ferris; 1931 Amblycera from, Bedford; 1932 Ishnocera from, Clay; 1938 Rhynchophthirina from Ferris, 1931).

*Ischnocera Suborder:* It comprises permanent, obligate ectoparasites with a cosmopolitan distribution with two main families (Trichodectidae and Philopteridae).

*Rhynchophthirina Suborder:* Only three known species are documented within the genus Haematomyzus (Family Haematomyzidae), which parasitize large mammals.

## MORPHOLOGY

The chewing lice (bird lice) are wingless, flat-bodied insects characterized by biting and chewing mouthparts and shortened front legs utilized for food transportation to the mouth. They typically measure between 1 to 5 mm (0.039 to 0.19 inches) in length with dorsoventrally flattened bodies, displaying colors ranging from white to black. The body is divided into three distinct parts: the head, the thorax, and the abdomen. Head: Compound eyes are absent without ocelli. The structures like antenna, mouthparts, and shape of the head vary depending on the suborder to which they belong. The thorax comprises jointed legs in the pro, meso, and metathorax. As a thumb rule, in all poultry lice, each leg has two tarsal claws. The elongated abdomen possesses sclerotized plates providing rigidity to the abdomen. In adults, the abdomen is 11-segmented (8 prominently visible segments and the last three telescoped) and terminates in the genitalia. The process of oviposition involves the female positioning herself on the host's hair or feathers and using her genitalia to carefully glue each egg to the substrate using secretions from her accessory glands. The abdomen is adorned with numerous setae. The male genitalia are relatively larger, and structured for efficient sperm production, storage, and transfer during copulation. The testes, vasa deferentia, seminal vesicles, and accessory glands work together to produce and store sperm, while the aedeagus serves as the primary organ for sperm delivery to the female [5].

The antennae of chewing lice in the suborders Amblycera and Ischnocera differ in both structure and significance, reflecting their distinct ecological adaptations and host interactions. Amblyceran antennae are typically short, clubbed and consist of 4-5 segments. They are located in recesses on the sides of the head, making them partially concealed. Concealing helps prevent damage from grooming by the host. Ischnocera: Antennae are longer, more filamentous, and consist of 3-5 segments. They are exposed, positioned more openly on the head, and often exhibit more mobility. This likely enhances the louse's sensory abilities, helping them navigate and feed on feather and hair debris. The Amblyceran head is typically broad and rounded, with a relatively large size compared to the rest of the body. Mandibles and maxillary palps are strongly oriented forward, aiding in anchoring to the host (Fig. **2**). Unlike other lice that often specialize in a particular host species, Amblycera can parasitize a range of host species. One of the representative species is *Menacanthus stramineus* (Chicken Body Louse): Found on chickens and other poultry, this species feeds on skin debris, feathers, and occasionally blood, causing irritation and potential harm to its host.

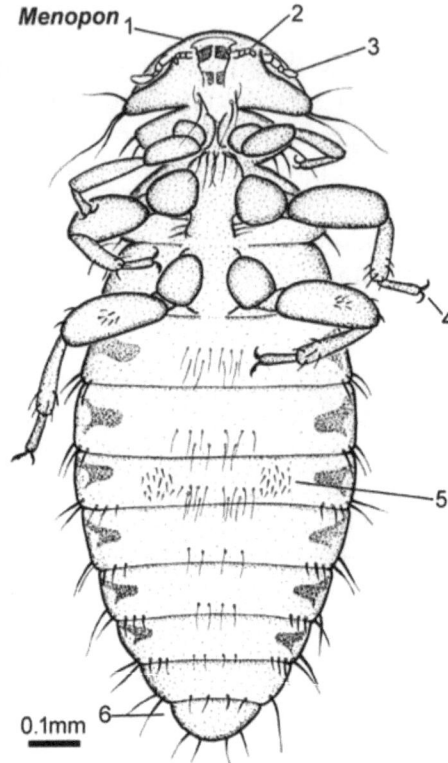

**Fig. (2).** *Menopon* female. 1- Head broad and rounded. 2-segmented palps. 3- concealed antenna in grooves. 4-Legs with two claws. 5- Abdominal segments have rows of setae. 6- The abdomen anterior broad and narrow posterior end. (*Source:*https://commons.wikimedia.org/wiki/File:Menopon_female_ventral.png).

*Lipeurus caponis (Wing Louse):* Commonly parasitizes poultry, particularly chickens and turkeys. Its presence can lead to feather damage and stress in birds.

*Trinoton anserinum:* Found on waterfowl, such as ducks and geese, this species is adapted to aquatic environments.

*Menopon gallinae:* commonly known as the Shaft Louse or Chicken Shaft Louse, is a chewing louse that parasitizes poultry, particularly chickens [6].

Ischnoceran lice have unique morphological and behavioral features that confine themselves to specific sites on the host body. They are more restricted to the concerned host species. The head is usually narrower and more elongated than in Amblycera lice. Mouthparts are adapted for feeding on keratinized material. The absence of maxillary palps distinguishes them from Amblycera (Fig. **3**). Further, they are sluggish movers and remain in specific regions on the host, making them less noticeable. Some representative species are:

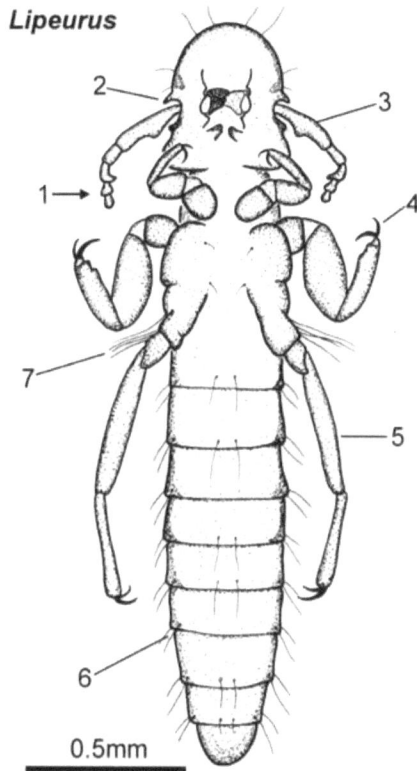

**Fig. (3).** *Lipeurus caponis* 1. Body elongate. 2. Head hemispherical in shape. 3. Antenna filiform.

• *Goniodes gigas* (Large Chicken Louse): Parasitic on chickens, this louse is often found at the base of feathers.

• *Goniocotes gallinae* (Fluff Louse): Another louse that parasitizes chickens, primarily found among the soft feathers near the bird's body.

• *Goniodes dissimilis* (Brown Chicken Louse): Found on the neck and back regions of poultry.

• *Cuclotogaster heterographus* (Head Louse): Restricted to the head of chicken.

• *Lipeurus caponis:* Wing louse of chicken

• *Anaticola anseris* and *A. crassicornis* are duck lice.

• *Columbicola columbae* (slender pigeon louse)

• *Goniocotes bidentatus* (pigeon louse)

• *Oxylipeurus polytrapzius* (slender turkey louse) and

• *Strigiphilus garylarsoni* (owl louse) [7].

• 4- Legs with two claws. 5 3$^{rd}$ pair of legs long and stout than the rest 6- Setae sparse          7-          long          setae          of          thorax (*Source:*https://commons.wikimedia.org/wiki/File:Lipeurus_male_ventral.png)

Few notable identification guides are available for chewing lice of the world [8, 9]. These publications provide information on steps to identify the species and detailed host-parasite checklists.

## LIFE CYCLE

Lice are hemimetabolous insects with no pupal stage. The entire cycle takes about 3 to 4 weeks to complete under optimal conditions, and each louse can lay several eggs during its life, contributing to rapid population growth. (Fig. **4**). Female lice attach their operculated eggs (nits) (Fig. **5**) firmly to the base of the host bird's feathers, usually close to the skin for warmth. The eggs are tiny, white, and often hard to detect. After about 4 to 7 days, the eggs hatch into nymphs. During a lifespan, the female lays about 200-300 eggs (Fig. **6**). Nymphs are immature lice, there are typically three nymphal stages (instars), and each instar molts to grow. Nymphs feed on the bird's skin, feathers, and dandruff for about 1 to 2 weeks as they mature into adults. Each nymphal instar lasts for 3-8 days. Adults remain on the host for several weeks but cannot survive without the host [10].

Host specificity aids in establishing specialized relationships with one or a few closely related poultry species [11]. Transmission or dispersal is very infrequent happening through direct contact with another bird.

## DYNAMICS AND ECOLOGY

Factors that drive the parasite prevalence, dispersal abilities, and biodiversity allow greater insights into the adaptability of lice to specific host species (Sweet and Johnson, 2016). The frequency and pathogenicity of bird lice differ among various host species and geographical locations. This diversity is associated with factors such as the health, morphology, habitat, and behavior of the host [12].

Bird-infesting chewing lice usually feed on small pieces of feathers, integumentary products, skin debris, and secretions. Some are facultative hematophagous (Ricinidae members of lice). As majority of them predominantly reside on the feathers or hair of the host, although one genus (Genus *Piagetiella*) resides in the throat pouches of pelicans and cormorants. Because of high reliance on host availability, lice have evolved robust host-attachment mechanisms: strong tibiotarsal claws (facilitating clinging to the feathers) and biting mandibles are seen as distinct holding appendages in chewing lice. However, the longtime survivability of lice without a host is quite a feat . Off-host survival is limited to 3 days to a maximum of 11 days in extreme cases. Amblycerans are seen off the host, many times crawling on bird cages or in unoccupied nests and crevices.

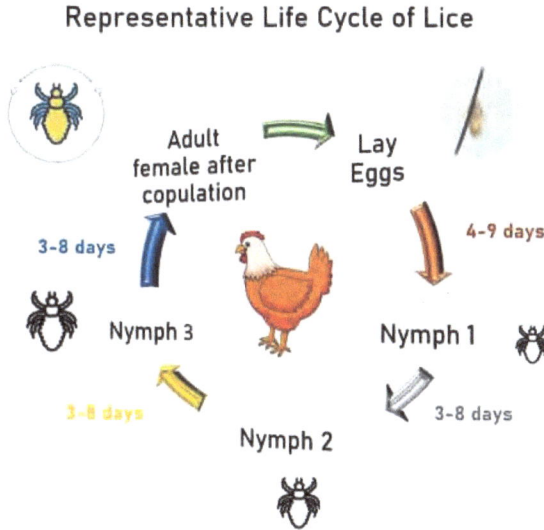

**Fig. (4).** Life cycle of Lice.

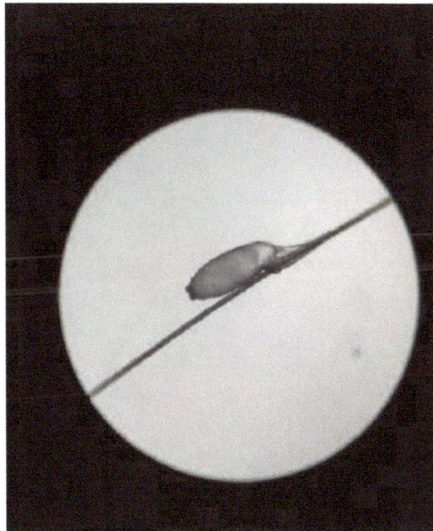

**Fig. (5).** Egg (Nit) glued to a hair follicle.

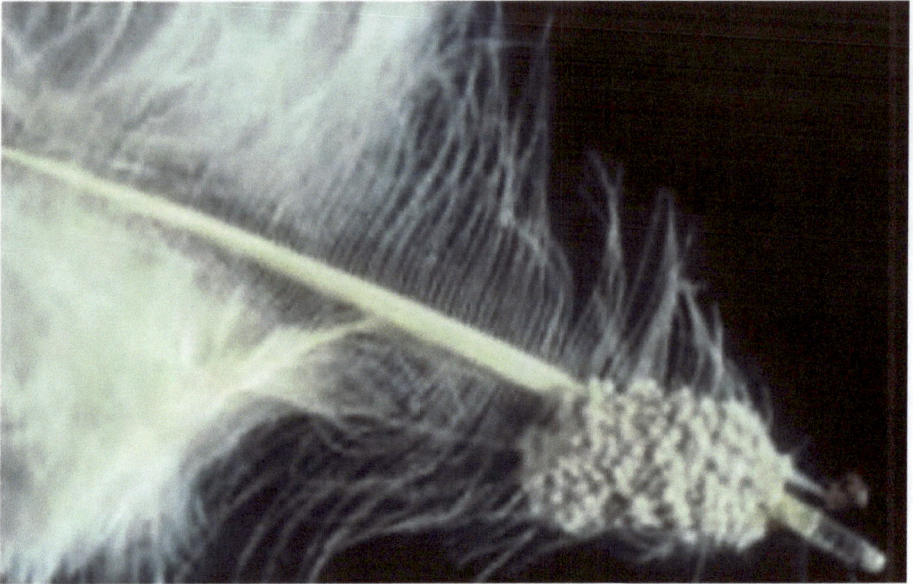

**Fig. (6).** Lice eggs at the base of feather shaft (source: Ohio State University Extension).

Direct host-to-host transmission appears to be the primary mechanism for lice infestation. Documented evidence of distribution *via* phoresy is encountered in ischnoceran lice. During phoresy, most lice attach to larger robust flies like hippoboscid or muscid members and are carried away onto their hosts [13].

Grooming and preening are the major means of reducing the lice population. Birds in poor health often with broken bills/beaks have intense parasite loads, possibly due to less grooming time. The incidence of bird lice is also influenced by the host's habitat, and they tend to be more abundant in humid climates [14]. Moreover, birds that flock more frequently have higher infestation rates compared to territorial, housed, or solitary birds [15]. These dynamics help to resolve many questions on 'why some species/hosts have higher louse prevalence than others' and thereby give us an insight into planning the control strategies.

**SIGNIFICANT POULTRY LICE**

Lice of veterinary significance fall under five families: the Boopiidae, Gyropidae, Menoponidae, Philopteridae, and Trichodectidae. As far as bird lice are concerned, at least ten-eleven species of chewing lice (distributed among four families- Menoponidae; Ricinidae; Laemobothriidae, and Philopteridae) infest birds.

## Suborder: Amblycera

*Menacanthus stramineous* (Previously known as *Menopon biseriatum*)

Commonly known as chicken body louse/yellow body louse is the most destructive louse in the poultry context. The host range is a wide group of birds (migratory birds/ game birds/ wild fowl) including chickens and turkeys. This lice has a worldwide distribution and it is found on the host's skin (particularly in the vent area of the bird) rather than on the feathers. Adults measure 2.8 to 3.5 mm in length. The head is broad, roughly triangular in shape with palps and 4 segmented antennae (Fig. 7). The concealed antenna appears like a club beneath the head. Spine-like ventral processes are often used for attachment. The ventral portion is armed with a pair of spine-like processes. The abdomen is generally broader than the thorax, giving the louse a slightly oval shape, with each segment bearing distinct setae (hair-like structures) that help it grip onto the host's feathers. (Fig. 8). It features a tough exoskeleton with dark transverse bands or sclerites across each segment. Eggs are laid in clusters at the base of feathers, especially near the ventral body and around the vent (Fig. 6). Eggs have distinct filaments on the anterior half near the operculum, the area where the nymph emerges (Fig. 9).

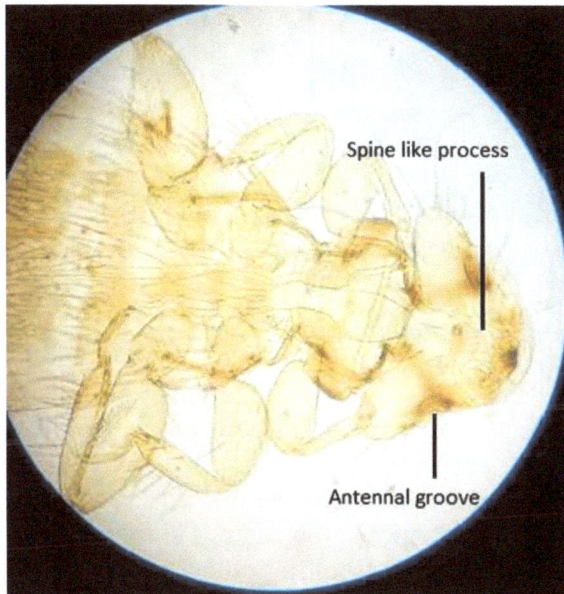

**Fig. (7).** *Menacanthus stramineous* -Head triangular with antennae lodged in a groove and a pair of ventral spike-like process.

The feeding activity of the louse leads to irritation of the skin, resulting in itching and discomfort. Affected chickens may scratch excessively, which can damage feathers, leading to feather loss and reduced plumage quality. These lice have chewing mouthparts and do not pierce the skin and suck blood. However, the gnawing action of the lice causes bleeding spots that attract the secondary flies. Infestation with this louse is linked to decreased feed conversion efficiency as the affected birds spend more time on preening and pecking than on feeding. Detailed effects of body louse on layers in caged and cage-free environments were documented by Murillo *et al.* [15]

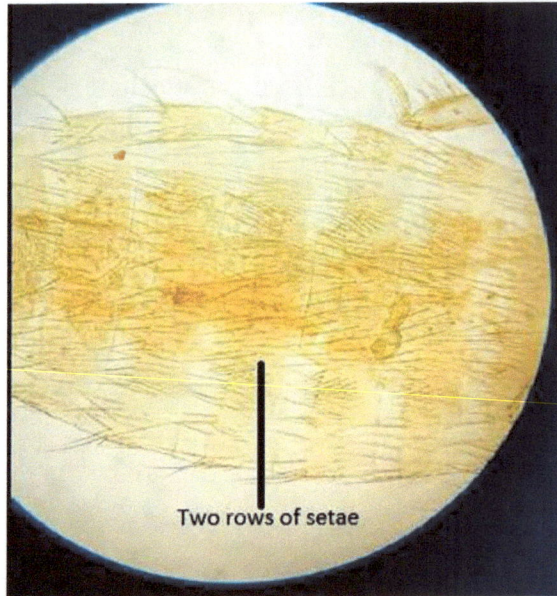

Two rows of setae

**Fig. (8).** *Menacanthus stramineus*- Flattened and oval abdomen with two dorsal rows of setae on each segment.

## *Menopon gallinae or Menopon pallidum*

Popularly known as "shaft louse" given due to their habit of resting feather shafts. They are super active and once disturbed will move rapidly to avoid the threat. Adults measure 1.7 – 2.0 mm in length with pale yellow body. Abdominal segments have a single row of bristles/setae that differentiates them from the body louse (Fig. **10**). Females strategically place eggs singly at the base of the shaft on thigh and breast feathers. The shaft louse besides causing serious irritation due to persistent scraping of skin also attribute to the death of young birds with heavy infestation.

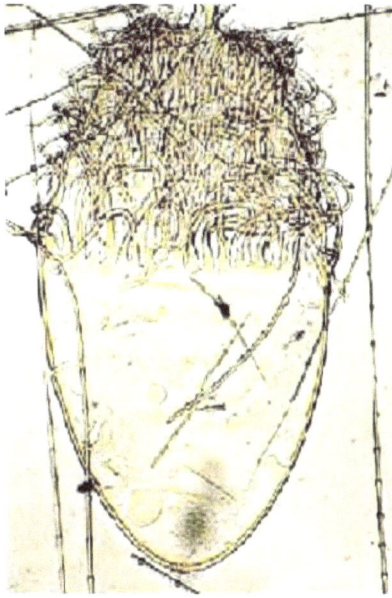

**Fig. (9).** *Menacanthus stramineous* Egg- with characteristic filaments on the anterior half of the shell and on the operculum (Source: http://www.icb.usp.br/~marcelcp/Imagens/piolho3.jpg).

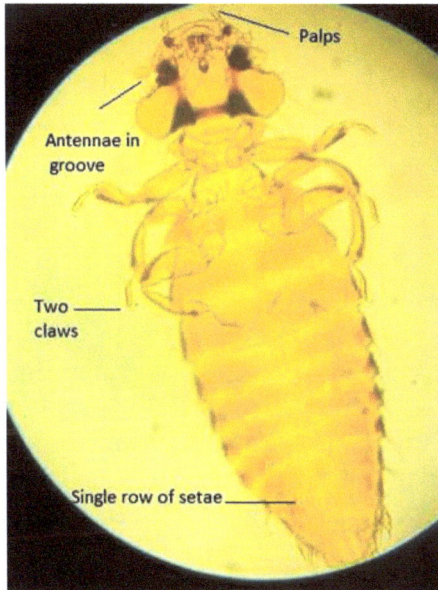

**Fig. (10).** *Menopon gallinae*- Head triangular with antennae lodged in a groove; Abdomen with single row of setae.

*Menopon phaeostomum* is the other known species found infesting peacocks.

### Holomenopon leucoxanthum

This shaft louse of duck is responsible for causing 'wet feathers'. Affected birds show soiled and tattered plumage, if large areas are affected, plumage no longer resists water and birds become wet and may die off due to pneumonia. The forehead is slightly conical with 2-4 segmented antennae and the abdomen is broadly oval in shape with equal segments. A detailed description of the morphology of these lice was documented by Ahmed *et al.* [1]

### Trinoton anserinum

Commonly known as the goose louse, it primarily infests waterfowl, particularly geese and ducks. *Trinoton* lice are the largest species which can reach up to 5–6 mm in length. They have numerous and diverse setae and possess strong legs with specialized claws for gripping [16]. Feeding behaviors among this species can vary, with approximately 22% of the population feeding exclusively on blood, while about 33% consume both blood and feathers. This louse species acts as an intermediate host of *Sarconema eurycerca*, a heartworm of swans that was investigated by Cohen *et al.* [8]. Conclusions from the study state that 9% of the lice possibly develop nematode larvae in their body.

### Suborder: Ischenocera

### Cuclotogaster heterographus

*Cuclotogaster* is a genus of ischenoceran chewing lice commonly known as "Head louse of poultry". They are short measuring about 2-2.5 mm in size. The body has a yellowish-grayish tinge. Fully exposed five-segmented antennae are seen on either side of the rounded head as plaits. In males, the first segment of the antenna is stout and long sexually demarcating it from females (Fig. 11). The abdomen is cylindrical and more elongated in the male with dark brown lateral tergal plates. It bears a row of dorsal hairs on each segment [17]. It is a dangerous parasite of chicken known for causing irritation and allergies, which affect the host's sleeping, reproduction, and deficiency in egg production. The female lays white eggs that glue to feathers or at its base.

Other less commonly documented species are *C. burnetii*, *C. eynsfordi*, and *C. pallidus*.

## Lipeurus caponis

*Lipeurus caponis*, the wing louse, resides more on the wing and tail feathers. They are sluggish lice measuring about 2.2 mm long with thin, grayish slender, elongated bodies. Predominantly the hind limbs are stronger and longer than the first two pairs of legs, and on each leg, there are two tarsal claws [18]. The eggs are deposited in clusters near the base of the feather, which hatch in 4 to 7 days. This louse is responsible for causing depluming in birds hence the name "Depluming louse". Other species are *L. maculosus*, *L. tropicalis*, and *L. variabilis* (Fig. **12**).

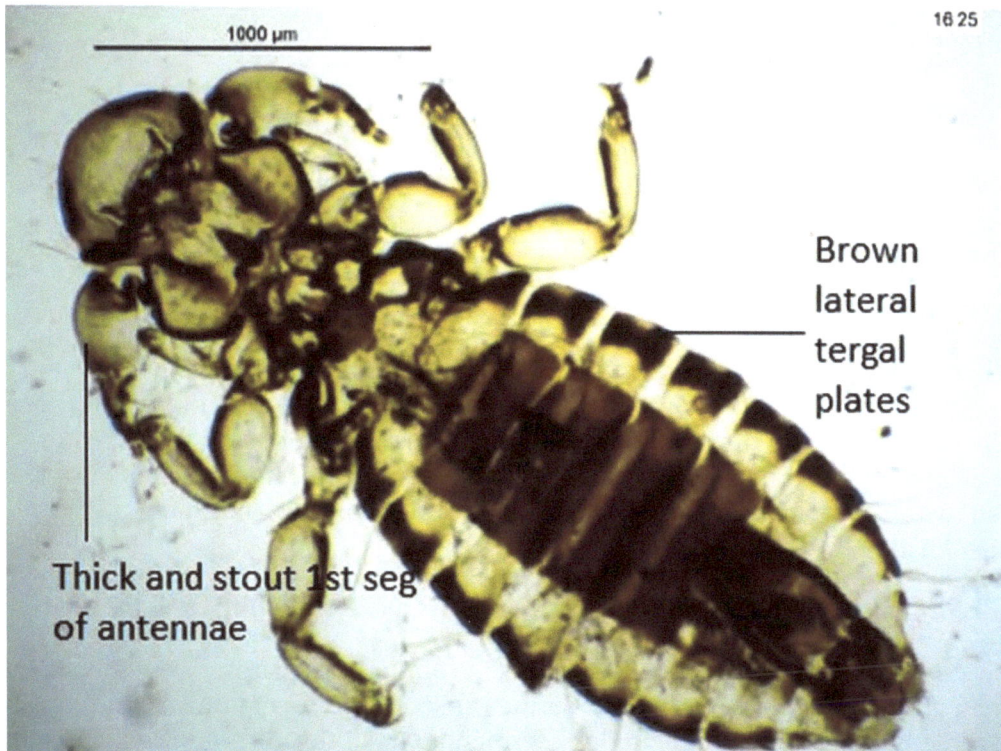

**Fig. (11).** *Cuclotogaster heterographus*: Head rounded, projected antennae, prominent lateral tergal plates. (Source: Kiraz Erciyas Yavuz, DOI: 10.3906/zoo-1411-45).

## Goniodes gigas

*Goniodes gigas* is often referred to as the "Large Chicken Louse/Giant Chicken Louse" with brown to reddish brown body color. It is found throughout the chicken's body roughly measuring 3-3.5mm [19]. The female lays eggs in clusters near the base of the feathers, providing protection and ensuring that the nymphs have immediate access to food upon hatching. There are three other known species: *G. dissimilis* ("Brown Chicken Louse"); *G. hologaster*, and *G. abdominalis*.

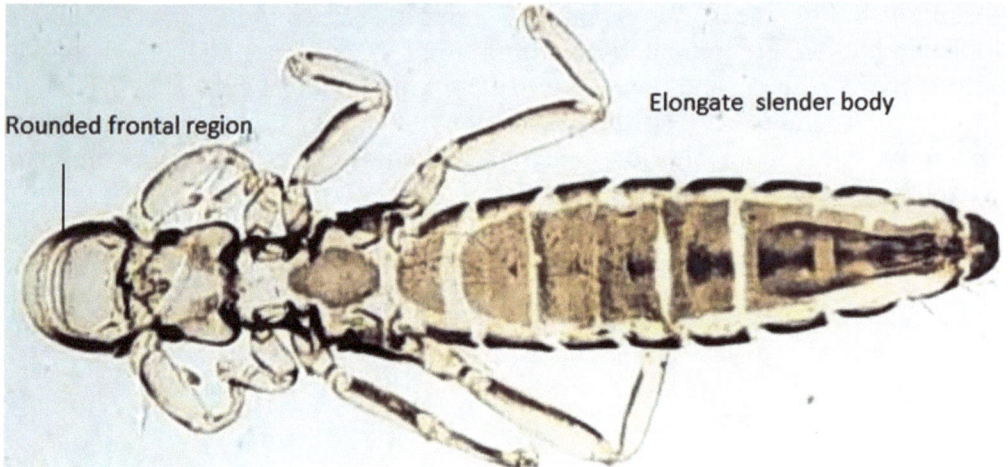

Rounded frontal region

Elongate slender body

**Fig. (12).** *Lipeurus caponis:* Frontal region rounded with slender elongate body. The third pair of legs is stronger and longer than the other two. (Source: http://www.icb.usp.br/~marcelcp/Imagens/u6.jpg).

### *Goniocotes gallinae*

This is commonly referred to as the "Fluff Louse", measuring about 1-1.5 mm in length with round, yellow bodies. The body is broad with a short head characterized by the presence of two long setae on the posterior margin of the head. These lice primarily feed on the keratin from feathers and skin debris. They can cause irritation and discomfort in infested birds. They are sluggish in movement.

### GENERALIZED PATHOGENESIS AND CONTROL OF POULTRY LICE

Lice infestation is termed as "Pediculosis" in animals and birds. Chewing lice that are parasitic on birds can cause serious discomfort. Symptoms of infestation include itching, irritation, pain, loss of appetite, and lowered egg production and also heavily infested young chicks may die. However, most infestations appear to have a little effect on their host [20]. The habit of dust bathing in domestic chickens is probably an attempt by the birds to rid themselves of lice. Additionally, ischnocerans can diminish the thermoregulatory function of the plumage, resulting in heavily infested birds losing more body heat compared to their less-infested counterparts. This can lead to increased susceptibility to cold stress and potential impacts on overall health and productivity. Lice can contribute to the spread of diseases within avian populations, and act as reservoirs and transmitters of pathogens causing fowl cholera, typhoid, and toxoplasmosis.

Some lice act as vectors of filarial nematodes, including *Pelecitus fulicaeatrae*, *Sarconema eurycera*, and species of *Eulimdana*.

Contact of domestic poultry with wild-infested birds should be avoided. When a new batch of birds is expected, it is important to remove all debris and the whole premises/cages should be flame singed to kill the nits. Classic control programs rely on synthetic insecticides, active ingredients include permethrin, pyrethrins, and ivermectin. Follow the manufacturer's instructions for application and dosage. Results suggest that their efficacy can be so strong. However, these pesticides are often toxic to human and animal health, and to the environment. They also rapidly lead to the development of resistance in targeted pest populations. Natural treatments such as diatomaceous earth can be effective in controlling lice populations by dehydrating them.

## CONCLUDING REMARKS

Lice can be found on the external surfaces of the body by the way of a thorough physical examination. The examination of the flock can help identify an early infestation and also can help protect a larger flock outbreak. Treatment of the environment is also necessary for controlling infestations of lice. Prevention as well as early detection of lice are the keys to successful treatment and control in poultry flocks.

## REFERENCES

[1]     Ahmad A, Gupta N, Saxena AK, Gupta D. First record of *Holomenopon leucoxanthum* on Domestic Ducks, *Anas platyrhynchos* (Anseriformes: Anatidae). Bioinfolet 2014; 11(2A): 364-6.

[2]     Bedford G A H. Trichodectidae (*Mallophaga*) found on South African Carnivora. Parasitology 1932; 24: 350-64.

[3]     Carrillo CM, Valera F, Barbosa A, Moreno E. Thriving in an arid environment: High prevalence of avian lice in low humidity conditions. Ecoscience 2007; 14(2): 241-9.
        [http://dx.doi.org/10.2980/1195-6860(2007)14[241:TIAAEH]2.0.CO;2]

[4]     Price MA, Graham OH. Chewing and sucking lice as parasites of mammals and birds. United States Department of Agricultured Agricultural Research Service, Technical. Bulletin 1997; 1849.

[5]     Clay T. New species of *Mallophaga* from Afroparvo congensis Chapin. American Museum Novitates 1938; (1008).

[6]     Clayton DH, Walther BA. Influence of host ecology and morphology on the diversity of Neotropical bird lice. Oikos 2001; 94(3): 455-67.
        [http://dx.doi.org/10.1034/j.1600-0706.2001.940308.x]

[7]     Clayton DH, Bush SE, Johnson KP. Coevolution of life on hosts: Integrating ecology and history. University of Chicago Press 2015.
        [http://dx.doi.org/10.7208/chicago/9780226302300.001.0001]

[8]     Poulin R. Variation in infection parameters among populations within parasite species: intrinsic properties versus local factors. Int J Parasitol. 2006 Jul;36(8):877-85.
        [http://dx.doi.org/10.1016/j.ijpara.2006.02.021]

[9]     Cohen S, Greenwood MT, Fowler JA. The louse *Trinoton anserinum* (Amblycera: Phthiraptera), an intermediate host of *Sarconema eurycerca* (Filarioidea: Nematoda), a heartworm of swans. Med Vet Entomol 1991; 5(1): 101-10.
[http://dx.doi.org/10.1111/j.1365-2915.1991.tb00527.x] [PMID: 1768889]

[10]    de Moya RS, Yoshizawa K, Walden KKO, Sweet AD, Dietrich CH, Kevin P J. Phylogenomics of parasitic and nonparasitic lice (Insecta: Psocodea): combining sequence data and exploring compositional bias solutions in next generation data sets. Syst Biol 2021; 70(4): 719-38.
[http://dx.doi.org/10.1093/sysbio/syaa075] [PMID: 32979270]

[11]    Delgado C, Rosegrant M, Steinfeld H, Ehui S, Courbois C. Livestock 2020: The next food revolution. Food, Agriculture and the Environment Discussion Paper 1999; 28.

[12]    Ferris GF. The louse of elephants *Haematomyzus elephantis* (*Mallophaga*: Haematomyzidae). Parasitology 1931; 23: 112-27.

[13]    Ikpeze OO, Amagba IC, Eneanya CI. Preliminary survey of ectoparasites of chicken in Awka, south-eastern Nigeria. Anim Res Int 2009; 5(2)
[http://dx.doi.org/10.4314/ari.v5i2.48745]

[14]    Koop JAH, DeMatteo KE, Parker PG, Whiteman NK. Birds are islands for parasites. Biol Lett 2014; 10(8): 20140255.
[http://dx.doi.org/10.1098/rsbl.2014.0255] [PMID: 25099959]

[15]    Durden LA. Lice (Phthiraptera) In: Mullen GR, Durden LA, Eds, Medical and veterinary entomology. 3rd ed. Academic Press 2019; pp. 79-106.
[http://dx.doi.org/10.1016/B978-0-12-814043-7.00007-8]

[16]    Murillo AC, Abdoli A, Blatchford RA, Keogh EJ, Gerry AC. Low levels of chicken body louse (*Menacanthus stramineus*) infestations affect chicken welfare in a cage-free housing system. Parasit Vectors 2024; 17(1): 221.
[http://dx.doi.org/10.1186/s13071-024-06313-6] [PMID: 38745229]

[17]    Price RD, Hellenthal RA, Palma RL, Johnson KP, Clayton DH. Illinois Natural History Survey Special Publication; Urbana-Champaign: The chewing lice: World checklist and biological overview 2003.

[18]    Sweet AD, Johnson KP. The role of parasite dispersal in shaping a host–parasite system at multiple evolutionary scales. Mol Ecol 2018; 27(24): 5104-19.
[http://dx.doi.org/10.1111/mec.14937] [PMID: 30427088]

[19]    Tomás A, Palma RL, Rebelo MT, da Fonseca IP. Chewing lice (Phthiraptera) from wild birds in southern Portugal. Parasitol Int 2016; 65(3): 295-301.
[http://dx.doi.org/10.1016/j.parint.2016.02.007] [PMID: 26899014]

[20]    Tuff D W. A key to the lice of man and domestic animals. Tex J Sci, 1977; 28: 145e159.

# SUBJECT INDEX

## A

Activation and signaling pathways 129
Activity 15, 23, 34, 35, 105, 124, 125, 126, 134, 139, 140, 141, 147, 311
  metabolic 23
  microbicidal 125
  phagocytic 124, 147
  potent cytotoxic 127
Air, trapping 119
Amoebotaenia cuneata infections 265
Animals, infected 185
Anthelminthic 180, 185
  effects 180
  medications 185
Anti-inflammatory cytokines 138, 139
Antigens, vaccinations transfer 192
Antiparasitic agents 17
Antiviral immunity 125, 127
Autoimmune processes 114

## B

Biomarkers, immunological 143
Boosting erythropoiesis 315
Bronchial-associated lymphoid tissues (BALT) 136

## C

Chemotherapeutic agents 39, 42, 72
Chemotherapy programs for poultry 214
Chicken(s) 5, 11, 21, 87, 152, 153, 189, 190, 191, 192, 193, 196, 198, 209, 216, 225, 234, 259, 264, 265, 266, 278, 285, 291, 329
  disease-resistant 285
  immunizing 192
  industry 190, 193
  meat production 21
  production 189, 191
  vaccinating 198

Chicks, infected 57
Conjunctival-associated lymphoid tissue (CALT) 136
Cryptosporidiosis 37, 190, 288, 289, 290
  respiratory 288
Cytokine(s) 15, 114, 115, 122, 132, 133, 139, 140, 141, 143, 145, 146
  feedback mechanisms 133, 139, 140
  production 132
  proinflammatory 122
Cytotoxic activity 127

## D

Damage 30, 82, 90, 93, 95, 96, 98, 101, 103, 115, 139, 233, 294
  erythrocytic 294
  mechanical 30
Debris 97, 107
  necrotic 97
  organic 107
Deficiencies, vitamin 142
Depression 87, 92, 238, 246, 250, 297, 315
Detection, direct microscopy 160
Diarrhea 26, 30, 37, 68, 78, 79, 81, 82, 84, 87, 96, 242, 249, 315
  bloody 82, 84, 96, 242
  severe greenish 315
Diarrhoea, watery 287, 301
Dietary supplementation 145
Disease(s) 24, 64, 65, 67, 74, 75, 78, 85, 100, 102, 125, 127, 130, 133, 138, 142, 151, 190, 280, 283, 284, 289, 293, 308, 328, 330, 315, 342
  hemorrhagic 280
  histomonosis 85
  life-threatening 308
  liver 284
  malabsorptive 280
  preventing autoimmune 138
  protozoan 190
  renal 289

www.ingramcontent.com/pod-product-compliance
Lightning Source LLC
Chambersburg PA
CBHW050801220326

41598CB00006B/88